Health & Social Care

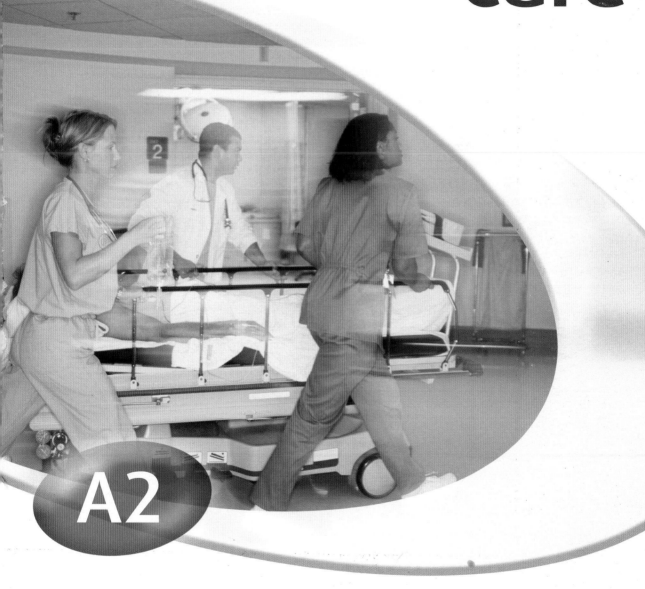

A2

Mark Walsh   Paul Stephens   Marilyn Billingham
Mary Crittenden   Alison Thomson   Douglas Thomson

Collins

William Collins' dream of knowledge for all began with the publication of his first book in 1819. A self-educated mill worker, he not only enriched millions of lives, but also founded a flourishing publishing house. Today, staying true to this spirit, Collins books are packed with inspiration, innovation and practical expertise. They place you at the centre of a world of possibility and give you exactly what you need to explore it.

Collins. Do more.

Published by Collins
An imprint of HarperCollins*Publishers*
77–85 Fulham Palace Road
Hammersmith
London
W6 8JB

Browse the complete Collins catalogue at
www.collinseducation.com

© 2006 Mark Walsh, Paul Stephens, Marilyn Billingham, Mary Crittenden, Alison Thomson and Douglas Thomson

10 9 8 7 6 5 4 3 2 1

ISBN-13 978 000 7200 405
ISBN-10 000 7200404

Mark Walsh, Paul Stephens, Marilyn Billingham, Mary Crittenden, Alison Thomson and Douglas Thomson assert their moral right to be identified as the authors of this work

British Library Cataloguing in Publication Data
A Catalogue record for this publication is available from the British Library

Commissioned and edited by Graham Bradbury

Cover Design by Blue Pig Design Limited

Cover image courtesy of Getty Images

Series design by Patricia Briggs

Book design by Ken Vail Graphic Design

Indexed by Joan Dearnley

Picture research by Thelma Gilbert

Production by Sarah Robinson

Printed and bound by Butler and Tanner Ltd, Frome

This high quality material is endorsed by Edexcel and has been through a rigorous quality assurance programme to ensure that it is a suitable companion to the specification for both learners and teachers. This does not mean that its contents will be used verbatim when setting examinations nor is it to be read as being the official specification – a copy of which is available at www.edexcel.org.uk

Health r Social Care
Diss High School.

Acknowledgements

The authors would like to acknowledge and thank everybody who has supported and helped us to write and produce this book. This includes Kay Wright at HarperCollins, Graham Bradbury, Emily and Sam at Ken Vail Graphic Design, Karen Seymour, Peter Billingham, Chris Walsh, Jim Dyson and the long list of other people who have contributed in various ways to improving our work.

Mark Walsh, Paul Stephens, Marilyn Billingham, Mary Crittenden, Alison Thomson and Douglas Thomson

The authors and publisher would like to thank the following for permission to reproduce photographs and other material:

p.9 Alamy/Janine Wiedel; p.10 SPL/Mauro Fermariello; p.14 (l) Alamy/Janine Wiedel, (r) Alamy/Medical-on-Line; p.24 SPL/BSIP,LSL; p.28 Alamy/AceStock; p.32 (t) Rex Features, (b) Alamy/Janine Wiedel; p.36 Photofusion Picture Library; p.51 Photofusion Picture Library; p.52 SPL/Ian Hooton; p.54 Cancer Research UK; p.56 Cancer Research UK; p.66 Alamy/Paul Doyle; p.67 SPL/Josh Sher; p.70 (l) Photofusion Picture Library, (r) Empics; p.72 Everyman Campaign/FA/PFA; p.78 Empics; p.80 Empics; p.86 Photofusion Picture Library; p.92 Chris Walsh; p.99 SPL/Samuel Ashfield; p.100 Roger Scruton; p.101 Douglas Thomson; p.106 (l) Alamy/Shout, (r) Alamy/PLC; p.112 SPL/Cornelia Molloy; p.115 SPL/Custom Medical Stock; p.118 SPL/Lee Powers; p.119 SPL/P. Marazzi; p.120 SPL/BSIP, Mendil; p.122 SPL/Lauren Shear; p.126 SPL/Mark Thomas; p.128 (l) SPL/Scott Camazine, (r) SPL/CNRI; p.129 (l) SPL/GCA, (r) SPL/Mauro Fermariello; p.130 SPL/Samuel Ashfield; p.132 Photos.com; p.133 SPL/Jim Varney; p.134 SPL/Mauro Fermariello; p135 Sally & Richard Greenhill; p.138 Advertising Archives; p.142 Photofusion Picture Library; p.144 Rex Features; p.150 SPL/Mark Clark; p.151 Roger Scruton; p.152 SPL/Antonia Reeve; p.157 SPL/John Cole; p.158 SPL/BSIP, Laurent; p.159 SPL/John Cole; p.160 Alamy/Phototake Inc; p.164 SPL/MFE; p.168 (l) SPL/Stanley Burns, (r) SPL/Ian Hooton; p.169 Alamy/Janine Wiedel; p.170 Empics; p.172 SPL/Victor de Schwanberg; p.174 Karen Seymour; p.176 Paul Stephens; p.178 SPL/BSIP, Keene; p.184 Alamy/OnRequest Image; p.188 Photos.com; p.190 SPL; p.192 Sally & Richard Greenhill; p.193 Corbis; p.194 Roger Scruton; p.196 Alamy/ Janine Wiedel; p.201 Photofusion Picture Library; p.202 Corbis; p.206 Photofusion Picture Library; p.210 Marilyn Billingham; p.212 Jim Dyson; p.213 Njampa Family; p.216 Sally & Richard Greenhill; p.222 Rex Features; p.226 Rex Features; p.230 Alamy/Photofusion; p.234 Photofusion Picture Library; p.239 Rex Features; p.240 (tl) Alamy/Lisa Dumont, (tr) Alamy/Photofusion, (bl) Alamy/Phototake Inc., (br) Alamy/Photofusion; p.246 Alamy/Photofusion; p.252 Photos.com; p.258 Alamy/PhotoNetwork; p.260 Ken Vail Graphic Design; p.264 Rex Features; p.270 Alamy/Peter Glass; p.271 SPL; p.276 Kay Wright; p.282 (tl) Alamy/Profmedia, (tr) Alamy/Aliki Sapountzi, (bl) Alamy/Bubbles Picture Library, (br) Corbis; p.288 Alamy/Photofusion.

Every effort has been made to contact copyright holders, but if any have been inadvertently overlooked, the publishers will be pleased to make the necessary arrangements at the first opportunity.

Contents

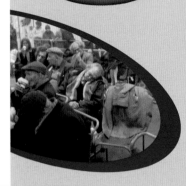
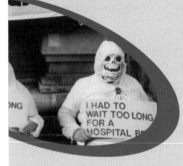
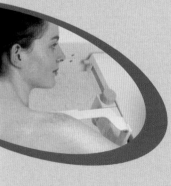

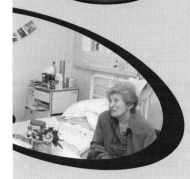

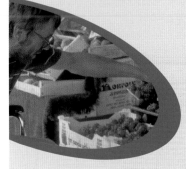

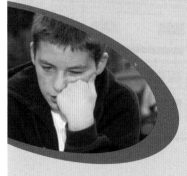

THIS UNIT IS ABOUT THE WAYS THAT CARE SERVICES IN THE UNITED KINGDOM ARE PROVIDED TO MEET INDIVIDUALS' NEEDS. It focuses on the organisation and provision of different types of care services that are available throughout the UK. It also considers how care practitioners use care planning to identify and respond to each individual's particular need for health and social care and support. The unit will provide you with the background knowledge that you will need to complete Unit 7 of the Edexcel GCE A2 Health and Social Care award. You will learn about:

- The structure and provision of care services in the United Kingdom
- The legal framework that care organisations and practitioners operate in
- How care services are tailored to meet each individual's particular needs
- The role of care practitioners in providing care and promoting a positive care environment
- The ways that the quality of care services are monitored and maintained in health and social care organisations.

Meeting Individual Needs

Key questions

By the end of the unit you should be able to use the knowledge and understanding that you develop to answer the following questions:

1 How are care services organised and provided in different parts of the United Kingdom?
2 How have changes in legislation over the past twenty years influenced the provision of health and social care in the United Kingdom?
3 How and why do care practitioners use the care plan process to meet individuals' particular care needs?
4 What factors affect the work of care practitioners in a care organisation?
5 What methods are used in health and social care organisations to monitor and regulate the quality of care service provision?

Understanding the UK care system

Getting you thinking

Natasha Bell is 37 years of age. She and her American partner, Charles, have been trying to have a baby for the past three years. Natasha and Charles now believe that some form of assisted conception, such as in vitro fertilisation (IVF), may give them the best chance of starting the family they long for. Charles knows very little about health and social care services in the United Kingdom. He is happy to pay for treatment. Natasha, on the other hand, believes that she may have a right to free IVF treatment which is available at her local hospital. Natasha and Charles have recently tried to find out about the availability of fertility treatment in Britain but have become confused and aren't sure what to do next.

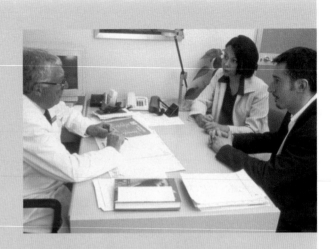

1 Which type of health care services offer fertility treatment to people who can afford to pay for it?

2 What other types of fertility service may be available to Natasha and Charles if they are unable to afford the fees involved?

3 Do Natasha and Charles need health care services or social care services? Explain the difference between these types of care service in your answer.

KEY TERMS

Commissioning
The acquisition or purchasing of care services on behalf of a local population of people.

Eligibility criteria
The requirements or standards that must be met before a person is provided with a care service.

Informal care/sector
Care that is provided by relatives and friends on an unpaid basis, outside of the professional care system.

Independent sector
A collective term for the private and the voluntary care sectors.

Internal market
A 'market' in care services that was introduced in the early 1990s to promote competition between statutory and other care providers.

Mixed economy of care
A care system that combines public (government), private, voluntary and informal sector provision. Each of these types of care is funded in a different way – hence the term 'mixed economy'.

Private care/sector
Care services that are provided to people who are willing and able to pay for them. Organisations and individual practitioners who sell care services in this way are collectively known as the 'private sector'.

Provider organisation
A care organisation that delivers care services directly to service users.

Purchaser organisation
An organisation that commissions or buys care services on behalf of an individual or group of people.

Statutory care/sector
Care services that have to be provided by law. They are usually provided by public or government-controlled care organisations, such as NHS Trusts.

Voluntary care/sector
Care services that are provided – free of charge or for a small, subsidised fee – by non-profit making organisations.

Ways of thinking about care services

A wide variety of health, social care and welfare services are currently provided to meet individuals' needs throughout the United Kingdom. In this first topic we will focus on the broad structure and provision of care services in the UK. To understand this, it is first necessary to think about the types of care and the different categories of care organisation that currently exist.

Types of care and categories of care organisation

In this unit we are mainly concerned with health care and social care services. Health care is typically medical, nursing or specialist paramedic or therapeutic care that is provided to treat a person who has a physical or mental health problem that affects their ability to function. Primary health care services are general or 'first contact' health services that are provided in community settings to treat everyday or less serious ailments, illnesses or minor injuries. Secondary health care services are more complex interventions, usually provided through a hospital or other health care institution after a person has been diagnosed and referred for treatment. Tertiary health care services are provided in both community and institutional settings for people who have chronic (long-term) or terminal (end of life) health care needs.

In the UK, health care is mainly provided through **statutory** health care organisations. The National Health Service is the main example of this type of organisation. However, **private sector** practitioners, care businesses and voluntary organisations can, in theory (but very rarely), also provide statutory health care if they obtain a contract and the funding to do so from the government. Instead, private practitioners and care businesses tend to provide a range of non-statutory health care services, like nursing home care, acupuncture and physiotherapy services, to people who are willing and able to pay for them.

Social care is any form of non-medical care that aims to provide support or assistance for vulnerable groups. The main groups of social care service users are children and families, older people, people with disabilities (physical, sensory and learning) and people experiencing mental distress. Social care services are also provided by statutory, private and voluntary sector organisations and through informal care provision.

We will look at the organisation and delivery of care services throughout the UK in more detail in Topics 4 and 5 of this unit.

Care sectors, the care system and the 'mixed economy of care'

So far we've looked at different types of care and at the different categories of care organisation that exist in the United Kingdom. However, to understand the 'big picture' of care provision in the UK, we next need to think about the ways in which care organisations are linked together into an overall care system. One way of doing this is to think about 'care sectors'. A care sector is simply a collection or group of care organisations that have something in common. In this case, the key, defining characteristic is the way in which services are funded in a particular sector. The UK care system consists of four different care sectors:

- The different types of government-funded statutory care organisations are collectively known as the **statutory sector**.

- The millions of ordinary unpaid partners, family members, friends and neighbours who provide care are known as the **informal care sector**.

- The diverse range of private practitioners and care businesses are collectively known as the **private sector**.

- Non-profit making voluntary care organisations are collectively known as the **voluntary sector**.

Because these last two sectors are independent of government, they are also some times known as the **independent sector**. The care system in the UK is also known as a '**mixed economy of care**' because of the different methods of funding that support each of the different care sectors. The UK care system could therefore be seen as being like a patchwork quilt made up from large national organisations, smaller local organisations and ordinary people – all combining in many different ways.

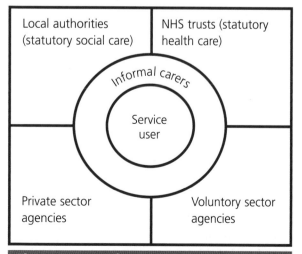

Figure 1 Types of care providers

Figure 2 *The four categories of care service*

Category	What this means	Example
Statutory	• A service that a person has a legal (statutory) right to receive • Funded by the government • Usually free to those who are eligible for services • Usually provided by a public care organisation	• Emergency care provided by an NHS Trust hospital • Social work services provided by a local authority
Private	• A service available to anyone who can pay for it • Funded by direct client payment or by the client taking out health care insurance • Usually provided by a private practitioner or care business	• BUPA private hospital care for cosmetic surgery • Home help service provided by a care services agency
Voluntary	• A service that is available to people who meet eligibility requirements • Usually free or low cost to service users Typically funded by voluntary donations or government grants • Usually provided by a not-for-profit, voluntary organisation	• MIND support groups for people with mental health problems • Age Concern advice and support services for older people
Informal	• Care interventions and support provided by a partner, relative or friend of a person in need of care • Typically practical, personal and non-technical forms of help and support	• Providing injections or prescribed medicine for a partner or relative • Going shopping and providing companionship for a friend or neighbour

Origins and development of care services

Understanding the origins of the care system, and the general way in which different parts of it have developed, will enable you to appreciate why the care system is organised and structured in the way it is today. The UK care system has a long history and is constantly evolving in response to social, economic and political changes in society. However, a key moment in the development of our present care system occurred in the late 1940s with the emergence of the 'welfare state'.

The emergence of the 'welfare state'

The birth of the 'welfare state' in the late 1940s was a watershed in British history. This was the moment when an organised, accessible and wide-ranging system of health and social care services first became available for all citizens. Before the welfare state system emerged, people had to pay for private care, or try to gain access to local voluntary care organisations and very basic state care services (where they existed), or – more commonly – rely on family and friends to help and support them. The pre-welfare state system provided quite limited and relatively poor quality services, and it favoured two groups – those who were very poor and entitled to

state services and those who were wealthy enough to afford to buy services privately. Before the welfare state, therefore, the system provided little care or support for the majority of the population.

The main architect of the welfare state was Sir William Beveridge. He produced a 'Report on Social Insurance and Allied Services' (now known as the Beveridge Report) which identified five 'evils' or 'giants' that he believed had to be overcome to improve the health and wellbeing of the nation. These were:

- 'Want' – poverty

- 'Disease' – ill-health

- 'Ignorance' – lack of education

- 'Squalor' – poor quality housing

- 'Idleness' – unemployment.

Beveridge suggested that the best way to tackle these problems was for the government to develop and fund a wide range of health, social care, education and social security services. A 'National Health Service' was one of his key proposals. This proposal was widely supported, and led to a range of health, social care and welfare services being set up across the country from the late 1940s. The decades that followed saw the state become the major source of funding for, and the biggest provider of, health and social care services that the United Kingdom had ever seen.

The period from the late 1940s to the late 1970s was the 'golden era' of the welfare state. During this time, many public hospitals, state schools and other care facilities were built and large numbers of people trained to become health, education and social care workers. They were needed because, for the first time, everyone in society was entitled to free statutory care and education services. During this time the cost of the welfare state was paid out of taxation and monies from a new 'National Insurance' scheme. However, despite the optimism and commitment that many politicians and the public had towards the welfare state, problems began to occur. By the mid-1970s it became clear that the welfare state was hugely costly, and the original principles of free and comprehensive services were being challenged. Charges for dentistry, prescriptions and glasses had already been introduced in the 1950s. More fundamental reforms were needed, however, to contain the costs of providing comprehensive health, social care and education services.

The National Health Service, local government and the education system all underwent successive reorganisations during the 1960s and 1970s, in an attempt to control costs and make the provision of care services more efficient. However, the most fundamental change occurred in the early 1990s with the introduction of an '**internal market**' in care services.

The internal market involved splitting parts of the NHS and local authority social services departments into separate **purchaser** and **provider** sections. The idea was that purchasing organisations would 'shop around' in the new care 'market' and buy care services for a local population from the provider organisations that offered them the best value deal. In effect, purchasing or **commissioning** bodies made contracts with NHS Trust, local authority, voluntary and private sector provider organisations for a particular volume of care. The Conservative government at the time believed that the internal market was a good idea because it would:

- create competition between providers

- create choice for purchasers

- cut costs, as providers tried to win contracts

- reduce inefficiency and save money.

The internal market was a very controversial development in the care system. The new Labour government, who were elected in 1997, modified it to reduce the 'competitive' element and promote cooperation between care providers. However, many of the innovations and effects it introduced still remain. In particular, the internal market in care had the effect of focusing care organisations on the costs of providing services. It also introduced a range of new financial management and contracting methods and changed the relationship between statutory, private and voluntary sector care providers. The result is that today, although central government is still the most significant source of funding for both health and social care services, the care system now relies heavily on private and voluntary sector care organisations and private practitioners to actually deliver care services. There are also much closer relationships between the different types of care providers, and a significant shift towards targeting care in a selective way at people who meet specific **eligibility criteria**.

Check your understanding

1 Identify the four different care sectors that exist in the UK care system.

2 Describe the origins of the statutory care system that exists in the UK today.

3 Explain the terms 'mixed economy of care' and 'internal market' in care services.

4 Identify the effects of the introduction of an 'internal market' in care services on the care system as a whole.

extension **activities**

1 Using a range of national newspapers, identify current stories about the health and social care system. After reading a selection of these stories, identify and summarise the main issues that seem to be of concern to care service providers and care service users.

2 The health and social care system in the UK is currently being 'modernised' by the new Labour government. Identify and discuss the effects that this is having on the provision, quality and availability of care services in your local area.

Getting you thinking

1 Identify reasons why legal rules and procedures might be needed in the health and social care field.

2 Describe the possible benefits of having clear laws affecting psychiatric and mental health care in the UK.

3 What legal rights and protection do you think children who are receiving care in the UK should have?

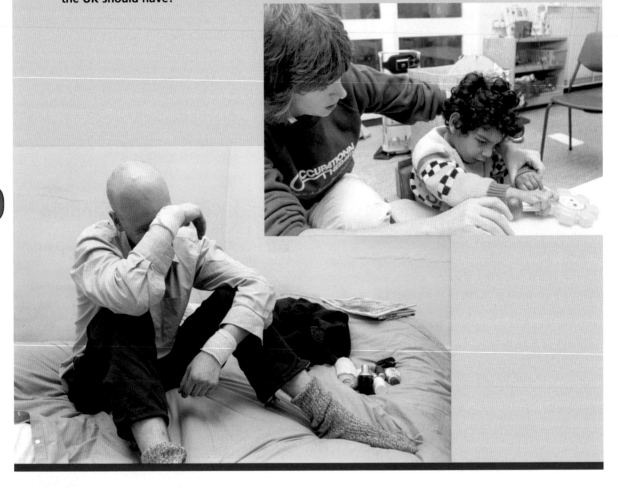

KEY TERMS

Legislation
A collective term for laws that are passed by Parliament.

Paramountcy principle
The principle of putting the welfare of the child first in all decisions affecting them.

Psychiatrist
A medical doctor who has specialist training and qualifications that allow them to work with people experiencing mental distress.

Regulatory
This refers to monitoring and control.

Statute
An Act of Parliament.

Legislation and the care system

We have already seen that the emergence of the 'welfare state' in the late 1940s was a watershed moment in the history of the UK care system. The proposals for a comprehensive system of health care, social security and education that were put forward by the Beveridge Report were translated into reality through an extensive programme of social **legislation**. The key pieces of legislation that helped form the basis of the welfare state in Britain were:

- *The Family Allowance Act 1945* – providing an allowance to families for all children except the first.

- *The National Insurance Act 1946* – a comprehensive contributory scheme designed to help cover people's loss of earnings because of unemployment, retirement, sickness, disability or widowhood.

- *The National Health Service Act 1948* – establishing a free health service that all people were entitled to.

- *The National Assistance Act 1948* – a safety net for those who were destitute (in total poverty) and not covered by the National Insurance scheme. It also allowed for local authorities to provide care services and other facilities.

These **statutes** introduced publicly funded health and welfare services in a comprehensive way for the first time in the UK. A large number of other care-related statutes have since been developed, debated and passed by successive governments since this watershed period in the middle of the twentieth century. Successive governments have used legislation to:

- Establish care organisations, enable service provision and set standards for service delivery.

- Create and maintain **regulatory** arrangements for monitoring care organisations.

- Provide service users with the right to access and receive public care services.

- Protect the rights of both service providers and service users in care situations.

Whilst various statutes have been important in gradually shaping the care system over the past fifty years, we will focus in more detail on a number of recent pieces of legislation that continue to have an impact on the provision and experience of care services in the UK today.

The Children Act (1989)

The Children Act (1989) is the most important piece of legislation currently affecting the provision of care services for children. Various childcare laws were brought together and simplified by this Act and by the Children (Scotland) Act (1995). These statutes have given children certain legal rights, whilst also imposing legal duties on parents and child care workers to promote each child's welfare and protect them from any form of abuse. The important principles introduced by the Children Act (1989) include:

- The welfare of the child is considered paramount (the most important thing) in any decisions relating to them. This is known as the **paramountcy principle**.

- Wherever possible, a child should be cared for and brought up by their own family.

- The parents of children 'in need' should be given help and support to bring up their children. Any help should be provided as a service to the child and his family and should be provided in partnership with the parents. It should also meet each child's identified needs and be appropriate to the child's race, culture, religion and language.

- Children in danger should be kept safe and be protected by effective intervention.

- Children should be consulted about decisions affecting their future and should be kept informed about what happens to them.

- Parents continue to have parental responsibility for their children even when their children are no longer living with them. They should be kept informed about their children and participate when decisions are made about their children's future.

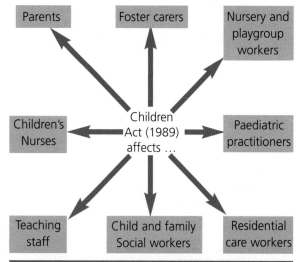

Figure 3 Who is affected by the Children Act (1989)?

The Children Act (1989) now has a profound effect on the work of all child care and education practitioners. Care practitioners employed by local authority social services, hospitals and education departments use and apply its principles on a daily basis to protect and promote the rights of children and their families.

Working with the Children Act (1989)

Sally Hughes is a Principal Social Worker. She is employed by a local authority and works for their social services department within the Child and Families team. Sally is responsible for managing the specialist child protection social workers. Sally tends to work on complex and often emotionally difficult cases involving children who are 'at risk' of neglect or abuse, or who have already been identified as having a clear need for care and protection.

Sally's daily work is heavily influenced by the provisions of the Children Act (1989). For example, she is responsible for ensuring that her social services team makes joint plans with schools and other areas of the local authority on child protection issues. Sally also plays a major role in managing the Child Protection Register. This is a record of all children in her local authority area who are considered to be at risk of abuse or neglect. Sally often attends child protection case conferences relating to children who are either being considered for inclusion on or are already listed on the child protection register. These meetings can be difficult and very emotional but Sally always has to ensure that the child's welfare is prioritised and seen as the main concern in any discussion or decision-making process.

The Mental Health Act (1983)

People who are experiencing 'mental disorder' are a second key group who require legal protection, because they are particularly vulnerable at the point where they require care services.

The Mental Health Act (1983) and the Mental Health (Scotland) Act (1984) are the key statutes affecting the care and treatment of people who are formally detained (compulsorily) on the grounds of their mental health problems. About 15 per cent of mental health service users are formal patients. This means that the majority of mental health service users are informal (voluntary) patients who have the same legal rights as anybody being treated for a physical illness. Formal patients do not have those rights.

The process of compulsorily admitting somebody to a mental health unit is known as **sectioning**. This is because the Mental Health Act (1983) is organised into ten different 'Parts' that are further divided into 'Sections'. Part I defines the scope of the Mental Health Act (1983) and states that it only deals with people who have a 'mental disorder'. This is defined in Section 1 as 'mental illness, arrested or incomplete development of mind, psychopathic disorder and any other disorder or disability of mind'. Part 2 of the Act contains what are known as the 'civil sections'. These are the sections that can be used to compulsorily detain people in hospital so that their mental disorder can be assessed and treated.

Sections of Acts allowing detention and treatment

Figure 4a Mental Health Act (1983)

Section	Purpose	Length of detention	Right of appeal
2	Admission	28 days	Yes, within 28 days
3	Treatment	6 months	Yes, at any time
4	Emergency	72 hours	No
5 (2)	Doctors holding power	72 hours	No
5 (4)	Nurses holding power	6 hours	No

Figure 4b Mental Health (Scotland) Act (1984)

Section	Purpose	Length of detention	Right of appeal
18	Admission (via Sheriff Court)	6 months	Yes
24	Emergency admission	72 hours, can be extended to 28 days	No

As you might appreciate, the process of sectioning is taken very seriously by all those involved. This is because it will result in the temporary loss of some of the person's legal rights. In effect, a person who is sectioned can be detained in a psychiatric unit against their will. Whilst under section, they are not allowed to leave the unit where they are detained without permission. In addition, they may also be required to accept treatment for their mental disorder. This could involve taking medication, participating in 'talking therapies' or receiving other treatments that they would ordinarily refuse to accept.

The Mental Health Act (1983) contains a number of provisions that are designed to protect and safeguard the rights of people during and following the sectioning process. For example:

- The sectioning process can only be carried out by qualified **psychiatrists**, or in limited circumstances by registered Mental Health Nurses, whose requests to detain a patient must be supported by an Approved Social Worker.

- The Act limits the length of time that a person can be detained, and provides individuals who are detained with the rights to appeal against their detention under a section.

- People who wish to appeal against their sectioning can apply for a hearing of their case to the Mental Health Review Tribunal. This consists of a panel of independent practitioners and lay people who have the power to rescind a section and discharge the person.

The Mental Health Act (1983) and Mental Health (Scotland) Act (1984) provide a legal framework for the care and treatment of people who are experiencing 'mental disorder'. This is seen as necessary because there is often a dispute between care providers and those who are identified as experiencing 'mental disorder' about the individual's need for care and treatment. In some cases the person or their relatives will dispute or fail to recognise this. Additionally, people who are experiencing 'mental disorder' are very vulnerable and may not be in a position to make decisions that are in their best interests or be able to assert their rights. The Mental Health Acts are therefore an attempt to provide a balance of care and control for those people deemed to be experiencing mental disorders.

Disability Discrimination Act (1995)

Disabled people are a third vulnerable group of care service users who now have their legal rights protected by legislation. The Disability Discrimination Act (1995) was passed to end long-standing discrimination against disabled people in:

- employment

- access to goods, facilities and services

- the management, buying or renting of land or property

- education.

Working with the Mental Health Act (1983)

Natalie Henry is the unit manager of a psychiatric emergency clinic at a large general hospital in London. People who need help or support for acute mental health problems can use the clinic as a walk-in service or are sometimes referred for help by their GP, or are brought in by the police.

Natalie needs to have a very good understanding of the Mental Health Act (1983) because patients at the clinic may present a risk to themselves or other people, and may have to be sectioned. On some occasions Natalie has used Section 5 (4) to detain patients who required an immediate assessment but who wanted to leave the clinic before a qualified psychiatrist could see them. However, this is an unusual occurrence. Natalie is more likely to be involved in arranging for appropriately qualified doctors and social workers to carry out Mental Health Act assessments and checking the sectioning forms to ensure that they have all been completed correctly. Advising patients on their rights to appeal against their sectioning and giving information to their families also forms an important part of her work. Natalie and her colleagues have to ensure that they are fully up to date with the Mental Health Act (1983) as this affects the type of care and treatment that they are able to provide for each patient.

Rights under the DDA (1995)

Virginia James has been a wheelchair-user for the last six years, after sustaining spinal injuries in a fall whilst diving into a swimming pool on holiday. Virginia has tried hard to adapt to her acquired mobility problems and has developed new skills and routines to enable her to carry out daily living and work-related activities. Despite having her home and workplace adapted to meet her new mobility needs, Virginia regularly experiences problems in her local town centre. Her biggest complaint is that many of the local retailers in her town have not adapted their premises to enable access by wheelchair-users. Virginia has written letters to several shop managers about this and has pointed out that their failure to modify their shops is contrary to the Disability Discrimination Act (1995). This places duties on shops and businesses to alter, adapt or remove physical barriers that make it unreasonably difficult for disabled people to receive fair treatment. Virginia has now consulted her solicitors with a view to suing these retailers. She believes that 'it is unacceptable to be put in the embarrassing position of having clothes brought to me on the pavement outside the shop because this makes it difficult for me to make choices and draws attention to my impairment. I have a right to be treated equally.'

The Act introduced new rights to reduce unfair discrimination on the grounds of disability. In particular, the Act now makes it unlawful for a provider of services to treat disabled people less favourably than other people, for a reason related to their disability. Since 1999, service providers have had to make 'reasonable adjustments' for disabled people, such as providing extra help or making changes to the way they provide their services. This includes adjusting premises to overcome physical barriers to access. As a result, public buildings and other facilities such as road crossings and toilets must be made fully accessible for all users.

Care organisations and practitioners working with disabled people now have to ensure that they work in ways that respect the rights of all disabled people. In addition, practitioners committed to anti-discriminatory practice should also challenge and try to change situations where people are being unfairly discriminated against because they are disabled.

Human Rights Act (1998)

The Human Rights Act (1998) is a recent addition to equality law in the UK. It is important in relation to care environments because it entitles people resident in the UK to seek redress for infringements of their human rights by a 'public authority'. A public authority is an organisation that has a public function or which operates in a public sphere. As such, the legislation covers, for example, all kinds of care homes, hospitals and social services departments. The Human Rights Act (1998) affects both the provision of care services and care practice.

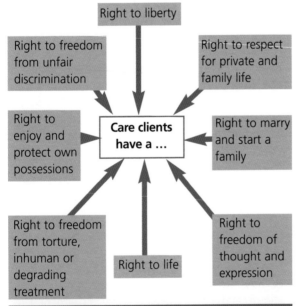

Figure 5 Example of clients' rights under Human Rights Act (1988)

Health and social care practice can, in some cases, affect the human rights and freedoms that are identified by the Human Rights Act (1998). For example, Article 8 of the Act states that 'everyone has the right to respect for his private family life, his home and his correspondence'. This does not change once someone enters a care setting. One consequence is that care practitioners have to be aware of their legal responsibility to respect service users' privacy – when gathering and using personal information, for example. Additionally, the right to life and the right not to be subjected to inhuman and degrading treatment have direct implications for health and social care practitioners. Under the Human Rights Act, people are able to challenge before the UK courts, what they consider to be unlawful interference with their human rights by health and social care laws, policies, practices and procedures.

NHS and Community Care Act (1990)

The NHS and Community Care Act (1990) introduced some of the biggest changes to public care services since the Second World War. These changes affected both the structure and practice of health and social care.

One of the most significant effects of the 1990 Act was that it ended a long-standing state monopoly (in the form of the NHS and local authorities) on the provision of statutory health and social care services. Instead it introduced an 'internal market' in public care provision. This meant that the state became an 'enabler', rather than the main provider, of public access to statutory and non-statutory care services. In effect, this boosted the role and influence of private and voluntary sector providers in the UK care system.

The internal market affected both health and social care provision. In the health care field, the Act created NHS Trusts. These were to be 'provider' organisations, making contracts with new GP fundholding practices and with commissioning or 'purchasing' bodies, to provide health care services for people in a locally defined area. In the social care field, local authorities were also restructured so that an internal market could operate in social care services. In effect, local authority social services departments were divided into purchaser sections and provider sections. The purchaser sections were required to carry out individual needs assessments and to then purchase a 'care package' from private, voluntary or statutory sector provider organisations.

The NHS and Community Care Act (1990) also radically changed the way that adult social care services were provided in the UK. In particular, it ushered in an era of community care for adults with social care and support needs. The idea of community care was that people with chronic or long-term care needs who would normally have lived in state-run institutions would be provided with sufficient support to live in their own homes or at least in a supported 'homely' or domesticated setting. Because of the NHS and Community Care Act (1990) every local authority is now legally bound to assess the care needs of any person with a physical disability, disabling illness, terminal illness, sensory impairment, learning disability or mental health problem. Following the assessment, the local authority must then decide whether the needs of the person call for the provision of any care services. Where this is the case, the purchasing section of the local authority must purchase a care package to meet these needs. As a consequence, the NHS and Community Care Act (1990) continues to support the provision of both community-based care and its delivery by a 'mixed economy' of care providers.

Check your understanding

1 Identify two examples of care legislation that seek to protect the rights of vulnerable groups of care service users.

2 Describe how the NHS and Community Care Act (1990) resulted in a restructuring of the care system in the UK.

3 Explain why care practitioners should be aware of the provisions of the Human Rights Act (1998).

extension **activities**

1 Carry out an internet search on the legal rights of a group of care service users, such as children, disabled people or people experiencing mental disorder. Produce a summary briefing sheet that outlines the key points that you discover.

2 Plan and take part in a discussion about how the rights granted to service users under the Human Rights Act (1998) may have an effect on the way in which practitioners work with people. You might want to select a specific client group to focus more clearly on the implications that this statute may have for care practice.

Patterns of service provision

Getting you thinking

1 Who do you think is responsible for planning and developing health and social care services for the UK as a whole?

2 Describe the difference between central and local government in the UK.

3 Explain how public health care and social services are provided in your local area. In particular, identify the public body that has responsibility for this

Local services to be cut for old and disabled people

Local authority pays for private care

KEY TERMS

Central government
The national, as opposed to the local, level of government.

Devolved system
A system based on the devolution of power – where central government grants power to government at regional or local level.

Informal care
Care that is provided by relatives and friends on an unpaid basis, outside of the professional care system.

Inter-professional working
Team working arrangements where care practitioners with different disciplinary backgrounds work collaboratively to meet and manage the care needs of a service user or client.

Local government
The local, as opposed to the national, level of government.

Mixed economy of care
A care system that is financed through public, private and voluntary sources of funding.

Multi-agency working
A situation where care practitioners employed by different care organisations ('agencies') collaborate to provide care for a particular individual or group of people.

The national provision of care services

As we've seen in Topic 1, health, social care and welfare services are provided by a variety of care organisations with the aim of meeting the individual care needs of the diverse population of the UK.

Health and social care services are organised differently in England, Wales, Scotland and Northern Ireland. Variations in organisation occur because the care systems in each country are controlled by different political institutions and because each country has its own population health needs and its own particular social and welfare history. However, even though there are national differences in care organisation, clear similarities can be seen throughout the UK in the way that care services are provided. For example:

- There is a **'mixed economy of care'** in each country.

- The statutory (public) sector is the largest of the professional care sectors in each country. Because of this, **central** and **local government** play a major role in the planning, funding and, to a lesser extent, provision of care services.

- Private and voluntary sector care organisations have become increasingly important suppliers of direct care services in each country over the past decade.

- Informal carers play a vital part in care provision throughout the UK. The **informal care** sector is, in fact, the largest of all the care sectors.

- Health care provision in each country is still mainly dominated by one large statutory organisation, the National Health Service (NHS), which has a clear national, regional and local structure. By comparison, private and voluntary organisations play a relatively minor role in health care provision.

- Social care is the statutory responsibility of **local government** authorities (councils) and is delivered by a mixed economy of care providers. Voluntary and private sector organisations and private practitioners now play a significant role in actually providing statutory and non-statutory social care and support services.

- The organisational structure of public or statutory sector care in each country is based around a tiered system of national, regional and local care organisations (see the following table).

Until recently, health and social care services have tended to be provided separately by distinct health or social care organisations. Each of these types of

Figure 6 Organisational tiers (levels) in the UK health care system

Country	National	Regional	Local
England	Parliament/ Department of Health	Strategic Health Authority	NHS trust/GP practices.
Wales	National Assembly	Regional government offices	NHS trusts/GP practices
Scotland	Scottish Executive	Health Boards	Primary care trust/local health care co-operative
N. Ireland	NI Assembly/ Department of Health and Social Services	Health and Social Services (HSS) boards	HSS Trusts/ Primary care co-operatives

Working together in care

Martin Jones is a community psychiatric nurse who specialises in working with adolescents. He is employed by an NHS Trust but works in a community-based youth offending team. Martin works alongside youth workers, social workers and education professionals as part of this specialist team.

Martin and his colleagues work with young people aged 13-19 years old who have been referred to the team by the Police, the local youth court or by the local authority education department. All of the young people who have been referred to the team have either committed a criminal offence, been excluded from school because of behavioural problems or have had an Anti-Social Behaviour Order (ASBO) imposed on them by the Courts. Martin and his colleagues aim to establish and develop effective relationships with the young people referred to them in order to help them to deal with personal problems, build up coping skills and self-esteem and modify their behaviour to avoid further contact with the police and the courts.

Martin tends to take the lead on any issues relating to substance misuse or mental health problems. He provides direct care for a number of young people in these areas and also provides information, guidance and support to colleagues where they require it. He thinks that this kind of multi-disciplinary collaborative working is the best way of working in complex areas such as youth offending. Martin believes that this approach will develop to become the norm in the near future.

Getting you thinking

1 Using the data table below, identify the country that has the highest rates of death due to lung cancer.

2 What factors might be responsible for the different mortality rates shown for Scotland and N. Ireland?

3 Describe how the statistical patterns of lung cancer death for Northern Ireland compare to those of other countries in the UK.

4 What kinds of health care and health promotion services should be developed and funded to deal with the mortality patterns in Scotland and N. Ireland?

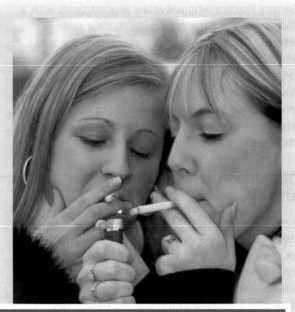

Figure 14 *Mortality due to lung cancer in UK*

Deaths	England	Wales	Scotland	N. Ireland	UK
Males	16,093	1045	2186	482	19,806
Females	10,912	683	1707	528	13,630
All	27,005	1728	3893	810	33,436
Crude rate per 100,000 population					
Males	66.7	74.1	90.0	58.1	68.8
Females	43.0	45.4	65.2	37.7	44.9
All	54.6	59.3	77.1	47.7	56.5

Source: Cancer Research UK website

KEY TERMS

DHSSPS
The acronym for the Department of Health, Social Services and Public Safety which has overall responsibility for health and care policy in Northern Ireland.

GP fundholding
A funding system where general practitioners are given a budget to spend on purchasing care for patients on their practice list.

Health and Social Services Boards
The main purchasing (commissioning) bodies in Northern Ireland.

Health and Social Services Trusts
The main providers of statutory care services in Northern Ireland.

Local Health Care Cooperatives
The bodies that have responsibility for primary care in Scotland.

Northern Ireland Assembly
The body (currently suspended) that is due to take on central government responsibilities in Northern Ireland.

Scottish Parliament
The body that has central government responsibilities in Scotland.

The care system in Northern Ireland

The care system in Northern Ireland has evolved over time into a mixed economy of care. As a result, services are provided through statutory (public), private and voluntary sector organisations and through informal care provision. The structure and organisation of care services in Northern Ireland is harder to describe than in other parts of the UK because of ongoing difficulties over the status of the Northern Ireland Assembly.

The Northern Ireland Assembly was created in order to give elected politicians in Northern Ireland law-making powers in their own country. However, these powers have not been fully implemented, and the Assembly is currently suspended. The Westminster Parliament in London is retaining control of law-making and public bodies until the conflict between sections of the Catholic and Protestant communities of Northern Ireland ends. When this occurs, the direct rule of Northern Ireland by Westminster (including control of the health and social care system) will cease, and politicians elected to the Northern Ireland Assembly will take over responsibility for the statutory care system.

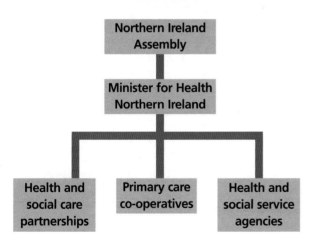

Figure 15 Diagram of proposed N. Ireland care system

One of the consequences of the current situation is that planned reforms of the health and social care system in Northern Ireland cannot go ahead. In the meantime, the statutory system is based around integrated health and social care services. This integrated approach differs to that of England, Wales or Scotland, and is delivered through different types of care organisation.

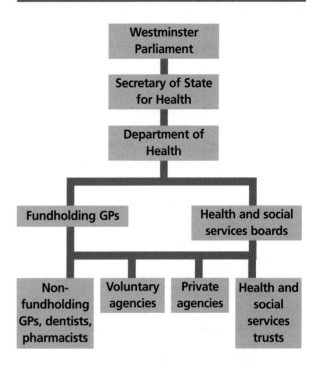

Figure 16 Diagram of N. Ireland care system controlled via Westminster Parliament

The statutory system in Northern Ireland

The Department of Health, Social Services and Public Safety (DHSSPS) – www.dhsspsni.gov.uk – is the central government department in Northern Ireland that is required by law to provide an integrated health and social welfare service for the population. The DHSSPS has three main strategic aims:

- to promote health and social wellbeing
- to target health and social need
- to secure and improve the provision and delivery of health and social services.

The Health and Social Policy Group of the DHSSPS is responsible for promoting wider health and social improvements. It does this by identifying the overall strategy for health and personal social services, and by taking the lead in targeting health and social need. It is primarily responsible for health promotion and protection, and for developing social policy and social legislation.

The four **Health and Social Services Boards** (Northern, Southern, Eastern and Western) are responsible for purchasing care services in Northern Ireland. In effect they act on behalf of the DHSSPS by planning and purchasing health and social services for residents in their areas. In deciding which services are needed, the Boards assess the population's health and social care needs by collecting information about patterns of death, illness and community care needs and by consulting local people. They also liaise with GPs and statutory and voluntary agencies to build up a picture of the health and social care needs of their residents.

Health and Social Services Trusts are the key providers of statutory health and social services in Northern Ireland. They are responsible for the management of staff and services at hospitals and other public sector establishments. There are twenty Health and Social Services Trusts in Northern Ireland, though mergers may reduce this number in the future. Like other parts of the UK, Northern Ireland also operates a mixed economy of care. As a consequence of this, voluntary and community organisations can also deliver health and care services on behalf of the Health and Social Services Trusts. Where these arrangements are made, they are monitored by the Health and Social Services Board for the area. One of the notable features of the care system in Northern Ireland is that it is the only part of the UK that, because of the integrated health and social services, has Trusts based solely on the delivery of community health and social services.

There are also a number of Health and Social Services Agencies and other statutory bodies that provide specialist care services. Examples include the Northern Ireland Health Promotion Agency and the Northern Ireland Blood Transfusion Agency.

Northern Ireland currently has **GP fundholding** arrangements. These allow GPs to purchase secondary and other specialist health care services on behalf of their patients. However, these arrangements are due to be abolished when the Northern Ireland Assembly takes control of the health and social care system. The aim is to replace GP fundholding with Health and Social Care partnerships. These will be made of primary care cooperatives, whose role it will be to assess the health and social care needs of their area (consisting of between 50,000 and 100,000 people) and commission the appropriate services.

Future developments in Northern Ireland

The proposed reorganisation of the statutory care system in Northern Ireland is outlined in a DHSSPS document, *Fit for the Future – A New Approach*, (1999). This indicates that health and social care services will be restructured so that:

- The Northern Ireland Assembly will take on direct control of health and social care services when certain political conditions are met.

- Health and Social Services Boards will be abolished.

- GP fundholding will be abolished.

- The number of Health and Social Services Trusts will be reduced.

These plans may or may not be implemented in the future, depending on political, economic and social developments in Northern Ireland.

The care system in Scotland

Responsibility for the organisation and provision of health and social care services passed from the government in Westminster to the new Scottish Parliament when it was formed in 1999. The **Scottish Parliament** makes fundamental policy decisions regarding health and social care services for Scotland. It delegates the practical, day-to-day work involved in administering care services in Scotland to a civil service body known as the Scottish Executive.

Figure 17 shows that the health service in Scotland is organised into a number of regional Health Boards. These organisations plan and commission health care services from a mixed economy of providers. This

Figure 17 The care system in Scotland

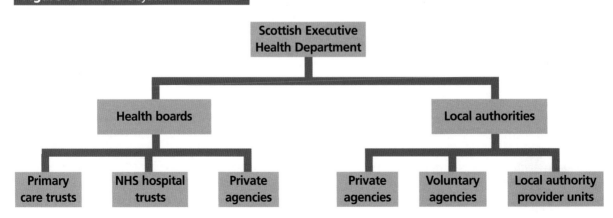

includes statutory NHS Trusts – providing primary and secondary health care services, private agencies and businesses, voluntary organisations and local health care co-operatives, consisting of GPs and other primary health care workers. The Health Boards themselves are responsible for strategic policy development and funding. They are also required to produce and monitor a 'Health Improvement Plan' to raise the quality of health care in their area.

Social care services are also provided through a mixed economy of care in Scotland. This means that local authority social services departments are the main planners and purchasers of social care services. Part of this role involves assessing individuals' care needs. However, whilst local authorities do also provide some social work and social care services themselves, they tend to purchase most of the care that people need from other organisations, such as private and voluntary sector providers.

Check your understanding

1 Identify the organisations that make fundamental policy decisions relating to health and social care in Scotland and Northern Ireland.

2 Describe how the internal market in health care works in Northern Ireland.

3 Describe how social care services are provided through the internal market in Scotland.

4 Explain the similarities and differences between *either* the Northern Ireland *or* the Scottish care system, and that of England or Wales.

extension activities

1 Review the latest organisational and policy developments in Northern Ireland and Scotland on the websites of the Department of Health, Social Services and Public Safety (www.dhsspsni.gov.uk), or the Scottish Executive (www.scotland.gov.uk).

2 Identify and explain some of the advantages of an integrated system of health and social care services, like the one that operates in Northern Ireland. You may want to compare and contrast this to the systems that operate in other parts of the UK, where health and social care tend to be provided by separate care organisations.

Getting you thinking

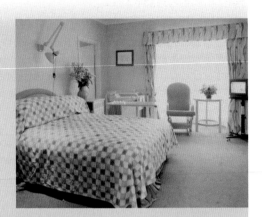

1 Which of these care services do you think is provided by a voluntary organisation?

2 If you wanted to use the services of the organisation in the right-hand picture, what kinds of financial criteria would you need to meet first?

3 How many voluntary organisations can you think of that work with (or on behalf of) children, older people, or disabled people?

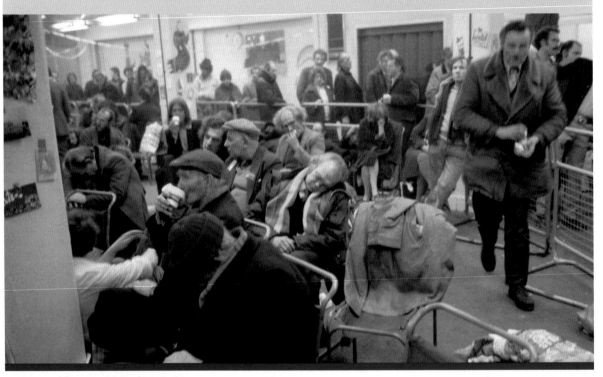

KEY TERMS

Commission for Social Care Inspection (CSCI)

A body that monitors, inspects and regulates standards of care in the social care sector.

Complementary and alternative medicine

A diverse range of health-focused practices and treatments that are not currently part of orthodox (conventional) medicine.

Healthcare Commission

A body that monitors, inspects and regulates standards of care in the health care sector.

Independent sector

The private and not-for-profit voluntary care organisations that are independent of government.

Informal care

Care that is provided on an unpaid basis, by relatives or friends of the person who has care needs.

Philanthropy

The practice of helping people who are less well off than oneself. It is associated with the charitable work of very wealthy people, and played an important part in the emergence of voluntary organisations in the Victorian era.

Independent and informal care provision

As we have seen, there is a mixed economy of care provision in the UK. A significant proportion of the care services available to people is provided by non-statutory organisations, private practitioners and by individuals acting as **informal carers**. The non-statutory organisations and private practitioners who provide care services are collectively known as the **independent sector**. This sector has become increasingly important as a source of care provision over the last twenty years. This is because:

- Conservative and recent Labour governments have deliberately encouraged independent sector provision.

- Demographic factors, including the ageing population, have created a growing demand for health and social care.

- A rise in the number of women in paid work, outside of the home, has increased the need for child care services.

- There is a lack of adequate public services in some areas.

It is also suggested that the growth in health consciousness and 'body-awareness' has partly been stimulated by a private sector that has marketed a variety of 'health' services and products to an increasingly consumer-oriented and image-conscious population. People are now much more willing to buy health and care services (including private dentistry, cosmetic surgery and home care services, for example) that link health to 'lifestyle' and personal choice in a positive way.

The private sector

The private sector identifies care as a 'market' in which profits can be made by selling services to 'consumers' of care. There is now a very diverse range of private care provision available throughout the UK. This includes everything from home adaptations and equipment for disabled people to private health screening, eye-testing and dentistry for people who take a preventive approach to their personal health. The market for private care services includes everything from life-giving fertility treatments to end-of-life terminal care. The key point about all of these services is that they are provided on a commercial basis. This means that the organisations and individual practitioners who provide them operate to make a financial profit.

Until recently, the people who used private care services had to either pay directly for services themselves or had to have private care insurance that covered the cost of the services they needed. However, it is now possible, in some circumstances, to receive publicly funded care in a private care setting, from practitioners employed by a private care organisation. This occurs in situations where a statutory (government-run) care organisation has agreed a funding contract with a private care provider. Nursing home care for older people, cataract operations and health screening have all been provided through such public–private partnerships. This is a good example of how the boundaries between care sectors have become increasingly blurred.

It is estimated that around 14 million people in Britain use private health of one kind or another. Many people do so because they don't want to wait for NHS treatment, because they want to choose when and where to receive care, or because they want a specific form of treatment or support that isn't available through the NHS – or isn't provided by their local authority. About 850,000 people have private operations each year. This accounts for 20 per cent of all routine surgery. In fact, almost a third of all hip replacements and almost half of all pregnancy terminations are carried out by the private sector.

The extent of private sector involvement in both health and social care provision is now significant. The private sector contributes to health and social care provision both directly and indirectly. It is also worth noting that whilst the private sector is increasingly involved in the health and social care field, the range of services offered by private providers tends to be more limited in range than those offered by the statutory sector. The private services available are limited to those for which there is a commercial market – that a sufficient number of people are prepared to pay for. These tend to be the specialist, lifestyle-related and less complex forms of care and treatment. In contrast, statutory organisations – such as the NHS and local authorities – provide a broader range of care services for people whose health, social care and support needs are often complex, critical and expensive to meet. Many of the diverse forms of care provided by statutory organisations are not commercially viable, because people are unwilling, and also unable, to pay for them.

The debate about whether, and to what extent, the private sector should participate in providing health and social care is a long and politically sensitive one. As well as being aware of the political and economics issues relating to private care provision, it is also worth noting that the debate involves major ethical questions too. These relate to the justice, fairness or ethical acceptability of making a person's ability to pay for care a condition for giving them access to services. In a fully privatised care system it is likely that poorer people would not have adequate access to care services, and that services which were not commercially viable would not be widely available – or would be poorly funded where they were provided.

Figure 18 *Forms of private sector health and social care provision*

Direct private provision
- Private fee-paying hospitals, nursing and residential homes, nurseries and clinics, for example.
- Drugs, surgical equipment, bandages, etc. sold to the NHS and local authorities.
- Low-cost treatments, non-prescription drugs, appliances and therapies purchased directly from private suppliers, such as chemists, opticians, dentists and private practitioners (including **complementary and alternative medicine** practitioners).

Private health insurance
There are a variety of different private health schemes, such as PPP, BUPA and Denplan.

Private funding
The Private Finance Initiative is used by government to fund some major hospital-building schemes and other projects that require large amounts of funding.

The voluntary sector

The voluntary care sector is both independent of, but interdependent on, the statutory health and social care sector. The voluntary care sector has a long history of providing health and, more significantly, social welfare services in the UK. The origins of the voluntary sector can, in fact, be traced back through the eighteenth and nineteenth centuries. It was during the nineteenth century, especially the Victorian era, that faith-based voluntary organisations like the Quakers and wealthy, socially motivated or **philanthropic** people, such as the Cadbury family, established the voluntary sector as a major provider of basic health care and welfare in the UK. However, even at this time the voluntary sector was only able to provide a small proportion of the social care and welfare services that people required. One of the main reasons for this was that services cost money to run, and voluntary services, at this time, relied almost entirely on donations of money and time to enable them to run.

The defining characteristics of voluntary sector services are:
- They have been established because an individual or a group of people has voluntarily decided to set up an organisation for a particular purpose. No law was required to create it.
- Voluntary organisations are usually (but not always) registered charities, and always operate on a 'not-for-profit' basis.
- They are partly staffed and run by unpaid volunteers. However, it is also very common for voluntary organisations to employ people to work in paid jobs within their organisation.

The voluntary sector has traditionally focused more on social care and welfare provision than on health care. This has often been provided on a 'safety-net' basis – to fill gaps in public (state-provided) services and to provide a basic level of provision for marginalised social groups, such as the very poor and homeless people. Additionally, most voluntary organisations, including the large national ones, don't necessarily offer their services in all localities. This is one obvious difference between statutory and voluntary organisations.

Inter-dependent provision of health and social care

As we have seen, the statutory, private and voluntary sectors are interdependent because, in reality, statutory organisations work closely with voluntary and private organisations. This usually occurs where a purchaser and provider partnership is established. Typically, a statutory body such as a local authority or NHS Trust will purchase care services from a private or voluntary sector provider organisation. In addition, the quality of services delivered by private and voluntary sector care providers are also monitored and regulated by statutory bodies, such as the **Healthcare Commission** and the **Commission for Social Care Inspection**. As a consequence, it is best to think of the different care sectors as being interdependent in various ways.

The informal care sector

The provision of health and social care services is often presented as the domain of qualified and highly skilled professionals. This is partly true, but this perspective fails to acknowledge the huge contribution that **informal carers** also make to care provision. According to the General Household Survey (1995), one in eight UK adults was providing informal care, and one in six UK households contained a carer. 'Carers' were defined as people who were looking after or providing some regular service for a sick, handicapped or elderly person living in their own or another private household. It is estimated that in the UK around 7 million people – mainly women – provide informal care on a regular basis (see examples, below).

Two-thirds of the people who are informal carers of working age have to combine their informal care role with paid employment. This can be exceptionally tiring and difficult. However, many of the people who receive informal care are wholly dependent on their carers for help and support. In some cases, this can mean adults being dependent on children. The Carers' National Association estimates that over 10,000 carers are young people aged 18 or under, generally caring for a parent. Data from the General Household Survey (1995) indicated that over a third of carers reported that nobody else helped them look after their dependants. A further 26 per cent did receive help, but spent more time looking after their dependant than anyone else, and just under 10 per cent shared the task of caring with someone else. Women were more likely than men to be caring unaided, while men were more likely to be 'non-main carers'.

It is evident that if no informal care was available then there would be no way the formal care sectors could fill the gaps.

Examples of informal care tasks:

- A relative helping with someone's personal care, washing, dressing, and so on.

- A neighbour doing shopping or collecting prescriptions.

- A relative helping with the cleaning.

- A neighbour walking a housebound old person's dog for them.

- A friend calling into give someone living alone some company.

- A granddaughter calling round in the evening to sit with her disabled grandfather, allowing her grandmother to go out.

Check your understanding

1 Identify reasons for the increase in independent sector care provision over the last twenty years.

2 Describe the main characteristics of the private health care sector.

3 Describe the main characteristics of the voluntary care sector.

4 Explain the role and importance of informal carers in the overall provision of care in the UK.

extension activities

1 To what extent are you either an informal carer yourself or the recipient of informal care from other people? Identify examples of the kinds of informal care that you give to others, and that you receive from others.

2 Find out about the work of the Healthcare Commission (www.chai.org.uk) and the Commission for Social Care Inspection (www.csci.org.uk). Try and find out about the inspections that they have carried out on health and social care services in your local area.

Planning care for individual needs

Getting you thinking

Geraldine is 85 years of age. She is the main carer for her husband Tom, aged 92. Geraldine is fiercely independent and has cared for Tom for the last ten years without any help from professional care workers, other than her GP. Tom has had *Parkinson's disease* for the last 10 years and has also become confused and disoriented since the onset of *Alzheimer's disease*, 5 years ago. Tom is now incontinent, has limited mobility and is unable to manage any of his personal care needs without Geraldine's assistance. Geraldine is becoming worried about Tom's health and his safety in the house. She says that she always does her best to look after him, but she is now willing to admit that she isn't able to do this on her own.

1 Identify the kinds of care needs that Tom and Geraldine each have.

2 What would you expect a professional care worker – such as a social worker or community nurse – to do if they were called to see Tom and Geraldine at home?

3 Explain why it is important that any professional care worker who is asked to see Tom or Geraldine avoids making any judgements about them and their situation until they have met and spoken with them both.

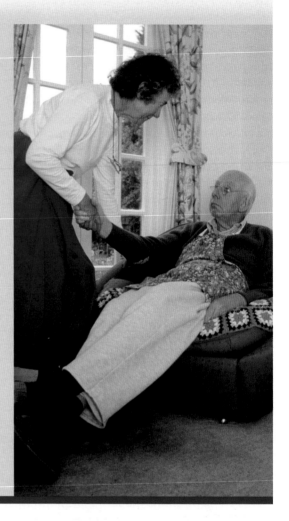

KEY TERMS

Alzheimer's disease
A disease that leads to progressive degeneration of the brain, and the commonest cause of dementia in people of all ages.

Assessment
The process of identifying and judging the importance of something.

Care planning cycle/process
A multi-stage cycle used by care practitioners to produce and implement individualised care plans.

Evaluation
The process of finding or judging the value or significance of something. For example, care practitioners evaluate the effectiveness of the interventions and treatments that they use.

Holistic assessment
An assessment that focuses on the 'whole person' rather than a specific or partial aspect of their functioning.

Individualised care
Care that is planned and delivered to meet the specific needs of an individual.

Parkinson's disease
A slowly progressing disease of the nervous system that results in involuntary tremors and the loss of muscular control and movement abilities.

Task-focused care
Forms of care that focus on carrying out a series of specified tasks for one or more service users, such as 'toileting everyone at 3 p.m.', regardless of the service users' individual care needs.

Care planning practices

Health and social care organisations employ a range of care practitioners to actually plan and deliver direct care services for individuals who have care needs. As an occupational group, health and social care practitioners have a very diverse range of skills and training. Depending on the type of care organisation and the area of care that they work in, these practitioners could specialise in medical treatment, nursing care, social work interventions or occupational therapy, for example. However, despite the differences in their skills and specialist knowledge, members of any care team are likely to take a similar approach to their work. This is because care practitioners tend to:

- Assess each individual's care needs.

- Develop an individualised plan of treatment, support or therapies to meet the person's particular care needs.

Individualised care is a very important feature of care practice today. It is now the preferred alternative to **task-focused care** (see opposite). Care planning is the key to providing high quality individualised care. Care practitioners are trained to follow and use a **care planning cycle** (see Figure 19) as a way of developing and delivering an appropriate, individualised care plan for each person they work with. This process is cyclical, in that one stage leads on to another (though there are overlaps), and a person's care plan is likely to go through several cycles of assessment, planning, monitoring and evaluation in response to either improvements or deterioration in their condition or personal or social problems.

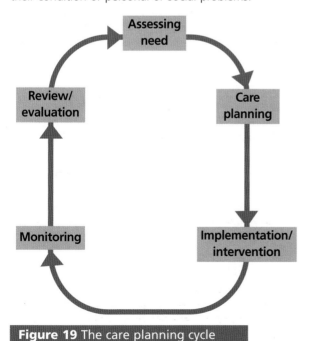

Figure 19 The care planning cycle

Task-focused care

Task-focused care was the dominant approach to care provision until the early 1980s. Until this point, care practitioners tended to deliver 'care' by routinely carrying out a series of specified tasks during their shift or working day. For example, a task-focused approach in a nursing home might involve making sure that every client was washed, dressed and taken to the toilet before breakfast. In task-focused settings, routines become more important than individual needs. As a result, care-giving can become an impersonal, ineffective and insensitive process. The effects and effectiveness of task-focused care were rarely questioned until individualised approaches to care suggested that it is better to recognise and adapt care provision to each individual's particular needs, strengths and abilities. Another criticism of the task-focused approach is that it tends to ignore the personal wishes and preferences of the individual, in favour of 'saving time' and 'getting the job done'. Individualised care is the modern alternative to task-focused care work.

Assessment of needs

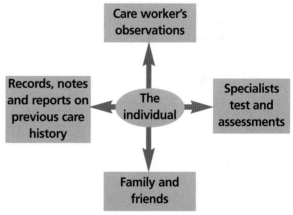

Figure 20 Sources of assessment information

As you can see from Figure 19, the care plan cycle has a number of stages or components to it. The first stage involves a thorough **assessment** of an individual's care needs. An individual who has complex needs or who requires ongoing care services may be assessed by a number of different care professionals. For example, a community nurse, social worker and an occupational therapist may each assess an older person who requires care and support to remain living in their own home. Whilst each of these practitioners should carry out a **holistic assessment**, they will also tend to focus on the individual's needs in a slightly different way. The differences will reflect their professional concerns, priorities and skills. However, a multi-disciplinary approach like this is also likely to lead to a more detailed and thorough assessment of the individual's care needs.

Tom Farmer, who is 92, currently lives at home with his wife Geraldine. She is his main carer. Geraldine, however, is 85 and has been finding it increasingly difficult to care for Tom on her own. Tom's GP has diagnosed him with Alzheimer's disease and Parkinson's disease.

Jason Greene is a staff nurse working in the accident and emergency department of a large general hospital. Jason recently met Tom for the first time after Tom was brought in with cuts and bruises to his face and scalp. Jason dealt with Tom's injuries and was then asked to assess Tom's mental and physical needs.

Jason asked Tom a range of questions to assess his mental state and also spoke with his wife Geraldine about Tom's current level of ability and self-care skills. He made a note that Tom's GP should be able to provide more information on his previous medical history and that he should be contacted. The outcome of the assessment was that Jason recommended that Tom should be admitted to an elderly assessment ward at the hospital for a more detailed period of observation. Both Tom and Geraldine were reluctant, but did agree to this.

Planning care

The second stage of the care planning cycle is the actual planning of care itself. The information obtained from the individual needs assessment should be used to produce an individualised care plan. The care plan should:

- identify the individual's particular care needs.

- set goals or objectives that care workers should aim to achieve by providing care.

- identify the type of care the person requires and the way it will be provided for them. Care interventions should be carefully selected to meet the individual's specific care needs.

Tom Farmer was admitted to Churchill ward from the accident and emergency department in the middle of the night. Jenny Neale, the nurse in charge of the ward at the time, read through the notes produced by Jason in accident and emergency and informed the duty doctor that a 92-year-old man had been admitted.

After showing Tom to a side room and settling him down to sleep, Jenny began completing the care planning documents that are used on Churchill ward. She recorded all of Tom's personal details and the contact numbers for his wife and GP. She then summarised the accident and emergency staff's notes in the section about 'Reason for admission'. Because Tom was now asleep and his wife had been taken home by her neighbour, Jenny could not complete any more of the care planning documentation. This asked questions about Tom's current levels of ability in a number of areas (such as mobility, feeding and washing and dressing) and about the types of support that he has at home. Jenny made a note in his records that the next shift of nurses should begin a full assessment of Tom's needs and abilities in order to produce an appropriate care plan for him.

Implementing care

The third stage of the care planning cycle is the implementation of the care that has been planned. This involves delivering planned care and monitoring its effects on the individual. The care provided should be monitored, and any changes in an individual's needs or condition should be documented in their care plan notes. This information is required for the final evaluation stage of the care plan cycle.

Figure 21 *Positive reasons for care planning*

- Planning individualised care is an effective way of recognising each person's particular care needs and preferences.
- Planned care is more likely to be targeted at an individual's priority needs.
- Planning care increases the consistency and efficiency of care delivery.
- Care plans provide a common focus and source of information for all care team members to use.
- Monitoring and evaluating planned care ensures that care interventions remain effective and appropriate to an individual's changing needs.

Evaluating care

The final stage of the care plan cycle is the **evaluation** of the care plan and the effectiveness of the care provided. In essence, a care practitioner or team of practitioners have to decide whether the care plan goals have been met and whether the current plan of care remains appropriate for the individual. A new assessment of need might be carried out if the individual's care needs have changed. This can happen because the person's condition or situation has either improved or deteriorated. Alternatively, the care that has been delivered may need to be changed because it has not been effective in meeting the person's needs. Care plans are not usually evaluated on a daily basis. It may, in fact, take months of care provision before any (even minor) changes occur in a person's needs, condition or situation. Despite this, care plans should be evaluated regularly to ensure that they remain up to date and relevant to the individual receiving care.

Involving service users in planned care

The person who has care needs should always be at the centre of care work. This is very much the case when planning and delivering care for individuals. Therefore, it is good care practice to involve an individual in the care planning cycle as early as possible and to find ways of maintaining this involvement in each stage of the care plan cycle.

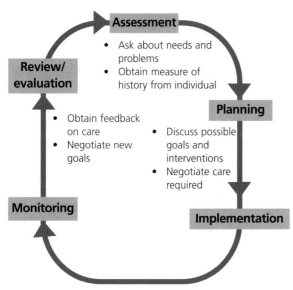

- Ask about progress
- Ask about possible changes required to change plan
- Involve and support self-care
- Assist during care delivery

Figure 22 Evaluating care

The assessment stage provides the first opportunity to involve an individual in planned care. Asking the person directly for information about their background, needs and preferences may provide a lot of relevant information that can be used to plan their care. It also provides the individual with a way of expressing their wishes and preferences and provides the ideal opportunity to negotiate about and gain the person's consent for the delivery of specific forms of care.

Wherever possible, you should discuss a *proposed* care plan with the individual. This discussion should be seen as an opportunity to describe and explain the care needs that have been identified, to negotiate some goals and to agree on care interventions. Discussing proposed care interventions is an important way of gaining consent and of preparing individuals for forms of care that may be intrusive or personal. It is also an opportunity to motivate and encourage people to maintain and make use of their existing self-care skills and abilities. Involving people at this

Following Tom's care plan experience

Tom Farmer spent six weeks as an in-patient on Churchill ward. During the first two weeks the medical and nursing staff carried out a range of physical checks and mental health tests on Tom. The nursing staff also spent time observing him and recording their impressions of his level of ability and his care needs. This period of assessment led to a meeting where staff discussed Tom's needs and discussed how these could be met. Jenny Neale took on responsibility for co-ordinating Tom's care and wrote a care plan. The goals of the plan were to maximise Tom's self-care and mobility skills, to put appropriate home care in place to support him and Geraldine when Tom was discharged and to use simple 'reality orientation' techniques to reduce Tom's confusion. These included using Tom's name and gaining his attention before asking him questions or giving him information, reminding him where he was and explaining when his wife would be visiting him.

The care plan was implemented by all of the nursing staff on the ward. A nominated person wrote brief notes about Tom's care and his progress at the end of each nursing shift. It gradually became clear that Tom was improving and was well enough to go home. Jenny and the nursing staff evaluated Tom's care plan and produced a new discharge plan a few days before he returned home with Geraldine.

Working in a care organisation

Getting you thinking

1 **Identify the biggest care profession working in the NHS.**

2 **What percentage of staff working in the NHS provide direct care services?**

3 **Which types of statutory care providers are not represented in these statistics?**

4 **Why do you think people choose to work in care occupations?**

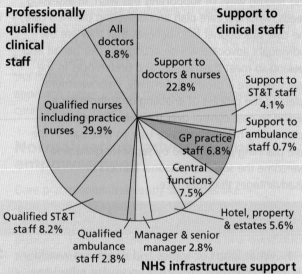

Figure 24 Care professions in the NHS

Professionally qualified clinical staff

All doctors 8.8%

Support to clinical staff

Support to doctors & nurses 22.8%

Support to ST&T staff 4.1%

Support to ambulance staff 0.7%

Qualified nurses including practice nurses 29.9%

GP practice staff 6.8%

Central functions 7.5%

Hotel, property & estates 5.6%

Qualified ST&T staff 8.2%

Qualified ambulance staff 2.8%

Manager & senior manager 2.8%

NHS infrastructure support

Figure 25 *Number of staff in the NHS in 2004, DOH (2005)*	
Occupational group	**Employed in NHS**
Nursing, midwifery and health visiting	397,515
Doctors	117,036
Qualified scientific, therapeutic and technical (ST & T) staff	128,883
Qualified ambulance staff	17,272
NHS infrastructure support	211,489
GP Practice staff	90,110

KEY TERMS

Accountability
Being responsible to someone or for something.

Mission statement
A formal statement of a care organisation's aims or objectives. It sets out the organisation's sense of purpose or 'mission'.

Organisational culture
The values, beliefs and assumptions that influence the practices, procedures, ways of working and 'atmosphere' of an organisation.

Private practitioners
Care practitioners who are either self-employed or who are employed by a private sector care organisation.

Role
The job, task, or function that a person has.

Team-building
The process of developing a group of employees into an effective work team.

Typology
A classification system that identifies 'types' of something.

Employment in the care field

As you can see from the statistics presented in Figure 24, a large number of people work in some form of care role in the UK. You should also note that these statistics only refer to people who work in *paid* health care jobs. There are, of course, a large number of social care employees and informal carers to consider too when thinking about the total care 'workforce'. People who are employed as care practitioners are either self-employed as **private practitioners** or are employed by a care organisation on a permanent or temporary basis. The vast majority of care practitioners are employed by care organisations. As we've seen, there are a variety of types of care organisation in the UK, including voluntary, private and statutory (public) organisations. Statutory organisations are the biggest employers. The NHS is, in fact, the largest employer in Europe.

Organisational culture

The ways in which employees work and practise care in the NHS, or any other care organisation for that matter, are influenced and constrained by the 'culture' of the care organisation they work for. **Organisational culture** is thought to be one of the most powerful influences on work practice in any employment setting. But what is organisational culture?

The culture of an organisation results from the values and beliefs of the people who control and work in the organisation. 'The way we do things around here' is one way of defining organisational culture. However, this is a little simplistic, as it doesn't draw attention to the powerful and critical role of the shared values, beliefs and assumptions on which an organisation's culture must be based.

An organisation's assumptions, values and beliefs about the best ways to carry out work tasks and treat both employees and users of the organisation's services are expressed through:

- the way care work is organised and experienced by employees and service users.

- the way power and authority are distributed and used in the care organisation.

- the attitudes to, and levels of, trust, risk-taking and anxiety in the care organisation.

- the ways employees are organised, rewarded and controlled in their work roles.

- the extent to which the care organisation adopts a formal or informal, standardised or flexible approach to relationships, communication and work-related matters.

- the extent to which the care organisation imposes rules, procedures and specific ways of working on employees or supports individual initiative and creative team-working.

Each care organisation has it own particular culture that affects the practice of people who work in it – and the clients' experiences.

Types of organisational culture

It might be argued that every care organisation has its unique working culture. However, it is also possible to identify common features in similar types of organisational culture. Organisation and management theorists, such as Charles Handy, have identified links between the structure of an organisation and its culture. Handy's typology (1985) is based on the claim that different organisational structures tend to establish different kinds of working conditions, in which particular organisational cultures emerge.

For example, a supportive and enabling culture may well be a feature of an organisation that has a democratic, participative and 'flat' structure. Care practitioners who work in this kind of culture may feel that they are able to contribute positively to decision-making, and that their views and concerns are taken seriously and responded to. In contrast, a formal, bureaucratic and rule-based organisational culture may emerge in an organisation that is autocratic and hierarchical. Care practitioners working in this kind of culture may feel that they have much less influence over their working environment or their ability to contribute to it in a personal way.

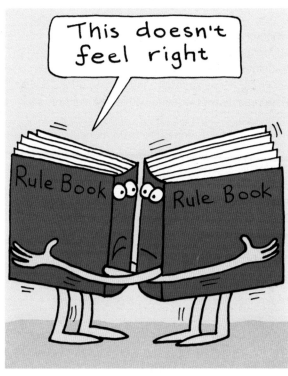

Charles Handy's own typology (1985) identifies four different organisational cultures:

The power culture

This is like a web with a ruling spider. Those in the web are dependent on a central power source. Rays of power and influence spread out from a central figure or group. In this organisational culture, power derives from the top person, and a personal relationship with that individual matters more than any formal title or position. This type of organisational culture may occur in small, owner-managed care settings and in support groups.

The role culture

This is often referred to as a bureaucracy. An organisation with a role culture tends to be controlled by procedures, role descriptions and authority definitions. Coordination of work occurs from the top. A person's job title or role position is central to their experience of the organisation. Predictable and consistent systems and procedures are highly valued in a role culture. As a result, care settings based around this type of organisational culture can be inflexible and find adjusting to change difficult. However, this type of organisational culture is also associated with highly structured, stable care settings in which people have clear job descriptions and are very aware of their work role.

The task culture

Care settings that are based around a task culture tend to adopt a small team approach to their work. Task cultures tend to focus on collaborations between people with specialist skills or knowledge, perhaps working as a network, who all contribute in a cooperative way in order to achieve a specific goal or to deliver a particular project. The emphasis is on achieving definable results and getting things done. Care practitioners working within task cultures are given a lot of personal control and discretion over how their work is done. The major benefits of this type of organisational culture are that it is flexible, adaptable and promotes collaborative problem-solving. The drawback is that there is less direct control and monitoring of individuals, and it works best where practitioners operate in specialist, highly-skilled small teams.

The person culture

The individual is the central point or focus of an organisation that is based on a person culture. If there is an organisational structure it exists only to serve the individuals within it. Organisations with this type of culture don't have bigger or more profound political,

social or moral goals. The individuals who are the focus of a person culture tend to have strong values about how they will work. They tend to have a great deal of professional autonomy, and control their own work. This makes them very difficult for the organisation to manage. A specialist medical or private psychotherapy practice may develop a person culture because organisations like these tend only to exist so that the practitioners who work through them can achieve their professional goals. These kinds of (often private) care practices cease to exist once key individuals leave them, because they have no broader or deeper social reasons for continuing.

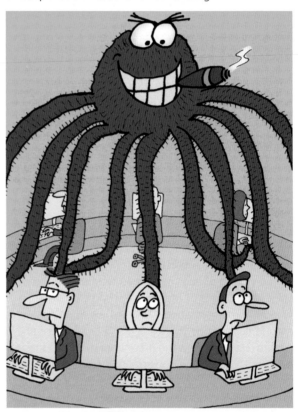

Typologies of organisational culture such as this shouldn't be interpreted too rigidly or literally. It isn't the case, for example, that a care organisation's culture never changes. Every organisation's culture is likely to develop and change over time, as the people who control and work in the care organisation move into and out of posts where they influence it. Moreover, elements of different types of culture may well exist and overlap in a large organisation, such as an NHS Trust, which has a lot of staff working in diverse roles and in specialist sub-groupings.

The effects of organisational culture

So, just as we are born into a culture that shapes our personal and social development, care practitioners enter into and are influenced by the 'culture' of the care organisation that they work in. In particular, the culture of a care organisation influences a care practitioner's:

- **decision-making** – because the organisation's processes and procedures must be followed.

- **management style** – because the distribution of power and authority, communication channels and personnel arrangements influence management approaches and opportunities.

- **accountability** – because managerial arrangements and the extent to which there is a culture of innovation and initiative or one of managerial monitoring and control will determine the way in which a care practitioner is held to be accountable for their care practice.

- **goals and objectives** – because these must be consistent with those of the organisation.

- **actions and behaviour** towards other people within the organisation and those they work with on behalf of the organisation.

An organisation's culture is the foundation on which it exists and operates in the care field. Because organisational culture is so powerful, care practitioners' decisions and actions may not always be 'their own'. This is because they are employees, and their decisions, approaches and objectives are shaped and constrained by the socialisation processes and cultural influences of the organisation they work for. This is one of the reasons why a care practitioner may say that they feel more or less comfortable working in a particular care setting. Where the culture suits them, and is conducive to their own expectations and ways of working, they will experience a better 'fit' – and vice versa.

Organisational culture and care practice

As we've seen, organisational culture is more complex than just 'the way we do things around here'. However, whilst assumptions, values and beliefs provide the foundations for organisational culture, the more visible and tangible consequences of an organisation's culture are seen in the policies, processes and care practices of the care organisation itself. For example, an organisation's culture will have a direct impact on its goals and objectives. These will be formally expressed through its **mission statement**. In practical terms, the organisation's admission policies and procedures, the models of care practice that are used, and the approach taken to issues such as unfair discrimination, equal opportunities and staff training and development – these will all be influenced by the culture of the organisation. The organisation's culture will pervade all of these areas and influence the collective response of the organisation's managers and care practitioners.

Check your understanding

1. Identify the care sector that contains the largest number of carers in the UK.

2. What does an organisation's 'culture' consist of?

3. Describe two contrasting types of organisational culture.

4. Explain how an organisation's 'culture' can affect the way care practitioners work.

extension activities

Different types of organisational culture tend to develop in different types of care settings. Which type of organisational culture do you think would be most suitable in each of the following circumstances?

- A multi-disciplinary team of health care practitioners working in a hospital accident and emergency department.

- A private counselling service where counsellors see clients for pre-booked individual appointments.

- A hospital ward staffed by registered nurses of different grades and levels of experience and expertise, and unqualified health care assistants.

- A surgical team working on complex operations in a hospital theatre.

Quality assurance issues in care

Getting you thinking

1 **Identify the problems or complaints that have led to the care practitioner in the extracts being exposed in the media.**

2 **Describe the standards of care that you expect your GP to offer you and other patients who go to your general practice.**

3 **Suggest reasons why establishing and monitoring specific standards of care practice and service delivery is an important part of service management.**

4 **Who do you think is responsible for establishing and maintaining acceptable levels of care services in the area where you live?**

GP struck off after 30 patients are infected with hepatitis B

A 70 year-old GP in London who served a jail term for obtaining illegal abortions was struck off the medical register for the second time last week after he admitted causing an outbreak of acute hepatitis B.

The General Medical Council found Dr S guilty of serious professional misconduct after causing 30 patients to become infected with hepatitis B.

The GMC's professional conduct committee said that he had a "cavalier approach" to the most basic medical procedures and had failed to take appropriate measures to protect patients from the risk of serious communicable diseases.

Source: BMJ. 2000 November 25; 321(7272): 1308.

KEY TERMS

Audit
A process of examining or checking activity or performance against a required standard.

Charters
Documents that set out the targets and standards of service that a care organisation seeks to achieve in its work with service users.

Clinical governance
The process of improving the quality of care services by controlling and improving work systems in a care organisation.

National service frameworks
Service standards for specific areas of care practice that are defined by government. Care organisations are expected to provide and achieve levels of service delivery that achieve these standards.

Quality assurance
A general process of monitoring and evaluating whether specified standards of service quality have been achieved.

Quality standards
Statements of performance or outcomes that define an acceptable level of service.

Total Quality Management
A management philosophy that seeks to integrate all of the functions of an organisation (marketing, finance, care delivery, customer service, etc.) in a way that focuses on meeting customer needs and the organisation's objectives.

'Quality' and national care policy

There has been a growing concern with the 'quality' of care services in the UK over the last 20 years, but especially in the last 5 years. The concern with improving the quality of care standards and care services has been a major focus of modernisation and reform efforts in the public (statutory) care sector in particular. Quality issues are now a major strand or theme of national care policy in the UK.

Efforts to achieve and maintain higher quality standards in care services really began in the 1980s. In particular, quality issues became a more significant focus in care policy in the mid-1980s when business principles were first introduced into the management of care services. At this time there was a new managerial focus on improving efficiency and reducing the cost of providing public care services. The introduction of **Total Quality Management** (TQM) methods into the public sector also led to a new focus in care organisations on:

- meeting customer needs

- defining what the standards of a quality service were

- monitoring and measuring the performance of practitioners and care organisations in quantitative ways.

Efforts to identify and monitor the quality of care work are not always popular with care practitioners, and many would dispute the way in which the quality of their work is evaluated (judged). However, despite the frequent criticisms that interpersonal services like care giving are difficult or even impossible to evaluate in a quantitative way, total quality management and other **quality assurance** methods such as **auditing** are now widely used throughout the health and social care field.

Quality assurance in care

The quality assurance system that operates in health and social care is complex, but can be understood by focusing on:

- the national system of care standards and service regulation

- organisational systems of governance and audit

- the accountability of individual care practitioners

Each of these areas of quality work contribute to the detailed systematic efforts that are now being made to establish, regulate and maintain high standards of professional practice and service delivery in all areas of health and social care.

National systems of care standards and regulation

The present-day concern of governments with establishing clear service standards for public sector organisations has its origins in the **Citizen's Charter** and **Patient's Charter** initiatives that were developed by a Conservative government in the early 1990s. The aim of the first Citizen's Charter was to maintain standards and improve 'every part of the public services'. Citizen's Charters are now an integral part of public sector care services. They are designed to encourage service users to judge whether the services that they receive match up to the targets that the charter sets out. As a result, they focus primarily on driving up quality and they make care organisations more accountable to service users. It is thought that by producing and working to achieve charter targets a care organisation will communicate with service users more often and seek to identify and meet their needs more effectively. Local service charters are supposed to incorporate national care standards, taking them as their starting point and seeking to improve on them.

The Patient's Charter, also introduced in the early 1990s, aims to put the Citizen's Charter into practice in the NHS by:

- listening to and acting on people's views and needs

- setting clear standards of service

- providing services which meet those standards.

Figure 26 *What a public service charter is designed to do*

- Help public organisations set out clearly what they are aiming to do.
- Clarify what their users need, and target resources in the way they want them.
- Encourage users to provide feedback on services, which can be used to raise standards.
- Explain to users the role they can play in helping public service agencies deliver the services they want.
- Explain how public services link together, to help drive and sustain a process of continual improvement in service quality.
- Encourage good relations with users, staff and other local service providers generally.

THIS UNIT IS ABOUT THE PROMOTION OF HEALTH AND WELL-BEING. It will enable you to develop your knowledge and understanding of the principles behind health promotion campaigns, including how and why they are carried out and how topics and target groups are identified. You will also develop skills in planning, carrying out and evaluating an activity. The unit will provide you with the information that you need to carry out your own small-scale health promotion activity. Evidence from this activity will provide the basis of assessment for Unit 8 of the Edexcel GCE A2 Health and Social Care award.

You will learn about:

- Why health promotion campaigns are carried out, and how topics and target groups are identified
- The different models and approaches that are used in health promotion
- The different agencies that are involved in health promotion
- How a health promotion activity is planned, delivered and evaluated.

Promoting Health and Well-being

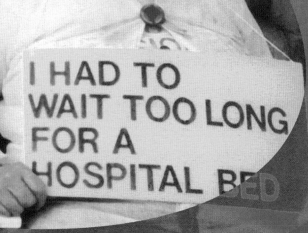

Key questions

By the end of the unit you should be able to use the knowledge, understanding and skills that you develop to answer the following questions:

1 What are the factors that influence the decision to launch a health promotion?
2 How would you describe the different models and approaches that may be used in health promotion?
3 What are the main stages in planning and implementing a health promotion?
4 How would you deliver a small-scale promotion to a specific target group?

Getting you thinking

Ten tips for better health

1 Don't smoke. If you can, stop. If you can't, cut down.

2 Follow a balanced diet, with plenty of fruit and vegetables.

3 Keep physically active.

4 Manage stress by, for example, talking things through and making time to relax.

5 If you drink alcohol, do so in moderation.

6 Cover up in the sun, protect children from sunburn.

7 Practise safer sex.

8 Take up cancer-screening opportunities.

9 Be safe on the roads: follow the Highway Code.

10 Learn the First Aid ABC – airways, breathing circulation.

(from *Saving Lives – Our Healthier Nation*, Liam Donaldson, Chief Medical Officer, 1999)

1 For each of the ten tips, why could following the advice lead to better health?

2 Identify which aspects of an individual's health and well-being each tip might influence.

3 If the advice is followed, who besides the individual might benefit?

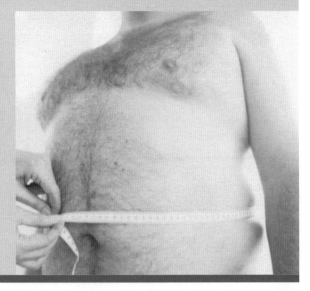

KEY TERMS

Need
Something a person requires or could benefit from. People have physical, intellectual, emotional and social needs.

Normative need
Needs defined by experts.

Felt need
What people feel they need.

Expressed need
What people demand or say they require.

Comparative need
Need in comparison with others in the same situation.

Pathology
The study of disease.

What do we mean by health?

Before considering how to promote health, it would help to know what we mean by 'health'. The answer can be all encompassing. The World Health Organization's definition is a positive view:

'Health is a state of complete physical, mental and social well-being, not merely the absence of disease or infirmity'

(WHO, 1946)

This statement can be expanded to identify a number of different dimensions of health, such as physical, mental, emotional, spiritual, social, sexual, societal and environmental. Physical health concerns the functioning of the body; mental health the ability to think clearly and make judgements, while emotional health relates to feelings and the ability to recognise and express them appropriately. Spiritual health is concerned with an individual's beliefs and values which may include religious beliefs and how they put them into practice. Social health is the satisfactory interaction with other people, and sexual health is the acceptance and expression of one's own sexuality. Societal health and environmental health are wider aspects which affect the individual. The way individuals are treated within a society will affect health, whether it is because of the lack of basic necessities or through racism, political unrest, war or inequalities between men and women, for example. Environmental health is the standard of physical environment in which individuals live, including housing, sanitation and pollution.

Although health can be divided into different aspects, it quickly becomes apparent that many of the aspects are interlinked. (When we are physically ill, for example, we often become depressed – which affects our emotional and mental health.) This realisation leads to the concept of a 'holistic' view of health, and health professionals need to understand the importance of treating an individual as a 'whole' and not merely concentrating on one aspect of health.

As health is seen as a positive, disease and illness are usually regarded as negative experiences. The diagnosis of a disease may be accompanied by symptoms of illness such as pain or loss of certain functions. However some individuals with long-term conditions would not classify their lives as unhealthy – people living with well controlled diabetes, for example, or someone who has been successfully treated for cancer.

Medical views have become very powerful in society, and health is often defined through a scientific concept linked with pathology – an understanding of the causes of disease – but as we have seen it can be viewed in a much broader light, and different aspects of health can be just as important to an individual as their physical health.

Health promotion and public health

The World Health Organization defined 'health promotion' as

'the process of enabling people to increase control over and to improve their health.... Health promotion is not just the responsibility of the health sector, but goes beyond healthy lifestyles'

(WHO 1996).

Another way of defining health promotion points to three distinct aspects:

- Health Education, which covers lifestyles, lifeskills and environmental education.

- Health Protection, which covers measures to ensure safety in housing, employment, food, etc.

- Prevention, which means specific preventative activities such as screening and immunisation.
  (from Tannahill (1990) 'Health education and health promotion planning for the 1990s', *Health Education Journal*)

Health can be promoted in a number of different ways, and promotion can be directed at any or all of the different aspects of health that have been discussed. Health promotion may aim to prevent ill health occurring – this is called 'primary health education'. 'Secondary health education' seeks to educate people about their current condition and what they can do about it – when an individual needs to lose weight, for example, to prevent further health problems. 'Tertiary health education' deals with conditions that cannot be cured but when education can help individuals or their families to deal with the situation and make improvements.

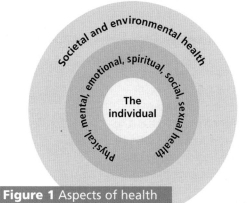

Figure 1 Aspects of health

Efforts by individuals to improve their own health (and that of their family) need to be supported by a healthy 'public' policy, which focuses on improving the health of a society, population or community. Public health focuses on social, economic and cultural factors, and the issues of health and illness that affect a local population. Environmental factors – such as clean water and air, social factors – such as income and employment, and physical factors – such as housing, can all affect an individual's health. We now take for granted that our tap water will not cause illness. In the UK and other western societies public health measures during the nineteenth century ensured that water was no longer a source of illness, but currently in the developing world an assessment by the United Nations reports that 4,000 children die *each day* as a result of diseases caused by drinking dirty water. However, in the UK air quality is still variable, and the rise in cases of asthma amongst children has led to further research about the effects of the atmosphere on the incidence of the disease.

The illness of an individual can affect a whole population. A case of meningitis in a school or college, for example, may lead to intervention from the public health professionals who would seek to prevent more cases through an immunisation programme directed at possible contacts. (More about public health can be found in Unit 6 where some of the main public health issues such as mental health, drugs and obesity were explored.)

Health promotion aims to improve health and reduce illness, which will not only benefit the individual but will have benefits throughout society – reducing costs to the NHS, ensuring a healthy workforce and reducing inequalities in society. Health promotion can be directed at individuals, groups or whole populations. It can use education, counselling, or changes in policy to influence behaviour or to make social, environmental or economic changes which will lead to improved health.

Looking after yourself

There are many ways in which we, as individuals, can take responsibility for improving our own health. Many of them are to do with choices that we make about our own lifestyle – whether we choose to smoke, for example, or take exercise. Good health is fundamental to all our lives, but many people still die too young from preventable illness, or they are ill for much of their lives. This is a cost borne not only by the individual but also by their family, the health and social services and the wider community.

The main causes of ill health in the UK are highlighted in the 'ten tips for better health' and we need to know how we can minimise our risks of becoming ill. At different times of our lives we need different information,

Look after your heart

'How much is the individual responsible for the health of their own heart? Are there any causes of heart disease outside an individual's control?'

and some groups will be more vulnerable than others to certain diseases. For these reasons, health promotion is a constant process which is regularly updated and targeted at appropriate groups according to their needs. In all areas of health and social care – whether you are working in health, with children, the care of older people or with individuals with specific needs – there are always opportunities to promote health and well-being.

Does health promotion work?

Health promotion takes many different forms, as shown by these examples:

- The NHS national cervical screening programme
- Legislation to ban cigarette advertising
- Free portions of fruit for primary school children
- World AIDS Day
- Advice on alcohol and health
- Promotion of awareness about breast cancer.

Some of the campaigns are directed at the individual, to persuade them to take personal action. Other forms of health promotion affect the whole of society. It is sometimes difficult to measure the effect of a particular intervention because many other factors may influence the outcome, including the personal choices an

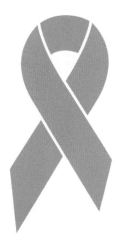

individual may make. For example, the national cervical screening programme is estimated to save 1300 lives each year through earlier diagnosis, but it depends not only on women knowing about the service but also on them being prepared to take part in it.

In addition to promoting knowledge, health promotion may also develop skills, so that an individual can act on their new understanding of the issues that affect them. In 2005 a report from Cancer Research UK on breast cancer showed dramatically improved survival rates (up 17–20 per cent) since the 1990s. This is attributed partly to better surgery, more radiography, and better chemotherapy – but also to the increasingly earlier diagnosis through the greater awareness by women of their breasts, the understanding of the importance of self-examination and the uptake of the breast screening services. All of this greater awareness and uptake can be linked to the health promotion activities over the past years.

Understanding health needs

Before starting a health promotion it is important to know what the needs are. This will mean analysing which individuals, groups or communities should be targeted, and which areas of health improvement should have the greatest priority. These factors need to be balanced with the resources that are available to carry out the activity.

A need may be identified in a number of ways. Professionals and experts can define a need which is matched to accepted (normal) standards. This may be against some external criteria, and may also include aspects, such as food hygiene, which have to meet legal requirements. This is called a **normative** need. A **felt** need is what people really want, although they do not always make a request for help. If these needs are demanded by individuals or groups they then become

expressed needs. Comparison between similar client groups can lead to the identification of a **comparative** need if, for example, there is a lack of services or resources for one group, compared with a similar group. The example of Mrs Jones, below, shows how the different types of need relate to each other.

Mrs Jones and her needs

Mrs Jones is expecting her first baby. Her midwife identifies that she needs routine (or normal) checks of her physical condition and that of her baby and a plan for the birth. After reading a newspaper article, Mrs Jones has become aware of different methods of checking her baby for any abnormalities. She feels that she would like to have her baby checked using the new methods of ultrasound. She meets with some other mothers at the ante-natal class, and they all agree that they would like the option of having the more detailed scan, so they express their requirement to the hospital. Their case is strengthened when they discover that, compared to their own experience, women in the next district all have access to the technology as a matter of course.

Check your understanding

1. Identify the different aspects of health that can affect an individual.

2. Explain what health promotion seeks to do.

3. Describe three different ways in which health is promoted.

4. Explain how health promotion needs can be assessed.

extension activities

1. Find out more about the government's strategy for health promotion in *Saving Lives – Our Healthier Nation*.

2. Find out about the local health promotion plans as part of the Health Improvement and Modernisation Plans (HIMP) developed by your local Primary Care Trust (PCT).

3. What does being healthy mean to you? Think of the different aspects of health. Which is the most important? Does it mean the same for others amongst your family and friends?

Identifying health and well-being issues

Getting you thinking

This one-year-old child has gone on holiday to Greece.

1 What health promotion message have his parents considered before letting him go into the sun?

2 How is this child being protected?

3 What conditions is this health protection trying to prevent occurring?

4 Why might the incidence of these conditions have risen in recent years?

5 How can the provision of sun-screening information make a difference to child health?

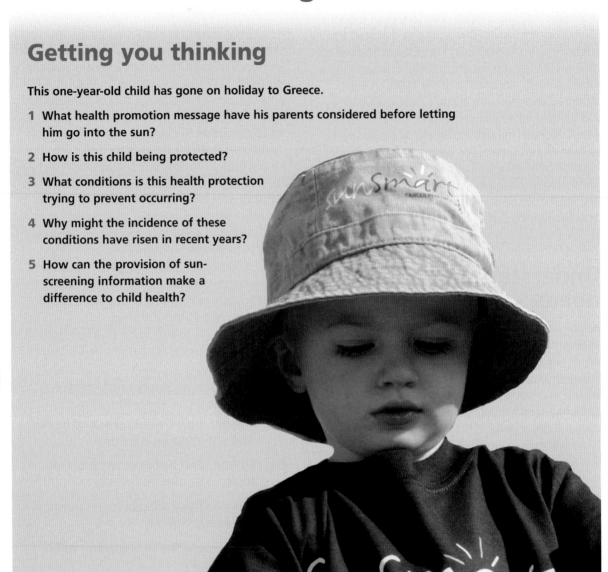

KEY TERMS

Epidemiology
   The study of patterns of disease and illness.

Target
   Something that is aimed for.

Endemic
   Regularly found in certain people or countries.

Mortality statistics
   Death statistics.

How health promotion needs and priorities are identified

There are a number of ways in which health promotion needs and priorities can be identified. These needs and priorities are used to decide whether to launch a health promotion – and which groups should be targeted. The study of how disease and illness is spread through society is called **epidemiology**, and it plays an important part in providing the scientific basis for planning a health promotion. Data is also collected on the risks associated with certain lifestyles or patterns of behaviour. Other factors include local **targets** set by professionals, national targets set by the government, or international targets that the UK has agreed to and are set by international organisations such as the United Nations or the World Health Organization. When targets are set in this way, they are usually time-bound and quantifiable, so that progress can be reviewed against them.

From time to time, particular health issues become important, and the government, the public or the media may express concerns which need a health promotion response. New scientific research and discoveries may also prompt a health promotion. Some organisations are founded to undertake health promotion around specific health issues, while other promotions may take place because of the particular interest of an individual.

Using and understanding data for health promotion

A good starting point for deciding whether or not it would be appropriate to launch a health promotion is to study the epidemiological data that is available.

Lifestyles and cancer risk in the UK population		
Cause	Attributable risk	Range of acceptable estimates
Tobacco	29	27–33
Diet	25	15–35
Reproductive hormones	15	10–20
Alcohol	6	4–8
Ionising radiation	5	4-6
Infection	5	4–15
Occupation	2	1-5
Pollution	2	1–5
UV light	1	1

Figure 2　　　　　　　　　*Source: National Statistics UK*

This will provide information on the health of the population, the causes and risk factors linked with ill health, and hence the possibilities of making improvements through health promotion.

Data may be collected internationally, nationally and locally and will be presented in a variety of statistical formats (see example below). The data may help to answer some important questions, such as 'How many people are (or could be) affected by an illness?', 'Who is most at risk?', 'Are certain groups more vulnerable than others?'

The types of data will include:

- **Mortality statistics**

- Childhood immunisation rates

- Disease register

- Uptake of screening services

- Main causes of admission to hospital

- Accidents

- Socio-economic data, including unemployment rates, crime statistics, leisure facilities, etc.

Another way of collecting data on health is through surveys which show lifestyle decisions and attitudes to health, such as smoking and participation in exercise.

Example of survey results

Percentage

Figure 3 Percentage of pupils aged 11–15 years who regularly smoked cigarettes.

Source: National Statistics UK

Many of these findings can be further analysed to link with social factors, ethnicity or geographical area.

An example of data related to ethnicity:

Figure 4 *Hypertension in ethnic groups in England*	
Hypertension is more common among:	**Hypertension is less common among:**
Black Caribbean men and women	Bangladeshi men and women
Black African men and women	Chinese men
Chinese women	Irish women
Irish men	Pakistani men
Indian men and women	
Pakistani women	

Source: Health Survey for England. The Health of Ethnic Minority Groups '99

Using data on which to base the need for a health promotion can be very helpful as it will give a scientific reason for the choice of target group and activity. This ensures greater credibility. It also gives a baseline, which can be used as a comparison to evaluate the success of the intervention. It is important, however, that the data used is up to date.

Comparison may also be made against other similar countries to see if the UK is in line with its international neighbours. The analysis of the reasons for any discrepancy could lead to specific health promotion activities to rectify any deficiency.

Targets for health and well-being

National targets

The health of its population is always of concern to a national government, and targets for improvement are set, sometimes with specific funding, to support initiatives. In 1992, *The Health of the Nation* strategy was published, with five key target areas: coronary heart disease, accidents, mental health, sexual health, and cancers.

The 'NHS Plan' launched in 2000 made commitments to radically improve the National Health Service. Amongst other reforms, it promised an expansion in cancer-screening services, a rise in the number of smoking-cessation programmes, and improved diet for children with the introduction of free fruit in schools.

Meeting national targets

Fred and Anne McCabe aged 64 and 62 have recently retired and moved to a bungalow near the sea. Many of their neighbours are also retired and take part in activities such as gardening, golf, bird watching and spending time with their grandchildren. Many of these activities involve some regular exercise which they enjoy.

Fred and Anne want to remain fit and healthy. Fred is Irish and knows that high blood pressure is more common for this ethnic group. However, he has always smoked. Anne enjoys cooking and eating good meals and is slightly overweight for her height. Fred and Anne have recently been to register with a new GP. The Primary Care Trust responsible for their local area has set the GP practice some health promotion goals in order to meet the national targets in Saving Lives – Our Healthier Nation. As a result, Fred and Anne were referred to the 'Well Persons' clinics to be given some advice about their health and lifestyles. The practice nurse identified that they were most at risk from some cancers, coronary heart disease and stroke. In addition to being booked into routine screening programmes, Fred and Anne were given advice about smoking, diet and exercise.

In *Saving Lives – Our Healthier Nation*, the UK government set the following key targets in 1999 to be achieved by the year 2010:

- Cancer – to reduce the death rate in people under 75 by at least a fifth.

- Coronary heart disease and stroke – to reduce the death rate in people under 75 by at least two fifths.

- Accidents – to reduce the death rate by at least a fifth, and serious injury by at least a tenth.

- Mental illness – to reduce the death rate from suicide and undetermined injury by at least a fifth.

These broad targets can then be broken down into more detail by different agencies, who often work together to tackle important health issues. The government has also issued strategy documents regarding other aspects of health that are not listed above. These include an 'Alcohol Harm Reduction Strategy' which seeks to improve treatment and support for people with alcohol problems, and provide better information to consumers about the dangers of alcohol misuse. The 'National Strategy for Sexual Health and HIV' seeks to reduce the rising prevalence of sexually transmitted infections and the rates of unintended pregnancies.

Alongside these targets are the standards set by the National Service Frameworks (NSFs) which have been developed for certain categories, including mental health, older people, diabetes care, renal services, children's services, coronary heart disease and the cancer plan. These set national standards for care, put in place strategies to support implementation, and establish ways to ensure progress with regular reviews. Aspects of these frameworks address health promotion possibilities. The standards for the 'NSF for Older People', for example, are focused on:

- Rooting out age discrimination

- Promoting person-centred care

- Intermediate care

- General hospital care

- Stroke services

- Falls services

- Mental health in older people

- Promoting health and active life in old age.

Local authorities, including councils and Primary Care Trusts, will have their own specific targets based on their local populations and resources. The government has Public Service Agreements (PSAs) with local and primary care organisations to meet targets. The target to reduce the number of under-18 year olds becoming pregnant by 50 per cent, by 2010, is an example that has been agreed between national and local government as part of the 'National Teenage Pregnancy Strategy'. Other commitments to increase the participation of teenage mothers in education, training or work by 60 per cent – in order to reduce the risk of long-term social exclusion – illustrates the way in which health overlaps with educational and social circumstances. Primary Care Trusts will respond to the specific needs of their local populations and increasingly work with other local agencies to identify and meet those needs.

International targets

As well as national targets, international bodies such as the United Nations or the World Health Organization have their worldwide ambitions to improve health.

Smallpox has been completely eradicated since 1980 through a WHO campaign, and currently polio is being targeted. By the end of 2003 poliomyelitis had been eliminated from all but six countries in the

Meeting international targets

Catherine Atieno lives in Kenya. Her family was displaced from their home and now lives in a slum on the outskirts of Nairobi. The only shelter that they have is a small hut made from old cement sacks. Catherine's father died three years ago. There are six children in her family. Catherine is 12 years old and attends a school with her brother Kelvin where they get their only meal of the day. Both of them are small for their age and get frequent illnesses. None of the other children attend school. The older boys try to earn money from begging or casual work. Her mother is living with HIV and most of the times she is very sick. The family lives in extreme poverty. They have no money for food, medicines or schooling. A charity is trying to help families like the Atieno's by setting up a feeding programme, supporting some self-help projects and funding a small medical centre. The charity believes that their goals match the Millennium Development Goals and Targets set by the United Nations in 2000.

world, as a result of the 'Global Polio Eradication Initiative'. However, one of the countries still experiencing cases of childhood polio was Nigeria, where one area of the country was suspicious of the vaccination process and refused to participate. This demonstrates the importance of knowledge and understanding going alongside a medical invention to ensure a successful health promotion. The advent of easy worldwide travel also underlines the importance of a global approach to health, because diseases can easily be spread across different countries and continents. UK residents travelling abroad must also

Figure 5 Millennium Development Goals and Targets

Goal 1 Eradicate extreme poverty and hunger

Goal 2 Achieve universal primary education

Goal 3 Promote gender equality and empower women

Goal 4 Reduce child mortality

Goal 5 Improve maternal health

Goal 6 Combat HIV/AIDS, malaria and other diseases

Goal 7 Ensure environmental sustainability

Goal 8 Develop a global partnership for development

be aware of the diseases that are endemic in other populations, and take appropriate precautions such as vaccination (see the following page).

Figure 6 *Health Risks around the World, and How to Avoid them*

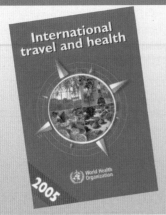

This health advice brochure, published by the World Health Organisation in 2005, covers such areas as:

- Eat and drink...safely

- Be safe outdoors

- Major diseases, and the precautions to take

- Immunisation summary.

In 2000 the UN published its Millennium Development Goals, most of which are health-related (see p.59).

The poorest countries of the world experience much of the worst health. The UK is the 12th richest country in the world and has an average life expectancy of 78 years. Zambia, which is the 14th poorest country, has an average life expectancy of 33 years. The top ten diseases in rural Zambia are:

- Malaria

- Respiratory tract infection

- Skin infections

- Diarrhoeal diseases

- Sexually transmitted infections

- Accidents

- Eye infections

- Ear infections

- Schistosomiasis (bilharzia)

- Worm infections.

How does this list differ from what you would expect a GP to see in the UK?

Other reasons for health promotion

From time to time a health issue may come to prominence through specific circumstances. For example, an outbreak of an infectious disease, an area of public concern, or publicity through the media may require a response in the form of health promotion.

Outbreaks of infectious diseases can occur for a number of reasons. They can be through a breakdown in hygiene, through a recognised annual cycle of raised infectivity, or because the level of immunity in the population has fallen. Influenza is commonly associated with the winter months and hence a programme of immunisation (flu jabs) starts in the early autumn every year. An increase in the number of cases of mumps amongst young people could be tracked to the gaps in the vaccination programme, while one of the risk groups for meningitis is university students starting their studies.

Public concern may be raised by the nature or severity of a disease and by the possibility of contracting it. Those who have previously experienced the disease will be more susceptible to any health promotion. The serious effects of polio and measles used to be well understood in the UK, but now that they are comparatively rarely seen, public concern has reduced, affecting the immunisation programme.

Mason, 5, dies after he and his brother get E.coli at school

'A boy of five died yesterday from the E.coli breakout that has swept through 38 schools.'

This story appeared in the *Daily Mail* in October 2005, following an outbreak of the bacterial infection in schools in South Wales. E. coli is a common bug which is present everywhere in the environment. Mostly it helps people to stay healthy, providing the body with many vitamins, such as vitamin K. But some strains – such as the O157 strain – are potentially fatal. Children and pensioners are especially vulnerable to E. coli 0157, which is normally found in the intestines of people and cattle and can be passed on by eating infected food and liquid.

Long journeys (more than 5 hours) by plane, train, etc. are thought to cause a slightly increased risk of DVT. This is probably due to sitting immobile and cramped for long periods. In plane journeys, in addition to the immobility, other factors which may possibly play a part (but are not proven) include: the reduced cabin pressure, reduced oxygen levels in the plane, slight dehydration caused by not drinking much water, and drinking too many alcoholic drinks – which are often freely available. It has to be stressed that the vast majority of travellers have no problems. The increased risk of DVT from travel is small. However, it is wise to try and reduce the risk, particularly if you are in any of the 'at risk' groups.

www.patient.co.uk/showdoc

New scientific discoveries may also lead to health promotion being needed because new information has been made available. Sometimes this may mean a change of advice. This can make for difficulties for the health promoter, whose credibility appears undermined. Advice about food and diet has changed over the years as new scientific discoveries provide greater understanding of the role of different foodstuffs and their contribution to healthy living.

The purpose of identifying and assessing health needs is to ensure that the health promotion is appropriate and sustainable. By researching the background it helps to direct the promotion, identify any specific need, target the 'at risk' groups, take notice of any public or professional views, and set priorities.

Check your understanding

1 Describe how epidemiology is used in planning health promotion.

2 Identify the national targets for health in *Saving Lives – Our Healthier Nation*, and describe how they could be met through health promotion.

3 Identify four international targets, and show how they are related to health.

4 Give two other reasons for developing a health promotion.

extension activities

1 Research the Millennium Development Goals, so that you can demonstrate how the targets are health-related.

2 How might health needs be differently prioritised in African countries or India, compared with the UK?

61

Topic 2 Identifying health and well-being issues

Getting you thinking

1 **What part do the different categories of agency play in promoting the health of populations or individuals?**

2 **How might some of these different types of organisation work together to promote health?**

3 **How does your school or college promote the health of the students and staff?**

4 **Think of an organisation or person that works to promote health in your local area**

International organisations – World Health Organization, United Nations and the EU.

Local government – Education authorities, social services, planning and housing, environmental health, recreation and leisure, police.

Mass media – national, local newspapers, radio, TV.

National Organisations – Department of Health, Ministry of Agriculture and Farming and Fisheries, Department of Education and Employment, Department of Transport and the Ministry of the Environment, and the Central Office of Information. NHS – including local services e.g. GPs, nurses, health visitors and other members of primary care team.

Voluntary organisations – at national level, local branches, local groups, churches and other religious groups, pressure groups.

Commercial organisations – manufacturers, retailers.

Work-related – trade unions, occupational health, Health and Safety Executive, professional organisations.

KEY TERMS

Mass media
The forms of communication designed to reach the mass of the people – television, newspapers, radio.

Pressure group
An interest group organised to influence public (especially government) policy.

Who promotes health?

Health promotion occurs both formally and informally. Health is discussed in a variety of informal settings, often with advice being exchanged – in the family, amongst friends or related to other experiences, such as the availability of new leisure facilities.

Formal health promotion is carried out in a wide variety of ways by various agents and agencies, ranging from very large statutory organisations, such as government departments, to small single-issue voluntary groups. Health, of course, is not an issue that is limited to any one organisation, and agencies with different areas of responsibility – education,

environmental health, social services, commercial groups and the voluntary sector – may all need to work together to address health needs. These are categorised as 'healthy alliances' and defined by the WHO in the document *Health for All* (2000):

> *'Health for all requires the coordinated action of all sectors concerned. The health authorities can only deal with a part of the problems to be solved and multi-sectoral cooperation is the only way of effectively ensuring the prerequisites for health, promoting health policies and reducing the risks in the physical, economic and social environment.'*

In the same way as health needs to be regarded holistically, so too do the solutions in seeking health improvement. The health services cannot work in isolation from other services, and they also need to respond to the needs identified by other agencies. A child suffering from repeated chest infections may be prescribed appropriate medication, but if his housing remains of poor quality and the income of his household is low, the chances of recovery are diminished. Older people are at risk of falls – a risk which might well be increased if the paving around their homes is cracked and broken. Health professionals are currently responding more flexibly to needs by going to the clients and undertaking a range of interventions. Mental health professionals working in the community have developed 'Crisis Assessment and Assertive Outreach' teams whose primary aim is to help clients in their homes by supporting them in undertaking their everyday tasks and keeping them out of hospital.

The main agencies promoting health can be grouped under the following headings:

- International organisations
- National governmental organisations
- Local government
- Voluntary organisations and pressure groups
- Commercial organisations
- Work-related promotion
- Mass media.

International organisations

The United Nations and the European Union have both issued directives which concern the health of the member countries. These include setting standards (or targets) and developing initiatives on issues which include cancer prevention, pollution, HIV/AIDS, diet and social inequalities. The World Health Organization has a role that is specifically aimed at monitoring and improving the health of all countries. It has been instrumental in shifting the emphasis from a medical base to primary health care. This meant promoting health in its broadest definition and directing action at ensuring that the environment supports healthy living.

National governmental organisations

The government is divided into different departments, each with a specific area of responsibility. The Department of Health naturally takes the lead on health. Within the Department of Health the National Health Service is the major agency for promoting health. It has been increasingly accepted that it cannot stand alone but must work with other government departments, such as Education and Science, Transport, Environment, and the Home Office – all of which also contribute to health promotion in a variety of ways. Recently the lead agency in health promotion – the Health Development Agency has combined with the Health Protection Agency under the banner of 'National Institute for Health and Clinical Excellence' (NICE) with the remit to provide national guidance on the promotion of good health and the prevention and treatment of ill health. The government also influences the structure of services that affect health, and there have been a number of different models over recent years. NHS Trusts are responsible for commissioning and providing health care, but there is an increasing use of the independent sector. A small number of care trusts have been set up which combine health and social services, but there is still no widespread structural integration of health and social care.

In primary care, GPs and other health professionals work to targets that are set to meet the specific needs of their populations. This group is known as the primary health care team, and may consist of GPs, Practice Administrator, receptionists, practice nurses, district nursing teams, health visitors, community psychiatric nurses and community midwives. The services provided in primary care are being expanded, and different professionals are joining the team. It is not unusual to have counsellors and therapists attached to practices and for specialist services to be offered. All members of the primary care team have a role in health promotion. The practice nurse may run 'Wellness Clinics' which promote healthy living as well as screening people with chronic conditions such as diabetes. The health visitor works with groups and on a one-to-one basis, but also with a network of other professionals in education and social services. The midwife provides information and support to mothers and their newborn children. The community psychiatric nurse works with those with mental health problems alongside the recently introduced STAR (Support Time and Recovery) workers. GPs provide medical services promoting health and, more recently, have the responsibility for ensuring that the practice is meeting government targets for immunisation, screening and checks for older people. Other professions allied to medicine and working with the NHS or independently include dentists, physiotherapists, occupational therapists and pharmacists. There are many opportunities for health promotion that are available to them throughout the course of their work through planned interventions and when the opportunity arises whilst giving advice. Pharmacists can offer further information to a client who is collecting a prescription, and may be asked for advice about appropriate medication or treatment.

Local government

The local authorities have responsibilities over planning, housing, recreation and leisure, and therefore have a pivotal role in promoting health. Education authorities, teachers and lecturers work through the schools and colleges, while social services staff are often concerned with improving the health of their clients, who include children, the elderly and those with mental health problems, as well as other vulnerable groups. The councils have agreed Public Service Agreements with the government, which set targets for health improvement. Increasingly, local government is joining together with local health organisations to plan and deliver health promotion.

Housing has already been identified as an important contributor to health, and the provision of good facilities for leisure and recreation are required for physical health – and for social health too. Good transport policies can contribute to preventing accidents and reducing pollution. Environmental health officers have statutory powers relating to food hygiene and pollution, and they are responsible for protecting the health of their local community from environmental hazards.

Social service departments have taken on an increasingly major role as more care is delivered in the community – and away from hospitals. Working closely with health professionals, social workers plan and deliver care and they have a responsibility to seek to provide health-promoting environments.

Services to young people include schools, youth clubs, residential homes and the specific responsibility for child protection – all of which provide opportunities for health promotion.

The police and fire service take a proactive role in accident prevention and other areas, frequently visiting schools and giving advice about personal and community safety.

Voluntary organisations and pressure groups

A huge range of voluntary organisations and pressure groups exist, including those which are categorised as 'non-governmental organisations':

- National organisations that work from a national base, such as the Royal Society for the Prevention of Accidents (ROSPA),or the Meningitis Trust.

- National organisations that work through local branches, such as Age Concern, or the National Childbirth Trust.

- Local groups may be set up to meet a particular need –a local hospice, for example.

- Community groups may come together for different purposes, some of which may be to support a particular aspect of health. Others groups, merely by providing social interaction will meet the emotional or social needs of their members. Churches and other religious groups will support spiritual health, but may also – through other activities – provide opportunities for recreation. The wide range of community activity that regularly takes place can quickly be discovered by looking at any local newspaper.

- Pressure groups may campaign on health issues –. Friends of the Earth, for example.

- Individually initiated groups may be started by an individual or a group who have experienced a specific disease.

Commercial organisations

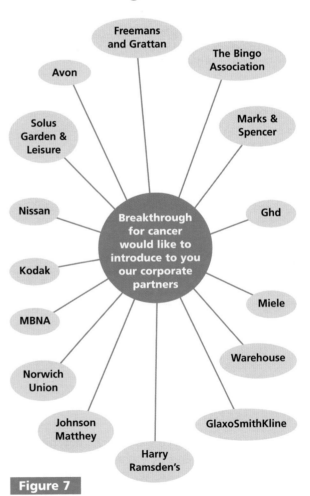

Figure 7

Commercial organisations include manufacturers and retailers who not only consider the health and safety aspects of their products but can influence shopping habits by making 'healthy options' more readily available. In addition, retailers may combine with health charities to promote awareness – through messages on packaging or through selling badges, wristbands and other goods with appropriate logos.

Commercial organisations also have the contracts for providing services that affect health – providing food for the NHS, for example, transport links, or waste disposal for local councils. As the interest in healthy lifestyles has increased there has been an expansion of commercial health facilities, with health clubs providing health checks and advice.

Work-related promotion

All employers are responsible for ensuring that their workplaces and practices comply with health and safety legislation. The Health and Safety Executive has wide-ranging statutory powers to inspect and require compliance with the standards set by law. Some employers offer regular health checks to their staff and have an occupational health scheme or provide private health insurance schemes. Trade unions and professional associations (UNISON, British Medical Association, Royal College of Nursing) are influential in promoting the health of their members through involvement in policy making and training.

Mass media

Messages about health are delivered through the media. Television, radio, newspapers and magazines may use features, advertisements or press releases to convey information. The mass media are the most powerful force raising awareness today, and they can have positive effects on health promotion, highlighting important health issues for the general public. The media can also have negative effects – especially by raising anxieties unnecessarily. Stories about the safety of vaccination, for example, have led to an increase in the incidence of some dangerous childhood diseases because parents have been too worried to have their children vaccinated.

As well as spreading the main messages, the media can convey health information within other storylines. For example, *EastEnders*, *Coronation Street* and other 'soaps' have tackled topics such as HIV, breast cancer, and mental illness. Professionals working in health promotion will frequently use the mass media to convey messages to a wide audience – such as reminders about 'National No Smoking Day' – but to be effective such approaches need to be backed up in other ways.

Check your understanding

1. Demonstrate how and why different organisations may come together in order to promote health.

2. Describe what role the NHS plays in promoting health.

3. Identify three categories of organisations that promote health.

4. Explain how the mass media can promote health.

extension activities

For each category of agency identified above:

1. Find a health promotion that has been developed.

2. Identify the aim of the activity and its target group,

3. Explain why the particular organisation would have been responsible for promoting it.

Approaches to health promotion

Getting you thinking

Mrs Brown is 85, and lives alone in a high-rise flat that has poor heating. She finds it difficult to get out, and therefore has little social contact. Last winter she was ill with flu and she has since become depressed. Her one pleasure is smoking and she smokes up to 20 cigarettes a day. Once a week she visits a day centre where she meets different health and social care professionals and discusses her situation with other elderly people. They all want to improve her health.

How might each of the following people promote the health of Mrs Brown?

1 Her GP

2 The staff at the day centre, including the social workers and health visitors

3 Her friends at the day centre

4 A local pressure group set up to improve the conditions for local people.

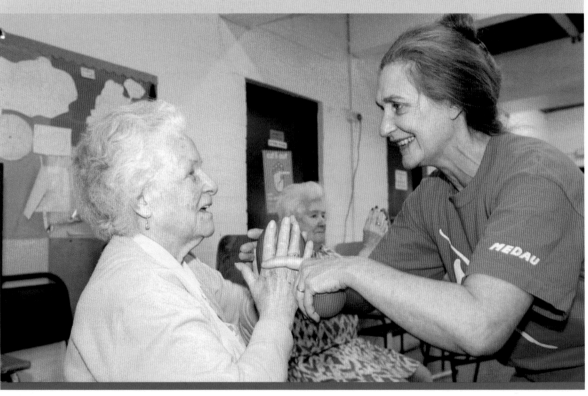

KEY TERMS

Behaviour change
Change in the way that someone acts and functions.

Empowerment
Enabling individuals or groups to exercise power.

Client-centred
Focusing on the individual needs, wishes and preferences of clients to maximise their involvement and control over their care.

Societal change
Changes in the structure and processes of a society.

Choosing the method

The main aim of all health promotion is, as we have seen, to improve the health of individuals in society. There is much debate, however, about the ways in which this might be achieved. Should, for example, individuals change their behaviours and lifestyle? Or would changing the physical or socio-economic environment be more effective? Smokers can be encouraged to give up individually, or smoking can be banned in public areas. The most appropriate and effective approach needs to be selected, and this will depend on a number of factors, such as:

- Aim of the health promotion activity
- The role and experience of the health promoter
- The circumstances in which the health promotion is to take place
- The target group
- The resources available.

A number of different models and approaches have been developed to give a framework indicating their main aims, values and activities. Although not an exclusive list, the following five approaches provide the basis for most health promotion activity:

- The medical approach
- The **behaviour change** approach
- The educational approach
- The **client-centred (empowerment)** approach
- The **societal change** approach.

The medical approach

The aim of this approach is to reduce medically defined disease and disability, using warnings and methods from the medical professions. The activity is targeted at scientifically identified high-risk groups or whole populations, and involves medical interventions – such as immunisation and screening – that will reduce ill health. It is an expert-led, top-down approach which values preventive medical procedures and encourages compliance by patients. It often relies on the availability of technology such as diagnostic facilities. Statistics of the uptake of the intervention and its results are collected and analysed. The results can be easily measured, and dramatic successes – like the eradication of smallpox – can be tracked and then confirmed. It is, however, easier to track the number of people participating in the programmes than the results of the intervention, because some may not be apparent for many years. In order to ensure that

patients should benefit in the long term, incentives have been given to GPs to undertake screening and immunisation with the target groups. This means that records can be kept of the number of people participating in the programmes and they will be compared against their health status in later years. Some methods of screening – such as simple routine tests for prostate or bowel cancer – are not yet seen as cost effective or reliable enough, and their implementation is still under review.

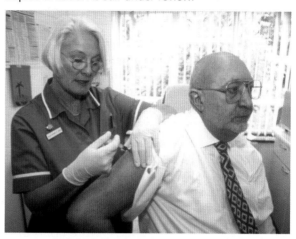

The behaviour change approach

The aim of this approach is to encourage individuals to adopt a 'healthy' lifestyle through changing their own attitudes or their behaviours. It expects individuals to take an interest in, and responsibility for, their own health. For example, campaigns will urge

Changing Mark's behaviour

Mark is 34 years old and smokes about 20 cigarettes each day. He is aware of the risks to his health that this implies and wants to give up smoking. He started smoking when he was at school because many of his friends also smoked. Mark continued smoking through university though he did try to give up a couple of times. Several of his non-smoking relatives are medical professionals and have actively tried to dissuade him from the habit. When he got married and had his first son Mark gave up smoking for nearly two years as he was aware of the damage that second-hand smoke poses to young children. However, following a move to a new more stressful job he started smoking again. He has found it impossible to give up since this time. Mark tried a number of different ways of quitting including acupuncture and several New Year resolutions. He is hoping that this year he will give up on National No Smoking Day with the help of the NHS Quitline and the fact that smoking is being banned in his favourite restaurants.

people to 'Look after your heart' putting the onus on the individual to adopt a healthy lifestyle by not smoking, eating a healthy diet and taking regular exercise. This approach, while appealing to the 'adult' in a person by not being imposed, does not recognise the difficulties associated with changing behaviour or the other influences that lie outside an individual's control. The decision to eat a healthy diet may also rely on the availability of healthy foods.

The educational approach

The aim of this approach is to provide knowledge, to ensure understanding of health issues, and to develop the necessary skills to enable an informed choice to be made. Information about health is presented in such a way that people are allowed to make up their own minds. This respects the rights of individuals to choose their own health behaviour, and assumes that greater knowledge will influence attitudes. It is often used when dealing with large groups, such as in schools when the information can be given within a set time. The educational approach covers three aspects of learning – the information that the target group needs to understand, an exploration of attitudes and feelings, and the development of appropriate skills. A health promotion to young people about alcohol would therefore first give them information about the effects of alcohol on their body and the results of alcohol abuse on them and others. It would explore

Promoting health at the youth group

'UR in charge' is a group of young people who meet regularly to chat and relax at the local youth club. They plan a number of activities that they enjoy and sometimes invite speakers to talk about issues that interest them. One of the group suggested that a local health promotion worker could come and discuss their health with them. On receiving the invitation Beverley James, the health promoter, was delighted to accept and saw it as an outstanding opportunity to address issues such as drug awareness. Beverley had planned a session to cover all the major aspects of substance misuse. She was therefore very surprised when the group indicated that they did not wish to hear about the topics she had suggested but chose the topic of exercise which she did not think was as relevant. They also wanted to investigate ways in which they could get involved and undertake more exercise. However, the discussion within the group was very lively and stimulating as they were all interested and engaged with the topic. Beverley was delighted to discover six months later that a number of the group had taken up regular activity.

attitudes to drinking amongst young people and society. It might then seek to develop skills in resisting peer pressure to drink, through such methods as role play. The problems associated with this approach include the difficulties in measuring whether it has been effective in changing behaviour. Generally, people dislike being told what to do, and may – despite having greater knowledge – ignore the information, exercising their right of free choice. This last outcome is often difficult for the health promoter to accept, because the whole object of giving the information was to influence a change in behaviour. The association with school experiences may also reduce the effectiveness of this approach.

The client-centred (empowerment) approach

The aim of this approach is to help people identify their own concerns and then to work with them in developing the knowledge and skills to take action. This is a 'bottom-up' strategy, where the clients are treated as equals and have the right to challenge and make changes. Self-empowerment is central to this approach, requiring the clients to develop skills leading to increased self-esteem and greater control over their lives. The role of the health promoter is therefore to provide support, helping individuals to identify their own needs and develop the knowledge and skills to attain the outcome they want. Most self-help groups, for example, use a client-centred approach. The participants themselves decide what they want to prioritise, and only require the health promoter to facilitate their choice. Evaluating the success of this approach is difficult because it is often a long-term process and other factors may influence any outcome.

The societal change approach

The aim of this approach is to make changes in the physical as well as the social and economic environment, by changing policies and attitudes in society rather than individuals. It seeks to 'make the healthy choice the easier choice' by ensuring that the environment in which an individual lives will support their aims to live more healthy lives. It makes healthy behaviours more acceptable, and the activity is usually on a large scale. Not all people will be happy about these societal change approaches and it may require the imposition of laws to enforce behaviour. A vigorous campaign to promote the wearing of seatbelts only finally succeeded when it became illegal not to wear one. More recently smoking in public has become less acceptable, although it is likely that smoking in public places will have to be banned legally to ensure complete adherence to the principle of a smoke-free environment.

Figure 8 *Approaches to health promotion*

	Aim	Activity	Values	Strengths	Weaknesses	Example (diet)
Medical approach	Reduce medically defined disease and disability.	Medical intervention to high-risk groups or populations.	Patients' compliance with the experts.	• Accurate scientific basis. • Expert knowledge. • Results easily measured.	• Authoritarian • Relies on infrastructure to support programme, e.g. screening. • People need to be persuaded to use facilities.	Aim: Freedom from diet-induced disease. Activity: Encourage people to measure weight regularly, attend dietician, and follow diet.
Behaviour change approach	Individuals to adopt a healthy lifestyle.	Activities aimed at changing attitudes and behaviours.	Knowledge about health lies with the promoter.	• Encourages personal change. • Not imposed by others. • Appeals to the 'adult' in a person.	• Behaviour not easy to change. • Client susceptible to other influences. • Intentions not always followed through.	Aim : To change individuals eating habits. Activity: Persuasive education to eat healthily and to adopt a weight-reducing diet.
Educational approach	Individuals to acquire knowledge, understanding and skills to make and act upon informed decisions.	Giving of information. Exploration of attitudes to health. Development of skills such as decision-making.	Respects rights of informed individuals to choose.	• Allows people to make up own minds. • Can be delivered to a large group. • Time constrained.	• People dislike being told what to do. • Bad school experiences may influence decisions • Difficult to judge if learning has taken place.	Aim: To enable individuals to make an informed decision about their diet. Activity: Education about healthy eating. Development of skills in making decision about healthy diets, e.g. shopping and cooking healthily.
Client-centred (empower-ment) approach	Clients to identify own health needs.	Facilitate the identification of needs and work with clients to develop their knowledge and skills.	Clients as equals. Clients are self-empowered to challenge and change.	• Greater engagement of clients with own choice of topic. • Better outcomes through self-empowerment.	• Health promoter may have little control of activity. • Outcomes difficult to measure.	Aim: Only to promote healthy eating if identified by client. Activity: Allow clients to request information and skills if they wish, and follow their agenda.
Societal change approach	Change physical, and socio-economic environment to support healthy lifestyles.	Political and social action, including legislation to improve environment for healthy living.	Choices about health by individuals need to be easy choices, through environments that support health.	• Healthy behaviour becomes more acceptable. • Reaches a wide group of people. • Some healthy behaviours become law.	• Social rebels may oppose change. • A range of approaches needed to effect social change. • Needs a large-scale approach.	Aim: To make healthy eating the easy choice. Activity: Legislation about the nutritional content of school meals.

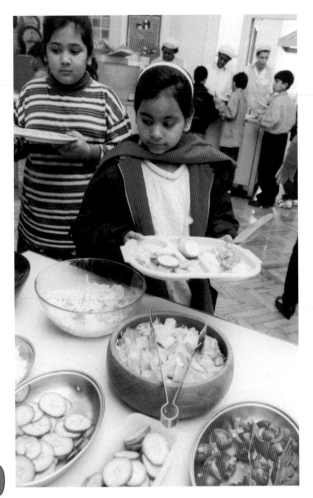

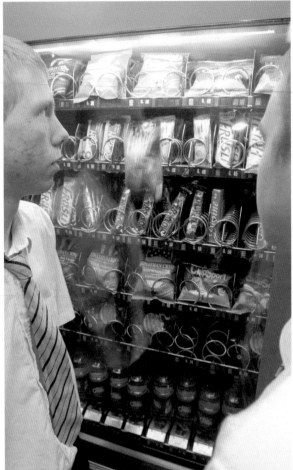

Taxation and other fiscal methods may also be used. The changeover to unleaded petrol from leaded (which had been shown to affect the development of children) was hastened by the government using the tax system to make leaded petrol cheaper.

Health promoters adopting the societal change approach need to have skills in lobbying, policy planning and political awareness. As with other imposed changes, there are certain 'rebels' who view compulsion as an erosion of individual liberty, and resist the changes, however sensible they are.

Applications of the different approaches

In practice, the five models identified may very well overlap. It is important to consider which approach is most appropriate to any given health promotion. Other researchers have developed different models in response to the requirements of health promotion. However the medical, behaviour change, educational, client-centred and societal change approaches encompass the main issues when analysing which approach is appropriate in any given situation.

The role and experience of the health promoter

The choice of model will also depend on the individual or group who are undertaking the health promotion. Each model requires different skills. The medical model needs professionally qualified individuals who understand the scientific basis of the health intervention, while other approaches require counselling, teaching or facilitation skills. A careful assessment of the skills available to undertake the promotion will influence the choice of method.

Circumstances, target groups and resources

Health promotion takes place in a wide range of different circumstances. Sometimes it is a carefully planned activity which is well resourced, and at other times it may be opportunistic. Major campaigns may take many months to plan while others may have to react quickly to a current issue.

The target group will also influence the choice of model. A small community group, for example, with a clear idea of what it needs will require a different approach from a group needing to access routine breast screening.

As with all activities, the amount and range of resources will always affect choice. Few campaigns have unlimited funds, but some undertaking a medical approach will require a large investment in technology while others can be delivered using no additional resources other than the individual doing the promotion. Some will require commercially produced resources while others will need highly trained and skilled professionals. An early review of the resources available for the health promotion is an important part of any planning, and may influence the choice of approach.

Check your understanding

1 Identify the five different models of health promotion and their main characteristics.

2 Describe how smoking would be discouraged, using an educational approach.

3 Explain how participation in exercise could be increased, using a societal change approach.

4 Describe how the health of children is promoted, and identify two different approaches.

extension**activities**

1 Identify two health promotions that have used different models or approaches.

2 Why were the particular approaches used?

3 Were they appropriate and, if so, why?

4 Which professionals were involved?

5 What resources were necessary?

6 In your view, how successful were the two promotions?

Health promotion methods and media

Getting you thinking

1 Which condition is this promotion raising awareness about?

2 Which target group is it aimed at?

3 Describe the approach that is being taken and explain why is it appropriate for this promotion.

4 What advantages might there be in having linked this campaign with football?

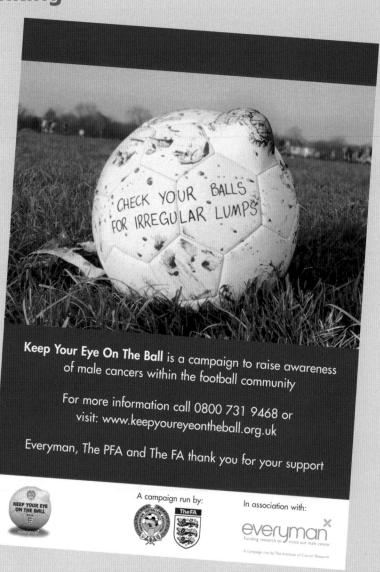

CHECK YOUR BALLS FOR IRREGULAR LUMPS

Keep Your Eye On The Ball is a campaign to raise awareness of male cancers within the football community

For more information call 0800 731 9468 or visit: www.keepyoureyeontheball.org.uk

Everyman, The PFA and The FA thank you for your support

KEEP YOUR EYE ON THE BALL

A campaign run by:

The FA

In association with:

everyman
Funding research to cross out male cancer

A campaign run by The Institute of Cancer Research

Unit 8 Promoting Health and Well-being

KEY TERMS

Equality
Having the same opportunities.

Format
Shape, colour or size of presentation.

Sponsorship
Support for a programme by an individual or organisation in return for advertising.

Mass media
Forms of communication designed to reach the mass of the people.

Selecting methods of health promotion

Ways of communicating health promotion are increasing in range. Traditionally, leaflets and posters were produced, but recently new technology – such as texting – has been used for conveying messages.

As well as the medium, the tone and style can vary in response to the topic. Some health messages can be seen as 'embarrassing' and ways of conveying vital information have included lively and light-hearted approaches. For example, a campaign aimed at raising awareness about testicular cancer has the slogan 'Keep your Eye on the Ball'.

Selecting health promotion methods

Sihan has been asked to undertake a health promotion in a nursery school about dental education. The class that she is due to teach is for 4 to 5 year-olds. Their teacher tells Sihan that the children are used to sitting and listening for about 15 minutes, enjoy colouring pictures and are used to doing some practical activities. The parents of the children have all given their permission for an activity involving cleaning their teeth. Sihan plans her lesson carefully by doing some research about the level of understanding the children will have and on what they already know. She visits her own dentist to get some up-to-date information about care of children's teeth. After checking with the teacher she prepares some brightly coloured posters to illustrate her talk and gives the children some pictures to colour in which show which foods are good for their teeth. The class ends with the children practising brushing their teeth with toothbrushes supplied by the dental practice.

Seven questions to ask yourself

1 **What is the most appropriate resource for conveying my health promotion message?**

- Are you directing it to an individual, to a group, or to a whole community, e.g. a school or college?

- Should it be paper-based so that people can read it, or take it away with them?

- Would visual images – photographs, videos etc. – enhance the message?

- Would an interactive activity be more challenging? Or is there a chance you could use a real-life activity?

- What is affordable or possible?

2 **What are the characteristics of the people with whom I am working?**

- Is the material relevant for the people to whom it is directed? Consider the age range, sex, ethnic group.

- What socio-economic backgrounds do they have?

3 **Does my work promote equality and diversity?**

- Does it promote equality of opportunity and celebrate diversity?

- Ensure that there is no stereotyping or unfair discrimination.

4 **Does it contain correct information?**

- Check that the information is up to date and accurate. New findings may alter advice over time.

- Is it unbiased?

5 **Is it understandable?**

- Is the information easy to understand?

- Is the language clear?

- Should it be in any other languages?

- Are your statistics easily understood?

6 **What is the best style or format?**

- What size of print, use of colour, etc.?

- What tone is appropriate? Fear tactics? A light-hearted presentation?

7 **Will it achieve my aim?**

- How do you intend to use the material?

- Will it have the desired effect?

Different types of health promotion media

The person undertaking the health promotion needs to consider the different media that can be used, and their advantages or disadvantages.

Figure 9 Different types of health promotion

Type of media	Use	Advantages	Disadvantages
Leaflets and handouts	• To give information • To support a presentation	• Information can be taken away for future reference. • Information can be shared with others. • Can give greater detail, e.g. statistics. • Handouts easily produced.	• Can be easily discarded or ignored. • Commercially produced leaflets can be expensive. • Mass-produced leaflets may not target a specific audience.
Posters	• To raise awareness	• Convey information. • Can have high impact through challenging images. • Can be made cheaply.	• Commercial posters can be expensive. • Poor-quality posters can distract from message. • Poor displays may be ignored.
Presentation	• To convey information to an audience	• Can be tailored to specific group. • Can go at the pace of the group. • Uses a range of methods to keep audience attentive.	• Requires presentation skills. • Needs careful planning to ensure audience remains engaged. • Presenter may need to answer unexpected questions on topic.

Characteristics of the group

Certain health promotions are directed at whole populations but, as we have seen, most have a particular target group which has been identified through analysis of epidemiological data or other sources. Other criteria which influence which group is to receive the information may be social or educational – such as pupils in a certain school year. Once the group is known, then thought needs to be given to their characteristics. The approach and methods appropriate for a group of young children being taught how to look after their teeth are completely different to those required for older people trying to prevent falls. Individuals from different ethnic and cultural backgrounds may have a variety of different values and attitudes to issues about health, while their socio-economic status will also have an influence. Material from different countries does not always transfer successfully because lifestyles may differ significantly. For example, attitudes and laws about young people drinking alcohol vary in different countries and according to religious beliefs. Health promotion may be targeted at either male or female groups – the sex-specific cancer prevention programmes, for example, such as prostate and breast cancer – although an understanding of such issues by both sexes is important in supporting the individuals affected. It has also been realised that only immunising baby girls against rubella – to prevent damage to their future unborn babies – was less than successful because boys were still able to spread the disease. Now, therefore, all babies are immunised.

Equality and diversity

It is essential that any health promotion should be seen as applying the principles of equality and non-discrimination. In fact it should promote equality of opportunity and celebrate diversity. Although some studies will indicate that certain racial groups are more vulnerable to some diseases than others, these differences should not be used in a racist manner – by suggesting, for example, that one race is inferior to another.

Stereotyping by sex can occur when it is assumed that only women should be targeted for messages regarding child care. Other areas of discrimination include sexual orientation, age and disability. Health promotions are able to actively encourage positive images regarding diversity by ensuring that any approach fully embraces the different physical, social and cultural differences that are present within any group.

Using information

As science advances, information about certain diseases may change. It is therefore important that facts are up to date. For example, the programme of immunisation for young children has changed over the years in the light of new research. The source of information also needs to be checked to ensure that it is reliable, unbiased and complete – some groups have been known to campaign using only 'half truths' in order to win their argument. Careful research from reliable sources must underlie the use of any information.

Understandable language

In addition to scientific and technical terms, which can cause barriers to understanding, it is a criticism of many official documents that they are written in 'official' language that cannot be easily understood. Consideration always needs to be given to the level of literacy amongst the participants – the age or abilities of the group, for example. In some areas, there may be many people whose first language is not English, and therefore arrangements need to be made to ensure that they can participate fully – either through the use of interpreters or the translation of written materials. Any statistics that are used should be clearly presented.

Style and format

The decisions about style and format will be based on a number of factors. One factor may simply be the style that the health promoter is most comfortable with. Although new skills can always be learnt, it would be pointless to expect an individual to undertake a task they were clearly unable to do – putting on a play, for example, when they had no

acting experience. However, other aspects will be influenced by the subject matter and the target group. Some will require a particularly sensitive approach while others lend themselves to a jokey and light-hearted approach. Fear tactics are sometimes used to reinforce messages. Examples of these are seen in some 'Give up Smoking' campaigns with graphic images of diseased lungs, or in Drink–Driving campaigns with real accident victims. Although having a very powerful effect – immediately gaining attention – their effect is often short-lived and quickly forgotten.

Other considerations of the use of colour, size of print, use of pictures and general layout should all be tailored to the promotion and target group.

Achieving your aim

When selecting what methods to use for health promotion, the aim must always be kept in mind, and continual checks made to ensure that any material or activity will have the desired effect. There is sometimes a temptation for an activity to be developed which fails to contribute to the aim of the promotion. For example, a video may be used which does not match the topic and only diverts or confuses the participants. Poor-quality materials will also detract from any impact they might have, and undermine the overall credibility of the message.

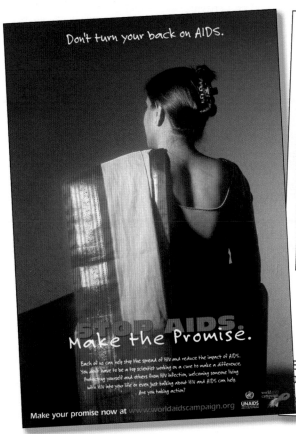

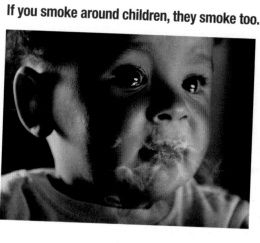

Using mass media

The 'mass media' refers to any printed or audio-visual material designed to reach a mass audience. This includes newspapers, magazines, radio, television, billboards, exhibition displays and widely distributed posters and leaflets. The media can convey uncomplicated information and raise the public's consciousness about health issues. As part of an integrated campaign the media can change behaviour, but they cannot teach skills or shift attitudes. There is no personal link with the mass audience. Some mass media campaigns have sought to shock people into changing behaviour but evidence has demonstrated that often the effects are short-lived or ignored, unless supported by other factors. Examples include the 'Eat less salt' campaigns and the annual 'World AIDS Day'.

Figure 10 How useful is the mass media?

Advantages of using mass media

- Raises awareness about health issues
- Puts health on the public agenda effecting societal change
- Increases knowledge
- Influences attitude and behaviour change
- Has immediate emotional effect

Disadvantages of using mass media

- Responses may be short term
- Cannot convey complex information
- Cannot teach skills
- May only change attitudes or behaviours if in combination with other enabling factors
- Some mass media stories may convey negative messages about health promotion.

Types of mass media campaign

- The major health promotion agencies use the mass media for their national or regional health promotion campaigns. These include television, radio, magazines or newspapers advertisements, and address issues such as influenza protection, healthy eating, and giving up smoking.

- Many commercial organisations sell their food products – fruit, wholemeal bread etc. – as health promoting. Other advertisements will highlight certain 'healthy' properties, such as 'low fat'. Companies may produce educational leaflets linked to their products – such as Flora and its healthy eating leaflets. Leisure facilities may emphasise the links between exercise and health, and restaurant chains advertise their 'healthy' options.

- Books, magazines, television and radio have articles, discussions and reports on health issues. Some magazines and books may be entirely concerned with health issues, while others have health amongst many other issues of interest to their readers. Television companies sometimes produce documentaries or whole series which promote health messages. Jamie Oliver, the celebrity chef, undertook a series on school meals, and the findings have resulted in major changes to nutritional standards in schools.

- Issues about health can be raised indirectly as part of storylines in television or radio. This most frequently occurs in 'soaps' such as The Archers or EastEnders or in programmes set in a medical context – such as Casualty. News items can reflect issues about health, and contribute to people's knowledge and understanding.

- The health experiences of media 'celebrities' and their behaviour can affect the behaviour and views of others, particularly if they are role models for certain groups. The attitudes of sports personalities towards alcohol and drugs may have an effect on young people who seek to emulate their lifestyle.

- A negative effect on health can be produced by the advertising and promotion of 'unhealthy' products. Sweets and food with a high fat content (such as burgers) can look very attractive, and encourage children to demand more and more of such foods – increasing the numbers of obese individuals.

- Many companies have realised the advantages of sponsorship linked with fitness and health, and have therefore sought to sponsor sporting events, teams and individual people. In the past, cigarette manufacturers were sponsors of sport but this has declined as it was accepted that the messages were contradictory in terms of good health, and therefore it was banned in most sports.

Government health promotion

Every year at Christmas there is a campaign in the mass media that seeks to reduce the number of deaths from drinking and driving. This is the announcement for the 2005 campaign. It suggests that the death of a young woman has been caused by two young men who have been drinking

'The campaign will incorporate TV advertising, cinema and cinema ambient advertising, radio advertising, partnership marketing, PR and will also be supported by a Police Christmas enforcement campaign to reinforce and extend the THINK! drink drive message.

The current '**Crash**' drink drive TV ad will air nationally for just over two weeks in December highlighting that 1-2 drinks can slow reactions and cause a crash. A new drink drive radio ad will be launched to complement the Police Christmas enforcement campaign. The radio ad aims to encourage young men to police their own drinking, before the police do it for them and if they risk drink driving this Christmas they will be caught. The radio ad will air nationally for four weeks throughout the festive season.'

Check your understanding

1. Explain what factors need to be taken into account when choosing a health promotion method.

2. Describe how and why the principle of promoting equality and diversity should be part of any promotion.

3. Identify which resources would be appropriate in three different situations, and why.

4. Describe the main advantages and disadvantages of using the mass media.

extension**activities**

Choose two health promotion campaigns, one of which has used the mass media. Analyse each one for its content, style, target group and likely impact.

Topic 5 Health promotion methods and media

Topic 6   Ethical issues in health promotion

Getting you thinking

The following situations may pose ethical problems for health promotion:

- A patient who is due to have heart surgery but continues to smoke.

- Sports equipment that has been sponsored by sweet manufacturers.

- A nursery that insists that all its children should be fully immunised before being admitted.

1 What dilemmas are illustrated by each situation?

2 Suggest how two health promoters might have differing views.

3 What do *you* think would be the appropriate action in each case?

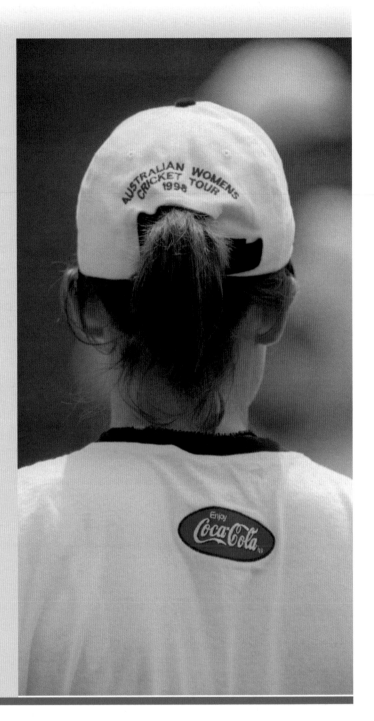

KEY TERMS

Ethics
The formal study of the principles on which moral rules and values are based.

Victim blaming
Being held responsible for one's own misfortune.

Ethical issues have to be considered

Health promotion is all about influencing the health of other people. As we have explored different approaches and methods it has become clear that not everybody has the same values and priorities. Principles such as promoting anti-discriminatory practice, maintaining confidentiality, supporting the rights of individuals, and acknowledging personal beliefs and identities are as applicable to health promotion as to all other aspects of health care. However, there may be situations when decisions have to be made – whether, for example, individual choice should take priority over the health of a whole community. Before commencing any health promotion, these questions of ethics need to be considered, and judgements have to be made about how to intervene and which strategies to adopt.

Informed choice or doing as you are told?

The intended aim or outcome of any health promotion will influence the approach taken by the health promoter. If it is expected that the client – whether an individual or a group – will make an informed choice and have the skills and confidence to carry it out, the health promoter will seek to ensure that all the facts and risks are understood, and be prepared to accept if the client declines to change their behaviour. On the other hand, if compliance is the aim, the health promoter might stress the risks of not changing – using a variety of persuasive techniques – and put pressure on the client to make the changes. A decision may need to be made as to how far to go in imposing values on individuals 'for their own good'.

Individual rights versus community good

The actions of individuals may have effects on others in their community, and a balance has to be struck as to whether their rights should take precedence. Smoking in public has been at the centre of such consideration, particularly since the understanding of the risks of passive smoking. Respect for an individual's rights to make decisions about their own health has to be weighed against the harm that might come to the wider community because of their actions. Immunisation is effective only if a high level of immunity is achieved in the whole population – which requires that *all* individuals should participate.

Victim blaming

An emphasis on the individual and their responsibility for their own health can lead to a situation when people can be blamed for their ill health. People with heart disease could be held responsible for their condition – and blamed for it – if they smoked or were overweight. This ignores the influence of other factors, such as economic or social conditions. A focus on high-risk groups can also lead to '**victim blaming**'. When HIV prevention was first developed there was much emphasis on targeting gay men. However, it is not *being* gay that is the risk factor but certain sexual activities.

Leading by example

We can all point to individuals who work in health promotion who set a poor example of healthy living. Nurses who smoke and doctors who are overweight do not give the 'right' message when trying to influence others about adopting a healthy lifestyle. Should health promotion only be undertaken by 'healthy' people, or can a realistic and honest debate help to gain the trust and understanding of clients?

Does 'do as I say rather than do as I do' carry as much weight?

Cost effectiveness

Health promotion, like all other aspects of health, has a financial cost attached to it. There will always be a finite amount of money and resources available, and it is the responsibility of the professionals to employ the most cost-effective methods of promoting health. This may require difficult decisions which have to balance the greatest good for the largest number of people and the return on any investment. For example, the use of universal techniques such as breast screening has been carefully assessed against the numbers of cancers diagnosed at an early stage. However, for each individual who has benefited from earlier treatment no cost would be too high.

Reliable research

Health promotion relies on research into the causes and cures for ill health. Over time, however, new research may become available that changes the experts' views and influences the messages about health improvement. For many years new mothers were encouraged to allow their babies to sleep on their stomachs until new research demonstrated that it was a contributory factor in Sudden Infant Death Syndrome (cot death). Other health issues may suddenly be publicised because of some startling –

but poorly researched – evidence and the media attention may have a major effect on individual behaviour. Health promoters have a responsibility to ensure that they are confident that their messages are factually and professionally based.

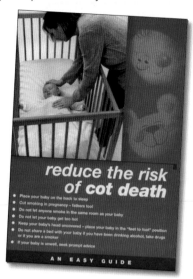

reduce the risk
of **cot death**

- Place your baby on the back to sleep
- Cut smoking in pregnancy – fathers too!
- Do not let anyone smoke in the same room as your baby
- Do not let your baby get too hot
- Keep your baby's head uncovered – place your baby in the "feet to foot" position
- Do not share a bed with your baby if you have been drinking alcohol, take drugs or if you are a smoker
- If your baby is unwell, seek prompt advice

AN EASY GUIDE

Sponsorship

With limited resources, the opportunity to use sponsorship is very attractive. In many cases it proves to be a very successful partnership between the health promoter and a commercial company. However, there are certain questions that need to be asked. Health is a subject that interests the general public and some manufacturers will try to link their brands with a 'healthy' image to counteract the unhealthy consequences of using their products – sweet manufacturers, for example, sponsoring sports equipment. Other problems may be that by accepting sponsorship from a particular company it may be seen as an endorsement of their product rather than its competitors. The independent credibility of the health promoter may be compromised, making it more difficult for clients to trust their messages.

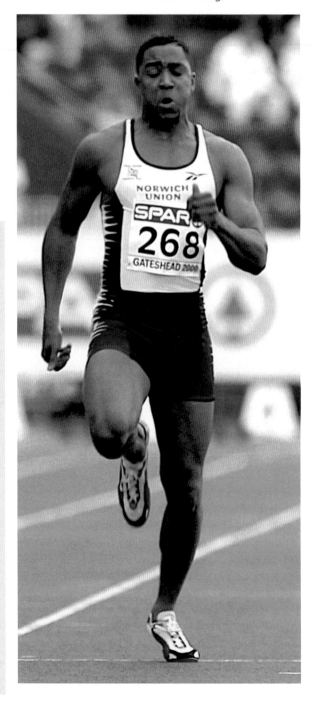

Chocolate and sport?

In 2003 Cadburys launched a scheme which involved collecting tokens in exchange for sports equipment. The scheme was called 'Get Active' and the publicity statement said "Cadburys is proud to offer up to £9m of free, unbranded sports equipment to help kids become more active." Cadburys was adamant that the scheme would not specifically encourage children to eat more chocolate. Instead they suggested that the scheme allowed the wider community to help schools. The Food Commission criticised the confectioner for a marketing scheme that involved collecting tokens from chocolate bars in exchange for school sports equipment. The commission said 'the scheme is absurd and contradictory. If children consumed all the promotional chocolate bars they would eat nearly two million kilos of fat and more than 36 billion calories'. It was estimated that it would take 170 bars to receive a basketball, 320 chocolate bars to receive a volleyball and 2,730 bars for a cricket set. To get volleyball posts it would require 5,440 bars costing £2,000 with 1.25 million calories. Cadburys argued that the chocolate would be eaten anyway and this would be an opportunity for everybody, not just children, to club together to get sports equipment.

Political control and vested interests

Political decisions sometimes involve health issues. Government departments may learn information that they do not wish to have released to the general public. In 1988, for example, the Department of Health was aware of the widespread presence of salmonella in eggs, but it was not publicised officially. Government may decide that releasing certain information may raise too many anxieties, but some people would argue for freedom of access to such information to allow the public to make their own choices. Decisions about health protection may affect other industries adversely. Farming interests may conflict with progress on food safety – as was the case with the BSE (Bovine Spongiform Encephalopathy) outbreak caused by farming practices and leading to the development of CJD (Creutzfeld–Jakob disease) in humans.

Professional codes of conduct

Most healthcare professions have codes of conduct, which members are expected to follow. The principles in public service are accountability, openness and probity. This means that workers in health should be accountable for their actions, open in their dealings and honest. They should not be open to persuasion away from their professional course. At times these principles may be challenging – when organizations or individuals seek to influence either the information or outcome of a health promotion.

Inequalities in health

The inequalities that are reflected in society – whether they be of income, education, resources or power – have an effect on health. Those with higher incomes are able to access a greater range of health resources, including private health care, while those who are better educated are more able to understand and apply the health promotion messages they hear. Parts of society experiencing social exclusion will suffer physical, mental and social health problems. The decision for health promotion is whether to provide an equality of health promotion across the whole of society or try to address the inequalities that exist through targeting those who are most in need. Programmes such as 'Sure Start' seek to provide support to parents who are in the greatest need, rather than to all families.

Ethical principles in research

Health promoters are frequently involved in undertaking research and evaluating their practice. When making decisions about their methodology, they need to follow certain principles – about informed consent, confidentiality and the right to privacy. Otherwise, there is a risk of compromising the standards which govern all professional interactions in health care.

Check your understanding

1 Explain what is meant by 'informed choice' and how it applies to health promotion.

2 Give an example of 'victim blaming' and describe why it might happen in health promotion.

3 Identify the advantages and disadvantages of having sponsorship.

4 Explain why inequalities in society can affect health.

extension activities

1 Choose two health promotion campaigns that have sponsorship. Analyse why the company might have wished to sponsor the campaign.

2 Review two recent press stories about health. Could any ethical issues arise from these articles?

Getting you thinking

This is a picture of a particular type of health promotion activity.

1 What message are the people in the protest picture trying to convey?

2 When would this form of health promotion action be appropriate?

3 Who might be influenced by this type of action?

4 What are the disadvantages of using this type of action?

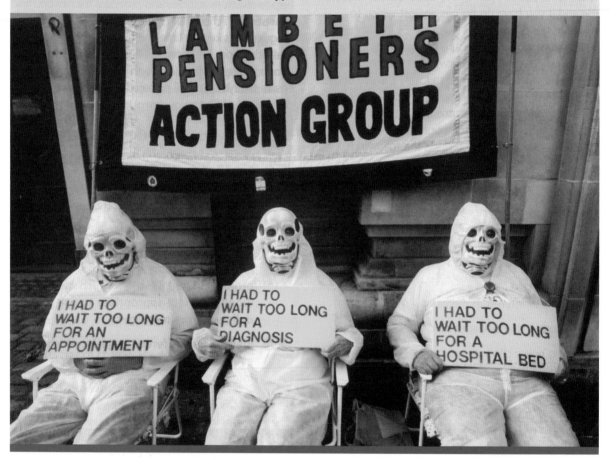

KEY TERMS

Action plan
Detailed plan of how a project will be managed.

Resources
Everything that will be required to undertake the project.

Time management
Using time effectively.

Communication
The process of sending and receiving messages.

Active listening
The process of listening to all aspects of a person's communication including verbal and non-verbal aspects.

Barriers to communication
Physical, social, emotional and other factors that restrict or limit the effectiveness of communication.

Time to put it all into action!

After all the planning, the time comes to put it all into action. You have identified what you plan to achieve, the best way to go about it, how you will evaluate it, and any resources that you need. You have considered what is the best setting for your activity. It may be a school or college, in the workplace, in primary health care – or even at home. Sometimes it is appropriate to go into leisure facilities, such as health clubs (or even pubs), or to attend meetings of the specific target group, such as parent and toddler groups.

Action plans

The action plan specifies the details of exactly **who** will do **what**, by **when**, and with **what resources**. This may require a few rough drafts to make sure everything is covered. It will be necessary to build in some 'reflection points' as you go along to ensure that the project is going to plan – and to be able to readjust if unforeseen circumstances affect the timing or content. Once you have worked out the details of your plan, the next stage is to review it to see if it is workable. Evaluating the plan before proceeding may save wasting effort, time and resources, and give you an opportunity for a rethink before too much is lost.

Who will do what?

An early decision will be as to whether the activity is to be undertaken by you alone or by a group working together. The advantages of working alone include easier decision making, control over your own time, and not having to rely on others. The disadvantages are that all the work falls on you – and, like anyone, you may not have the full range of skills needed to undertake all aspects of the promotion. If working alone, an honest assessment of your own skills is important. For example, are you artistic or able to produce good quality posters or will you need to rely on commercially produced material? Will your speaking skills need practice?

Working in groups demands good coordination and teamwork, and an early discussion is required to allocate roles and responsibilities. Good team communication will lie at the heart of a successful project. The characteristics of a successful team are:

- Shared aim – agreed by all
- Specific individual skills that are recognised and utilised

- Roles and responsibilities of each member known and understood by all
- Members support and trust each other
- Good communication between members
- Clear leadership that is recognised by all.

Communicating, whether with members of your team, other colleagues, those in official positions or your clients, will take up time which needs to be built in to your planning. It may be necessary to write letters – to request permission to hold an event, to approach sponsors, or to order literature. Team meetings need to be structured into the plan, and records kept of any decisions. When writing the action plan it is important to indicate who has agreed to do what.

Identification of what needs to be done – either by the individual or by the group – will link very closely to the objectives that have been set in order to achieve the overall aim of the project. There may be some preliminary stages to go through. For example, permission may be required to carry out the activity, such as parental consent in schools. Questionnaires may need to be piloted before finally being handed out. Resources will need to be obtained or made, etc. When working in a team it is appropriate to divide up the tasks according to individuals' interests and capabilities. However, this means that the team will be reliant on each other to complete the project – so regular assessment of the progress of the project is essential. It can be useful to draw up a list of key actions that need to be undertaken, with dates by which they should be completed – and keep the list under regular review.

Managing your time

Time is a resource that should be used efficiently and cost-effectively. It needs to be planned and organised in the same way as any other aspect of the health promotion. But how good are you at managing time? Ask yourself the following questions:
1 Do you always hand in your work on time?
2 How often have you stayed up late to complete work to meet a deadline?
3 Do you tend to do the things you like first, and leave the more difficult tasks?
4 Do you manage to work without breaks? If not, what sort of breaks to you take?
5 At what time of day do you find it easiest to work?

To assist effective time management, the following two questions need to be answered: When does the work need to be done by? How long will the work take? Then the times can be incorporated into the

Analysing and evaluating a health promotion activity

Getting you thinking

A local sports coordinator has put up some posters advertising a new range of activities which he hopes will appeal to the local young people and increase their participation in exercise.

1 What ways could he use to evaluate the success of his campaign?

2 What are the positive benefits in the coordinator undertaking the evaluation himself?

3 What advantages and disadvantages would there be in using an external researcher to evaluate the success?

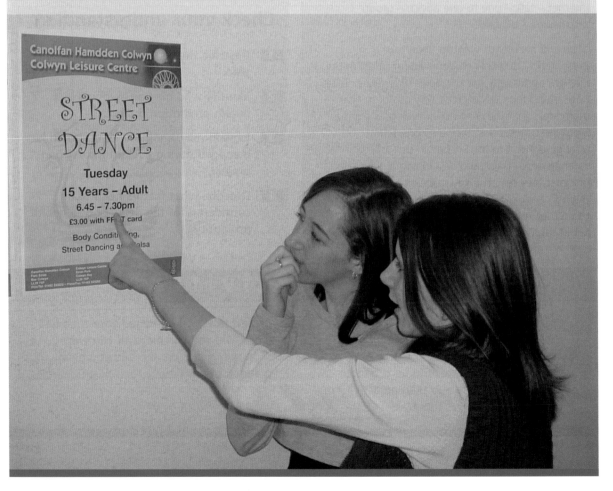

KEY TERMS

Qualitative data
Data that describes the outcomes in words, rather than numbers.

Quantitative data
Data that is numerical.

Analysis and evaluation

Evaluation takes place on a regular, but informal, basis when health promoters appraise and assess their work as a matter of course. However, a more systematic approach is explained in the World Health Organization's definition:

> 'Evaluation implies judgement based on careful assessment and critical appraisal of given situations which should lead to drawing sensible conclusions and making useful proposals for future action.'
>
> WHO, 1981

The success of a promotion must be related to the aim and objectives that had been set, but might also be influenced by unforeseen circumstances. An evaluation seeks to cover these aspects, as well as measuring the effectiveness of the promotion, the cost and any benefits that can be directly linked to the activity.

The size of any health promotion activity will influence to what extent its findings can be generalised to other contexts. Small-scale activities can really only provide an illustration of findings already demonstrated in larger-scale promotions.

Process, impact and outcome evaluation

'Process' (formative) evaluation means looking at what goes on during the process of implementing the health promotion.

'Impact' evaluation means understanding the immediate consequences of the health promotion.

'Outcome' evaluation means an assessment of the longer-term effects, matched to the aim and objectives of the activity.

Self-evaluation

As well as an assessment of your own personal contribution, self-evaluation may also encompass the way in which your team worked. An assessment of how the team worked together, the strengths or weaknesses of each member, and whether the appropriate expertise was available could be discussed within the group. As an individual, you may want to reflect on what you did well (and what you did not do so well), anything you would change, what you have learnt from the activity – and what you have learnt about yourself. This can all be written up as part of the project or as part of your record of personal development.

Evaluative data

The collection and analysis of data should be planned into the project. It will be needed to demonstrate the outcomes of the activity and to measure any change. This can be by using **qualitative data** which will give a descriptive (and probably personal and subjective) view, or by using **quantitative data** which gives a numerically measured account, such as *how many* changed their views or *what percentage* difference in knowledge can be demonstrated.

All data collection must pass the two tests of reliability and validity. Reliability concerns the consistency of the data. The data is reliable when the same results would be achieved if the activity were run again and again, if all the other variables were the same. Validity is the appropriateness of the research method. The data is valid when the method used measured what it was intended to measure, and the link between cause and effect can be shown.

Methods of collecting data include interviews, reflective accounts, oral questioning or using

	Characteristics	Advantages	Disadvantages
Process evaluation	• Notes reactions to activity. • Identifies other factors affecting activity. • Uses interviews, diaries, observation.	• Involves participants. • Responses from particular target group.	• Not scientifically rigorous. • Unable to predict what would happen in different circumstances.
Impact evaluation	• Review at end of promotion. • May use pre- and post-questioning.	• Easy to undertake. • Involves participants. • Immediate results.	• May not reflect longer-term result.
Outcome evaluation	• Assessment of longer-term effects. • Collection and analysis of data.	• Measures sustained changes. • Credibility of data.	• Complex and costly. • May need a control group.

Figure 15 Types of evaluation

questionnaires. All methods need to work to a planned structure, with careful recording of the results. In interviews, for example, it is useful to have a number of structured questions to ensure that all aspects requiring evaluation are covered.

If measurements can be taken before and after an intervention (pre-testing and post-testing) then the specific effects of the programme can be demonstrated. If, for example, the same questionnaire about healthy diets is used before and after a presentation about nutrition, the change in knowledge and attitude can be measured.

Designing a questionnaire

Questionnaires are used to get information, but they need to be carefully designed to ensure that the required data is actually obtained. Here are some basic questions to think about when constructing a questionnaire:

- What information do you require, and from whom?
- How is the information to be collected – completed by the participant on their own or by interview?
- How many people do you need in the sample?
- When will the survey take place?

- Does the questionnaire need to be pilot tested?
- How will the data be analysed and reported?

The introduction to the questionnaire

The introduction to a questionnaire should indicate to the respondents the reasons for undertaking the survey. It should also reassure them regarding the confidentiality of their answers. Below is an example of a good introduction.

The content of the questionnaire

Careful thought needs to be given as to what information is essential to collect. Is it necessary to know the age or sex of the respondents? Do you need to know their ethnic background ? This will require thought about the results and how they will be analysed.

When designing the questions, remember that the way a question is worded is very important. Interesting questions will hold attention. But, more importantly, questions should be clear and as specific as possible. They should be easy to understand and respond to. The most important principle is 'keep it simple'.

Health in your community

Please take some time (approximately 20–25 minutes) to complete this questionnaire.

What this survey is for

This survey provides you with an opportunity to share your thoughts about what you feel about sport and the facilities available. Your responses will provide important information which will demonstrate what is required to improve participation in sport.

Confidentiality

You do not have to complete this survey if you do not wish to do so. However, everyone's views are important and the more participation we receive, the better the results will be.

Please understand that this questionnaire is completely confidential.

1 Do not write your name on the questionnaire.

2 Seal your questionnaire in the envelope provided.

The envelope will *only* be opened by the team entering your responses into the computer system. It will be placed with many others, and there will be no way to identify individual respondents. The results of *all* the questionnaires will be added together and reported back.

Any term that is used must have the same meaning for both the questioner and the respondent. The term 'exercise', for example, might be intended by the questioner to refer only to organised activity, while a respondent might think it encompasses all aspects of physical movement – including walking to the shops.

Care should be taken to ensure that only one question is asked at a time. For example, 'Do you plan to leave your car at home and walk to work?' asks several questions rather than one.

Getting the answers you need

There are different ways of asking for the answer to simple questions, such as *How many cups of coffee did you drink yesterday?*

Example 1: _____ (*specify number*)

Example 2: *none 1 2 3 4 5 6 more than 6 (circle one)*

When using the second method, every eventuality needs to be covered.

When using numerical responses, the numbers given should not overlap.

How many portions of chips do you eat in a month?

   None   1–5   6–10   11–15   16+

(**Not:** None   0–5   5–10   10–15   15+)

There are two types of question: 'closed' and 'open'. Closed questions give the respondent a choice of answers from which they select one, while open questions give the respondent an opportunity to answer in their own words.

For example, *What do you think is the most important problem facing today's youth?* is an open question. It could provoke as many answers as there are respondents. If it were framed as a closed question, it might be:

Which of the following do you think is the most important problem facing today's youth?

Unemployment   ☐

Environment   ☐

Youth violence   ☐

Drugs in schools   ☐

Analysing the responses to closed questions is much simpler because they fit into a simple structure and are consistent, but they are limited to the options given and may not give sufficient breadth.

Questions that might be sensitive or self-incriminating are best avoided – questions about drug taking, for example, breaking the law or personal issues such as abortion. If, however, they are essential to the activity they must be handled with an unbreakable code of anonymity.

Questions should be applicable to all those questioned, if possible, and they should flow naturally from one to another. They should not ask for the same information more than once, even in a later context.

Often it is a good idea to end with an 'any other comments?' section which allows the respondent to record any other relevant information. All questionnaires should end by thanking the respondent for taking the time to answer the questions.

Pilot testing, sample size, timing

Whenever possible, questionnaires should be pilot tested on a number of people who are relevant to the activity (but not those who will eventually form the survey group). This often reveals that some of your carefully thought-out wording is, in fact, ambiguous and can easily be 'taken the wrong way' – leading to unhelpful responses. This process allows adjustments to be made to the wording or structure of the questionnaire before it is distributed to the actual target group.

It is obviously complex and expensive to undertake large surveys that truly represent a population. But with small surveys the numbers involved mean that differences and swings can be greatly exaggerated. For example, if one person out of ten people surveyed disagrees with an idea, then it is reported as '10% of those surveyed'. If, however, that same person were surveyed in a group of five it would be reported as '20% of those surveyed'. Care therefore needs to be exercised when seeking to apply findings from small surveys to a more generalised principle.

The value of undertaking pre-activity and post-activity surveys has already been discussed, but further thought should be given as to the timing of the second survey. If given immediately following the health promotion it will capture the immediate impact, but it may not reflect longer-term changes in attitudes and behaviours.

Analysis of the findings and presentation

Once the research has been collated and the findings analysed, conclusions can be drawn. By comparing 'before' and 'after' data, the health promoter can demonstrate the success or otherwise of the activity, and may make suggestions as to how any future programme could be improved. Evaluation is most useful when it shows what difference can be made in the future by demonstrating the effectiveness of the health promotion or by showing where changes need to be made.

There is also the opportunity to reflect on the appropriateness of the evaluation methods used. For example, was a questionnaire the most useful method and was it well constructed? Was the baseline of knowledge established prior to giving a presentation so that any increase could be measured?

Findings from evaluations can be presented in a range of formats. Some will need to be reported in a descriptive manner, while others can be reported statistically, using a variety of charts including bar charts, pictograms, histograms or pie charts, depending on the method of evaluation that has been chosen.

The final stage of a health promotion is to write the report. This will include your knowledge and understanding of the topic addressed by your health promotion, how and why you chose your target group, and a summary of the research undertaken prior to the activity which supported the need for a health promotion. The planning of your promotion will be demonstrated by stating your aims and objectives, by identifying and discussing the health promotion models that you chose and by describing how you intended to measure the success of the health promotion. The implementation of your health promotion will be shown by an account of the methods by which the promotion was delivered, including the use and development of appropriate media and materials – and how and why they were chosen. An analysis of the success of the promotion should include an understanding of the process and method of analysis as well as the outcomes. Finally, there should be conclusions from the analysis of the findings and well-argued recommendations for the future. These should be based on evidence, and be clear, well-reasoned and detailed. Whenever possible, they should show independent thought and initiative. Acknowledgements of individuals and organisations who have given support should be included, as a matter of courtesy.

1 Evaluating how the presentation went

There are a number of factors that help or hinder learning and understanding and it is useful to evaluate how your presentation might be received. Think of two occasions when you were taught new knowledge or skills. It may have been in a class or as an individual. It could include practical skills such as cooking or driving as well as learning in college or school.

Analyse each of these occasions to establish which factors helped your learning and which hindered. Consider factors such as:
- The environment (temperature of room, any distracting noise, comfortable surroundings)
- The individual doing the teaching (what sort of personality – friendly/strict)
- The presentation (length, interest level, understandable, use of supporting material etc)

Make a list under each heading showing what helped and what hindered.

You can evaluate your own presentation in the same manner.

2 Getting feedback

You can ask the class to whom you have done your presentation to give you some feedback. One way is to give them an evaluation sheet. A ' Field of words' (see following page) is an interesting way for them to evaluate. What disadvantages might it have?

Circle all the words that apply to your view of the presentation

challenged

interesting

helped

boring

confusing

positive

okay

well presented

great

too long

good fun

relevant

irrelevant

varied

too much information

right length

enjoyable

Check your understanding

1 Identify the different types of evaluation, and describe when they are most appropriate.

2 Describe the difference between qualitative and quantitative data, and show when they may be used.

3 Identify the main points of designing a questionnaire.

4 Explain the main points that should appear in a report on a health promotion.

97

Topic 9 Analysing and evaluating a health promotion activity

extension activities

Examples of process, impact and outcome evaluation are shown below. Which type of evaluation is easiest to do? Which will give the most accurate and useful results?

1 Rates of falls amongst the elderly, a year after a 3-month falls-reduction campaign.

2 Review of uptake of healthy food options in a college canteen, 3 months after the introduction of a 'Healthy Eating' policy.

3 Take-up levels of a flu immunisation programme.

4 Questionnaires testing knowledge before and after health education lessons in school.

5 Number of leaflets handed out during a health promotion.

6 Study of no-smoking policies in local restaurants.

THIS UNIT LOOKS AT DISEASES AND HOW THEY ARE DIAGNOSED, TREATED AND PREVENTED. It also considers the factors that affect these aspects. We begin by looking at how health and disease are defined. These are not easy terms to define and there are no particularly correct ways of doing this. We then consider epidemiology, and see how learning about the patterns of disease in society can help the treatment of an individual.

You will have to choose one 'communicable' and one 'non-communicable' disease to compare for your portfolio. To help you make your choices, we cover more detail about a variety of communicable diseases in Topic 3, and about non-communicable diseases in Topic 4.

Different methods of diagnosing diseases are then introduced, and we shall see that there is a variety of methods, including biochemical detection and imaging techniques. Treatment may be at different levels – individual, in local health practice, in a local hospital, in a specialist national centre or a combination of all of these.

'Prevention is better than cure' is a common saying. We shall look at disease prevention and consider some of the factors that affect the prevention of diseases.

Finally, to help you draw all the ideas together, we shall consider some case studies. We shall make comparisons between communicable and non-communicable diseases – an important aspect in the assessment of this unit.

...estigating Disease

A02 dishbuhon

Key questions

By the end of this unit you should be able to use the knowledge and understanding that you develop to answer the following questions:

1 What are some of the different ways in which health may be defined, and why does 'being healthy' may mean different things to different people?

2 What is meant by epidemiology, and how can a study of epidemiology aid the diagnosis and treatment of diseases?

3 What are some of the differences between communicable and non-communicable diseases?

4 How can different diseases be diagnosed?

5 Who treats diseases, and what factors might affect the treatment and support of people who have a particular disease?

6 What strategies can be employed to reduce the risk of developing a disease, and what are some of the factors that may interfere with disease prevention?

Understanding health and disease

Getting you thinking

1 What does being healthy mean to you?
2 What does being healthy mean to the person sitting next to you?
3 Look at the picture and explain who you think is the most healthy.
4 Describe a time when you were not feeling well.

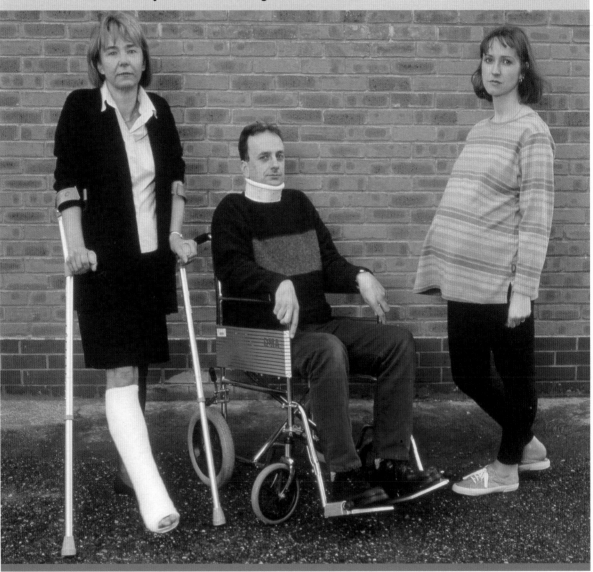

KEY TERMS

Communicable disease
A disease, caused by a micro-organism, that can be transmitted from one person to another.

Non-communicable disease
A disease that is not caused by a micro-organism, and that cannot usually be transmitted from one person to another.

What is 'health'?

You are studying a course called 'Health and Social Care', so you should know what 'health' means – or should you? Health can mean different things to different people.

Different definitions of health

Blaxter (1990) examined how people defined health. She carried out a survey of over 9,000 people. Figure 1 shows some of the ways these people talked about their health.

Figure 1 Different ways people talked about their health

'Health is when you don't have a cold'

(man of 19)

'Generally, it's being carefree, you look better, you get on better with other people'

(single woman of 20)

'Health is having loads of whumph'

(married woman of 28)

'Health is when you don't feel tired and short of breath'

(man of 51)

'Health is being able to walk around better, and doing more work in the house my knees will let me'

(woman of 70)

Source: M. Blaxter (1990) Health and Lifestyle, London: Tavistock.

Some people defined health in a 'negative' way, and some in a 'positive' way. What do we mean by negative and positive definitions of health? A negative definition might be ' Health is being free of symptoms of illness – for example, I don't have a headache or a backache' or 'Health is not having a disease or disability – for example, I have no medically diagnosed condition such as a broken leg or arthritis'.

A positive definition might be 'Health is psychological and social well-being – for example, I feel emotionally stable and able to cope with life' or 'Health is being physically fit – for example, I am physically fit enough to play sport'.

Blaxter concluded that there is no single agreed definition of health. It means different things to different people.

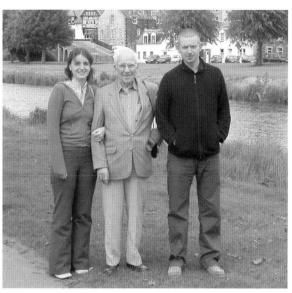

This photo shows two 20-year-olds out for a walk with their 80-year-old grandfather. Think about what being healthy means to someone who is 20. How would this differ from someone who is 80? If you are 20, you would hope to be reasonably fit and be able to take part in various forms of sport. If you are 80 years old, you might expect to be fit enough to carry out your daily tasks and to be able to walk a reasonable distance.

Relating health to PIES

Throughout your study of AS Health and Social Care you will have become aware that our development is in four different areas: physical, intellectual, emotional and social (PIES). It would seem natural then that health applies to all these four areas of development. You could say that we could categorise 'health' as physical health, intellectual health, emotional health and social health. The question is, do we need to have good health in all these areas to be healthy overall? Can we be healthy if we feel miserable most of the time? Can we be healthy if we cannot easily interact with other people?

Suppose you wake up one morning happy, full of energy, and confident about your day ahead. You might wonder why you are feeling so healthy. Is it because:

- you slept well the night before?

- your headache has gone?

- you solved a difficult crossword the night before?

- you are on holiday for the next few days?

- it is your birthday?

- you have just passed your driving test?

- the results of your blood test the day before were normal?

- you are going out with some friends later?

- you are in love?

Now, decide which area of your development each of these explanations applies to. This is not an easy task. For example, going out with some friends later relates to your emotional and social development – and may even relate to your physical or intellectual development, depending on what you are going to do.

The point here is that being healthy may be influenced by all areas of our development. Physical, intellectual, emotional and social aspects all act simultaneously in a dynamic way to produce a feeling of being healthy.

What is 'disease'?

Disease, like health, is a difficult term to define. The Oxford dictionary defines disease as 'morbid condition of the body, illness, sickness; deranged or depraved state of mind or morals'. We can see then, that disease can affect our body, our mind and the way we act. This means that, just like health, there are physical, mental (psychological) and social aspects to diseases.

What does having a disease mean?

Think of the word disease. Break it down to dis-ease and think of this as 'not at ease'. When was the last time you were 'not at ease'? It might have been when you had a cold, or you were depressed. For someone else, it might have been when they had chicken pox, or schizophrenia, or had a drug addiction. The list is endless.

Feeling 'not at ease' can mean different things to different people. It can arise from having different conditions and being in different situations. It may be simply thought of as ill-health, or not being healthy. The important thing to remember there is that, like health, there is no one correct definition.

How can diseases be classified?

There are many different ways of classifying diseases, some of which are very basic and some of which are very comprehensive. When trying to classify anything, we look for similarities and differences – putting things together that are similar. This is not as easy a task as it might seem.

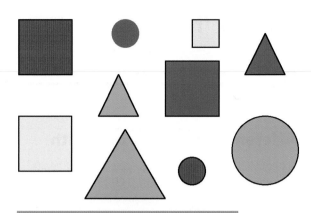

Figure 2 Ten shapes

Look at Figure 2, which shows objects of different sizes, shapes and colours. Try to group them together, using their similarities. You will find that there is more than one way to do this. You might have grouped the shapes by colour, by shape or by size. There is no right or wrong way. Similarly, diseases may be grouped together in various ways.

The International Classification of Diseases

In 2003 the World Health Organization introduced the 10th revision of the International Classification of Diseases (ICD –10). This is a comprehensive classification of diseases (see Figure 3). There are twenty main chapters; with each one subdivided many times. Each disease has its own identification code. For example, breast cancer (neoplasm) is C50. This category is subdivided further, depending on which part of the breast is affected by the cancer.

The WHO International Classification of Diseases system is used when recording diseases and other health problems on numerous types of records, including hospital records and death certificates. These records provide the basis for the compilation of national morbidity and mortality statistics by WHO member states. You will learn more about morbidity (illness) and mortality (death) in the next topic.

Simpler methods of categorising diseases

Sometimes it is useful to have simpler methods of categorising diseases. We shall discuss two ways of grouping diseases here:

- Grouping linked to the area of development the disease affects – physical, mental (psychological) or social.

- Grouping depending on whether the disease is caused by a micro-organism or not – that is, communicable or non-communicable.

International Statistical Classification of Diseases and Related Health Problems

10th Revision   Version for 2003
Tabular List of inclusions and four-character subcategories
Chapter List

Chapter	Blocks	Title
I	A00-B99	Certain infectious and parasitic diseases
II	C00-D48	Neoplasms
III	D50-D89	Diseases of the blood and blood-forming organs and certain disorders involving the immune mechanism
IV	E00-E90	Endocrine, nutritional and metabolic diseases
V	F00-F99	Mental and behavioural disorders
VI	G00-G99	Diseases of the nervous system
VII	H00-H59	Diseases of the eye and adnexa
VIII	H60-H95	Diseases of the ear and mastoid process
IX	I00-I99	Diseases of the circulatory system
X	J00-J99	Diseases of the respiratory system
XI	K00-K93	Diseases of the digestive system
XII	L00-L99	Diseases of the skin and subcutaneous tissue
XIII	M00-M99	Diseases of the musculoskeletal system and connective tissue
XIV	N00-N99	Diseases of the genitourinary system
XV	O00-O99	Pregnancy, childbirth and the puerperium
XVI	P00-P96	Certain conditions originating in the perinatal period
XVII	Q00-Q99	Congenital malformations, deformations and chromosomal abnormalities
XVIII	R00-R99	Symptoms, signs and abnormal clinical and laboratory findings, not elsewhere classified
XIX	S00-T98	Injury, poisoning and certain other consequences of external causes
XX	V01-Y98	External causes of morbidity and mortality
XXI	Z00-Z99	Factors influencing health status and contact with health services
XXII	U00-U99	Codes for special purposes

Figure 3 Summary of the WHO International Classification of Disease

Physical, mental (psychological) and social diseases

We saw earlier that disease can affect our body, our mind and the way we act. It makes sense then to group diseases depending on how and whereabouts in the body they affect us. Figure 4 shows examples of physical diseases, mental (psychological) diseases, and social diseases.

You may be able to see a problem with this way of categorising diseases. The categories are fairly broad,

Type of disease	Examples
Physical	Tooth decay, arthritis, influenza, AIDS
Mental (psychological)	Schizophrenia, depression, dementia
Social	Alcoholism, drug addiction, malnutrition

Figure 4 Types of diseases and some examples

and they overlap, so diseases may fall into more than one category. For example, AIDS could be considered as both a physical and a social disease, as it affects so many people in some societies. Alcoholism is a social disease but it might lead on to cirrhosis of the liver, and this could be considered a physical disease.

It is impossible to classify diseases precisely, as there are no rigid boundaries between the disease categories we generally recognise. For example, a genetic predisposition to a certain disease, such as cardiovascular disease, may combine with lifestyle factors to trigger the appearance of the disease. The relationship between the mind and body in disease is also very important.

However, there is one simple way of classifying diseases we have not yet considered. This is to distinguish whether diseases are communicable or non-communicable.

Communicable and non-communicable diseases

Communicable diseases are caused by micro-organisms, such as viruses and bacteria, and they can be transmitted from one person to another (see Figure 5). Non-communicable disease, such as cardiovascular disease or deficiency diseases, are not caused by living organisms and are not usually passed on from one person to another (see Figure 6). Although this way of classifying diseases is not foolproof, it gives us a reasonably clear basis for thinking about them. This is the classification you will use in your portfolio, and you will learn more about communicable and non-communicable diseases in Topics 3 and 4 of this unit.

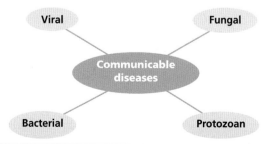

Figure 5 Communicable diseases

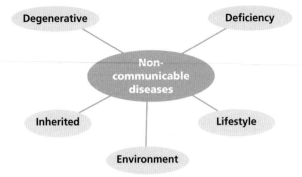

Degenerative

Deficiency

Non-communicable diseases

Inherited

Lifestyle

Environment

Figure 6 Non-communicable diseases

Emily, a children's nurse

Emily works as a nurse at a Children's Hospital. She qualified last year and only started work at the hospital last month. Her friend, Kay, would like to train as a nurse, and she meets up with Emily one evening to ask her all about her work. Emily tells Kay that she thoroughly enjoys her work, although some days she feels really tired at the end of her shift. Kay wants to know all about the children Emily looks after. Emily says that she can't say much as she has to respect the confidentiality of the patients.

She tells Kay, however, that there are 'highs' and 'lows'. Kay asks her what she means. Emily says, 'Well, last week we had good news about a little boy who has had a rare form of cancer of the blood. He was only six months old when he was diagnosed with the cancer and he has spent much of his life in hospital. He was given a bone marrow transplant seven weeks ago and has now made a good recovery. 'That's great', says Kay. 'Yes, isn't it?', says Emily, 'But it's not always like that'. She tells Kay about a baby born with a serious heart condition who is not expected to live long. This baby is being cared for in the Cardiac Intensive Care Unit where she can have one-to-one nursing care. Emily says she would like to work in that unit one day, although she would be sad if a child she cared for died.

Kay asks Emily if children with infectious diseases are treated in hospital. Emily says they are if the diseases are serious enough. She tells Kay that infectious diseases usually treated in hospital include:

- Meningitis
- Hepatitis
- Diphtheria
- Polio.

Kay asks Emily if she is not worried that she might catch any of those diseases. Emily says that there are very strict procedures to be followed to stop the spread of the infectious diseases. When she was young, like most people, she was immunised against most of the childhood infectious diseases, like polio, diphtheria, whooping cough and measles.

Emily says she must go home now and get an early night, as she is on an early morning shift. Kay thanks Emily and says they must keep in touch. She says she has found it fascinating talking to her, and maybe one day she might be a nurse like her.

Check your understanding

1. Look at Figure 1. For each of the different ways people talked about their health, decide whether it matches a negative or a positive definition. Once you have done that, see if you can be more precise about which negative or which positive definition it matches best.

2. Describe how being healthy may mean different things to a 20-year-old, a 50-year-old and an 80-year-old.

3. Who uses the WHO International Classification of Diseases, and for what purpose?

4. Give an advantage and a disadvantage of categorising diseases as physical, mental (psychological) or social.

5. Give an advantage and a disadvantage of categorising diseases as communicable or non-communicable.

extension activities

1. Ask ten people what being healthy means to them. Depending on their answers, decide what type of definition each person has for health. Discuss your findings with the rest of your class.

2. Visit the WHO website and find out more about the International Classification of Diseases. Write a paragraph outlining the advantages and disadvantages of such a classification.

3. Explain why health and disease are both difficult to define precisely.

Getting you thinking

1 **How can studies of large groups of people help someone who is ill?**

2 **How can we get information about the health of a large group of people?**

3 **Why is it important that a study should include men and women, old and young?**

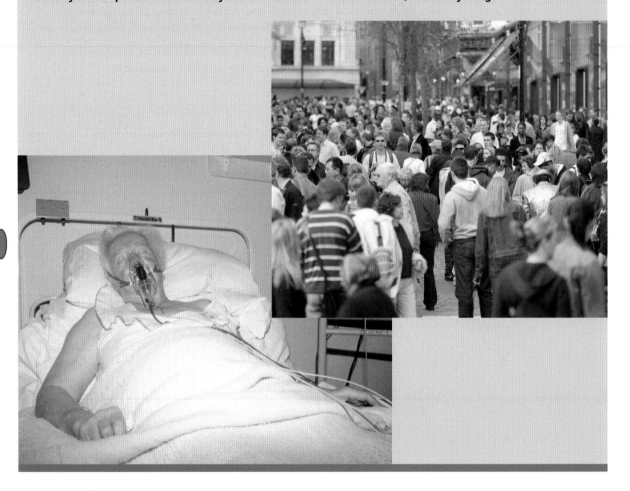

KEY TERMS

Aetiology
The study of what causes a disease.

Demography
The systematic study of the growth, size, distribution, movement and composition of human populations.

Epidemiology
The study of the spread of disease and causes of death and disability in a population.

Incidence
The number of new cases of a specified disease occurring in a given period of time.

Morbidity rate
The number of people who have a particular disease in a given population and time period.

Mortality rate
The number of people who have died from a particular disease in a given population and time period.

Prevalence
The total number of cases of a specified disease occurring in a population at a particular point in time.

What is 'epidemiology'?

Epidemiology sounds as if it should be the study of epidemics. It does include this, but the term is much wider. **Epidemiology** can be defined as the study of all factors which affect disease in human populations. It involves identifying the cause of the disease and all the factors which contribute to its appearance in a given population.

OK, you might say, but how does that help someone who is ill? Let's suppose that someone called Bob has just been diagnosed with heart disease. What would Bob want to know? He might ask his GP the following questions:

- How did I get this?

- What treatment will I get?

- What can I do to stop it getting worse?

- How could I have prevented this in the first place?

Bob may be surprised if his GP starts talking about how many people in the area had the same disease, where they lived and what they ate. Bob may wonder why the GP is doing this, rather than being interested in 'curing' him.

The point is that studying large groups of people often provides valuable information that helps manage an individual person's ill-health. For example, if Bob lived in a part of the country where many people developed heart disease, it may be linked to pollution, limited opportunities to exercise or to too many fish-and-chip shops. The GP will be able to use this information to advise Bob how to improve his condition.

Epidemiology's three areas of study

Epidemiology can be divided into three main areas of study. These can be summarised as three questions:

- Who gets ill?

- Why do they get ill?

- How should they be treated?

Who gets ill?

This area of epidemiology involves looking at *patterns* of disease in populations. It includes counting the number of people who get a particular disease (morbidity) and the number of people who die from the disease (mortality). We shall come back to this later.

Epidemiologists need to know about **demography**. Demography is the study of populations. Demographers are interested in details about populations, such as how many people live in an area, how many males there are and how many females, how old they are, how many are married, and how many are born and die each year.

Why do people get ill?

This area of epidemiology involves looking at *causes* of disease. As you might expect, studying the cause of a disease has its own term – **aetiology**. Sometimes the cause of a disease may be quite specific – the bacterium Streptococcus causing a sore throat, for example. Another example is the Human Immunodeficiency Virus (HIV) which causes Acquired Immunodeficiency Syndrome (AIDS). Sometimes the cause of a disease is not so clear, like in the case of Bob and his heart disease. There may be many factors involved, interlinking with each other to cause heart disease.

Studying the aetiology of a disease is sometimes like solving a mystery. There have been many examples of this in the past, including a famous study on cholera, undertaken by John Snow in the mid-nineteenth century (see below).

How should people be treated?

The third area of epidemiology looks at how people should be treated after they are diagnosed as having a disease. It is important to know the effectiveness of different methods of treatment. There is little point in having a particular treatment – especially one with painful side effects – if there is very little chance that it will be successful. Think of Bob and his heart disease. He might be given a new drug to reduce his blood pressure, but will it work, and what might the side effects be?

Here are some of the questions that an epidemiologist might ask about a treatment:

- How many people does it cure?

- If it is a new treatment, is it better than an existing one?

- Will the disease that is being treated shorten the person's life?

- How should the National Health Service be organised to cope with the treatment?

What are these questions all designed to achieve? They are designed to evaluate the *effectiveness* of the treatment, to see if it is worthwhile.

In 1854, death and despair engulfed London. In the Soho district, six hundred people died from cholera in just ten days. At that time there was no known cure for cholera and people started to panic. The local people had many different ideas about what was causing the disease. Some believed that 'vapours' were coming from corpses buried in a nearby cemetery– many of whom had died from cholera a century before.

John Snow, a physician, knew that they would have to identify the source of the disease in order to stop it spreading. He believed that the cause of the cholera was the drinking water. At that time, people got their drinking water from pumps in the streets. Snow produced a map showing the location of the pumps and the homes of the people who had died from cholera (see right).

Snow concluded that the pump that was the source of the problem was the one in Broad Street. Can you think how he proved this? He removed the handle of the pump, so that no one could use it anymore. And guess what? The number of cases of cholera decreased significantly. Although this does not prove conclusively that the pump contained infected water, it strongly supported the hypothesis that the disease was transmitted by something carried in drinking water and that the infected water came from that pump.

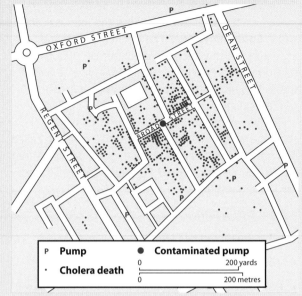

| P | **Pump** | ● | **Contaminated pump** |
| · | **Cholera death** | | |

0   200 yards
0   200 metres

Although Snow was concerned about the individuals in Soho, his study did not concentrate on them as individuals. He was interested in the patterns of where the victims lived and where they got their water, and of where the people who escaped the disease got their water. Yet his study led directly to a better understanding of the disease at the individual level, and ultimately to the control of the disease.

Dealing with data

When researching the diseases that you will choose for your portfolio, you will come across information presented in the form of tables and graphs. At first sight, the data may seem daunting, but do not be put off. Tables and graphs can help us see patterns and relationships more easily than if the information was just in words. This section will introduce you to some of the forms of data you will come across. It should help you feel more comfortable when interpreting data.

Population pyramids

One of the most important and useful sources of demographic information is census data. An official census of the population is carried out in the UK once every 10 years. A census is a way of counting people, and it provides a 'snapshot' of the national population on a particular day. One of the strengths of the census is the large amount of data about the UK population that is collected and then published. However, censuses are not completely accurate, because some people fail to provide information, and others make errors.

Figure 7a Table and Population pyramid for the United Kingdom in 2001, (data from official census report)

Age Range	Total	Males	Females
0–4	3486253	1785688	1700565
5–9	3738042	1914727	1823315
10–14	3880557	1987606	1892951
15–19	3663782	1870508	1793274
20–24	3545984	1765257	1780727
25–29	3867015	1895469	1971546
30–34	4493532	2199767	2293765
35–39	4625777	2277678	2348099
40–44	4151613	2056545	2095068
45–49	3735986	1851391	1884595
50–54	4040576	2003158	2037418
55–59	3339004	1651396	1687608
60–64	2880074	1409684	1470390
65–69	2596939	1241382	1355557
70–74	2339319	1059156	1280163
75–79	1967088	817738	1149350
80–84	1313592	482707	830885
85–89	752035	226520	525515
90 and over	372026	83492	288534
Totals	58789194	28579869	30209325

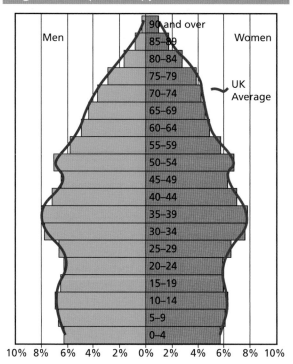

Figure 7b Population pyramid

Figure 7 shows the total number of people, males and females in different age ranges, provided by the census carried out in 2001. The information is given in two forms – in a table and in a graph, known as a population pyramid. Look at the two different ways the information is presented, and consider which is clearer. The population pyramid is an immediate way of comparing the numbers of males and females at different ages. The length of each bar represents the proportion of the total population that is in that particular sex–age group. The bottom left-hand bar, for example, indicates that at the 2001 census, 6% of the total population consisted of males aged 0–4 years.

Counting births and deaths

How do demographers count births and deaths? How do they compare numbers of births and deaths at different times and different places?

There is a national system of registration of births, marriages and deaths in the UK. Knowing the number of people who have died from a disease (the 'mortality' due to the disease) is important. However, it is much more useful to know the **mortality rate** (death rate) from a disease. Knowing death rates enables fair comparisons to be made between numbers of deaths at different times and places, taking account of the size of populations.

An example will help you understand this. Supposing there are two towns – A and B. In town A, 20 people died from strokes last year. In town B, 50 people died from strokes last year. You might think that the situation was more serious in town B. However, if you are told that the population of town A was 1,000 last year and the population of town B was 100, 000, you might change your mind. The death rate from strokes in town A would have been 20 per thousand, whereas the death rate from strokes in town B would have been 5 per thousand.

Mortality rates from different diseases

Figure 8 is a table showing the mortality rates from different diseases in England and Wales in 2002. The information given is the number of deaths per 100,000 population, and is shown for males and females, as well as for different age ranges.

You can see that the mortality rates by cause of death vary with age and sex. For young people aged 15–29, mortality rates were highest for injury and poisoning (41 per 100,000 population for men and 10 per 100,000 for women). For those aged 45–64, cancers were the major cause of death, and for older people, aged 65–84, circulatory diseases were the leading cause of death.

England & Wales	Rates per 100,000 population					
	0–14	15–29	30–44	45–64	65–84	85 and over
Males						
Infectious diseases	2	1	3	6	30	142
Cancers	4	6	23	245	1,403	3,422
Circulatory diseases	1	4	27	232	1,861	7,982
Respiratory dseases	2	2	5	41	566	3,610
Injury and poisoning	4	41	45	36	59	299
All causes	28	71	139	654	4,427	18,806
Females						
Infectious diseases	1	1	1	4	24	115
Cancers	3	5	32	218	921	1,858
Circulatory diseases	1	3	11	88	1,269	7,016
Respiratory dseases	1	1	4	30	403	2,654
Injury and poisoning	3	10	12	15	45	294
All causes	21	28	80	416	3,155	15,983

Figure 8 Mortality rates from different diseases in England and Wales in 2002

Figure 9 shows how the mortality rates from different diseases in England and Wales have changed over that past 90 years. Note that mortality rates from circulatory and infectious diseases have both decreased, whereas mortality rates from cancers have remained much the same. Cardiovascular diseases (which include heart disease and strokes) have remained the most common cause of death in England and Wales over the last 90 years. Cancers are now the second most common cause of death. Death rates for infectious diseases declined rapidly in the first half of the twentieth century and have remained low since. Can you think why this might be the case?

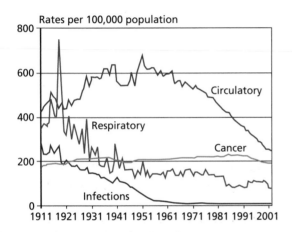

Figure 9 Mortality rates from different diseases in England and Wales over the past 90 years

Morbidity statistics

Thankfully, not every disease results in a death. Yet, we still want to have information about the numbers of people who suffer from different diseases (morbidity). The total number of cases of a specified disease occurring in a population at a particular point in time is known as the **prevalence** of the disease. We can work out **morbidity rates** if we know how many people have the disease over a specific period (usually a year) and divide this by the number of people in the population. Information about prevalence and morbidity rates may come from hospitals, GPs or disease registers. An example of a disease register is the national cancer register started in 1962. This depends on local doctors reporting the incidence (the number of new cases) of cancer arising.

Some infectious diseases – such as measles, meningitis and tuberculosis – are 'notifiable' (see Figure 10). This means that they must be reported. Public health practitioners collate and produce data on 30 such diseases in the UK. They do this so that they can identify and monitor trends, and respond to outbreaks when they occur. Recent examples of outbreaks include meningitis, measles and whooping cough.

Risk of measles epidemic

The Health Protection Agency said that outbreaks of measles in England and Wales had increased in recent years as fewer parents vaccinated their children because of fears about side-effects. Scientists have predicted that outbreaks of the viral disease will get worse as the proportion of unvaccinated children in the population increases. The latest study, by scientists at the Health Protection Agency and Royal Holloway College in London, is published in the journal *Science*. The new research warns that if the number of unprotected children continues to grow at the present rate, a national epidemic is inevitable.

Researchers say each measles outbreak in the UK now affects an average of ninety people, compared to ten people 4 years ago.

Complications from measles can cause permanent damage or death. The proportion of children vaccinated has fallen from 92% in 1996 to 79%, as a growing number of parents fear that the triple measles, mumps and rubella (MMR) vaccine can cause autism. The study suggests that there will soon be so many unvaccinated people that an outbreak will spread continuously.

Source: www.careworld.net, August 2003

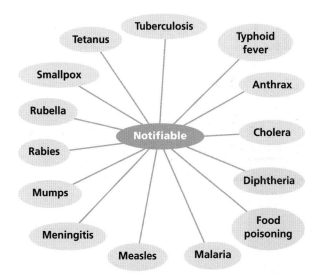

Figure 10 Some of the common notifiable diseases

Check your understanding

1 What is epidemiology, and why is it important?

2 Summarise the three main areas that epidemiologists study.

3 Explain, in your own words, what a population pyramid shows.

4 Describe how morbidity statistics are compiled, and suggest why they may be useful to epidemiologists.

extension**activities**

1 Find out where your local registrar of births, marriages and deaths is located. If possible, arrange a visit or a talk from a registrar to find out how registrars contribute to population health data through their work.

2 Using the internet or your local library, obtain some official statistics on mortality rates in your area. See how these compare with statistics for the country as a whole. Summarise your findings and present the material to the rest of the class.

Topic 2 Exploring epidemiology

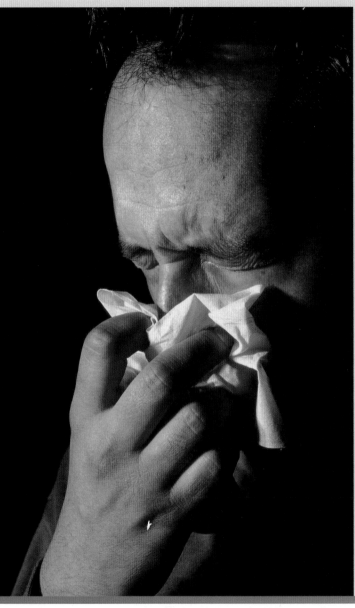

Getting you thinking

1 Can you remember being like the person in this picture? What did you feel like?

2 Where did you 'catch' your last cold from?

3 Why does using a handkerchief help prevent the cold spreading?

KEY TERMS

Bacterium
Single-celled micro-organism, capable of reproducing on its own.

Communicable disease
Disease caused by a micro-organism, caught from another person.

Fungus
Usually a multi-cellular micro-organism with a thread-like structure, e.g. mould, but sometimes exists as a single cell, e.g. yeast.

Transmission of disease
The passing of a disease from one person to another.

Vector
An organism that transfers a disease-causing micro-organisms from one person to another, e.g. mosquito or rat.

Virus
A very small micro-organism with a simple structure.

What do all communicable diseases have in common?

Communicable disease are those that you 'catch' from someone else. They are caused by micro-organisms. Most communicable diseases can affect us during any life stage. Usually we recover from them fairly quickly, although this may depend on how fit we are, and how old we are.

For your portfolio, you need to compare a communicable disease with a non -communicable one. This topic will introduce you to some communicable diseases and the micro-organisms that cause them. You will not be expected to learn everything about every communicable disease, but working through the topic will allow you to make an informed decision about which communicable disease you might choose. You might like to choose a communicable disease you have had yourself, or one that someone you know has had, or you might prefer to choose one you had not heard of before, but interests you, having now read about it.

Before reading on, make a list of as many communicable diseases as you can. Your list might start with the common cold and influenza (flu).

Micro-organisms

Micro-organisms are very small organisms. Most are so small we cannot see them, except under a microscope. Some micro-organisms are 'friendly' and useful to us – such as yeast, which is used in the production of bread and beer. However, many micro-organisms are 'harmful' and cause diseases. Their effects were known long before micro-organisms themselves were discovered. Can you think why? We had to wait until the invention of the microscope before their existence was known.

Micro-organisms can be divided into four main categories:

- Viruses (singular virus)
- Bacteria (singular bacterium)
- Fungi (singular fungus)
- Protozoa (singular protozoon).

We should therefore be able to divide communicable diseases into four categories, too – according to the type of micro-organisms that cause them: those diseases caused by viruses, those caused by bacteria, those caused by fungi and those caused by protozoa.

But there are some diseases, such as meningitis, that may be caused by both a virus and a bacterium. Don't worry though. Most diseases are just caused by one type of organism. Influenza, for example, is caused by a virus, and tuberculosis is caused by a bacterium.

Viral diseases

So far, no 'friendly' viruses have been discovered. All viruses cause diseases in other living organisms, including animals, plants and bacteria. In this course, we are interested only in viruses that cause diseases in humans. Below is a list of some viral diseases, and the viruses that cause them.

Figure 11 Some of the common viral diseases and the viruses that cause them

Viral disease	Virus responsible
Influenza	Influenza virus
Measles	Measles virus
German measles	German measles virus
Mumps	Mumps virus
Chickenpox	Varicella-zoster virus
Rabies	Rabies virus
Poliomyelitis	Polio virus
Warts	Human papilloma virus
Smallpox	Smallpox virus
Cold sores	Herpes simplex virus
Glandular fever	Epstein–Barr virus
AIDS	HIV (Human immunodeficiency virus)

What do you notice about the names of the viruses? Most of them have the same name as the diseases they cause, even those that do not appear to do so at first glance. For example, cold sores are sometimes called 'herpes simplex infections', and an alternative name for chickenpox is 'varicella'.

The structure of viruses

Viruses can cause devastating diseases. So, you might be surprised to know that they are the smallest of all the different types of micro-organisms – and they have the simplest structure.

Figure 12 The influenza virus

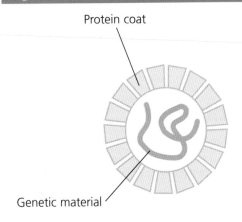

Protein coat

Genetic material

Figure 12 is a diagram representing the influenza virus. This structure is similar for all the viruses that cause diseases in humans. There is some genetic material in the centre (RNA – ribonucleic acid) surrounded by a protein coat. There is an outer lipid (fatty) envelope with some protein spikes.

There doesn't seem much to their structure, and you might wonder, in fact, if they are living organisms at all. They do not move, feed or respire, but they do reproduce. To reproduce, however, they need the help of a living cell. So they get inside our cells to reproduce. The way that the new viruses get out of our cells is by destroying them. Imagine this destruction of our cells happening many, many times. That is one of the reasons why viruses make us feel unwell.

Bacterial diseases

Have you ever had a sore throat? Or food poisoning? If you have, then you have had a bacterial disease. Have you ever had 'antibiotics'? If you have, then you have had a bacterial disease. Antibiotics only work against bacteria and not against viruses. (We shall hear more about antibiotics in a later topic.) Some of the common bacterial diseases and the bacteria that cause them are listed below.

The names of the bacteria are in Latin. Many organisms have Latin names. The first name is the genus and the second name is the species. You may have heard of *Homo sapiens*. That is the Latin name for modern man. *Homo* is the genus we belong to and *sapiens* (meaning wise) is our species. Notice that pneumonia and pharyngitis belong to the same genus – *Streptococcus*, but they belong to different species within the genus. (This may seem a bit confusing, but you will need to pay attention to detail like this if you want a high grade in your portfolio.)

You may have heard of many of these bacterial

Figure 13 Some of the common bacterial diseases and the bacteria that cause them

Bacterial disease	Bacterium responsible
Tuberculosis	*Mycobacterium tuberculosis*
Pneumonia	*Streptococcus pneumonia*
Diphtheria	*Corynebacterium diphtheriae*
Pharyngitis (sore throat)	*Streptococcus pyrogenes*
Whooping cough	*Bordella pertussis*
Food poisoning	*Salmonella species (caused by different species)*
	Escherichia coli
	Staphylococcus aureus
Cholera	*Vibrio cholerae*
Typhoid	*Salmonella typhi*
Boils	*Staphylococcus aureus*
Meningitis	*Neisseria meningitis*
Tetanus	*Clostridium tetani*
Syphilis	*Treponema pallidum*

diseases. Try to remember which parts of the body each affects. For example, food poisoning affects the digestive system, tuberculosis and pneumonia affect the respiratory system and meningitis affects the nervous system.

The structure of bacteria

A bacterium has a cell-like structure (see Figure 14).

Cell wall

Cell membrane

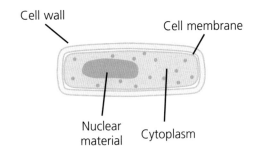

Nuclear material

Cytoplasm

Figure 14 Bacteria structure

Bacteria have a rigid cell wall – to maintain their shape, and for protection. Outside the cell wall of some bacteria is a slimy layer or capsule. Capsules protect the bacteria, too, but they also allow them to attach to things. Some bacteria exist as single cells, some exist in pairs, some in chains and some in clumps. The shape of the cells may differ – some bacteria are rod-shaped, and some circular, whilst others are shaped like spirals or commas (see Figure 15).

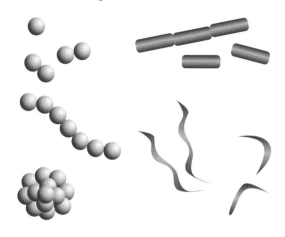

You can see that *Staphylococcus aureus* (which causes boils and food poisoning) is circular-shaped, and the circles are arranged in clumps. On the other hand, *Salmonella typhus* (which causes typhoid fever) exists as a single rod.

Bacteria are capable of living and reproducing on their own. Unlike viruses, they do not need to reproduce inside other living cells. So why do bacteria make us feel ill? Many of them produce 'toxins' (poisonous substances) that cause damage to our tissues, such as the lining of our throat.

Fungal diseases

Fungal diseases are not usually serious, but they can be a nuisance and take a long time to get rid of. A common fungal disease is ringworm, caused by a

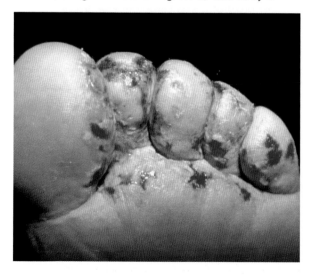

fungus called *Tinea*. You may have heard of the form of ringworm called 'Athlete's foot'. Athlete's foot usually affects the skin in between our toes. A mild form of the infection will make the skin itchy and a bit scaly. Fortunately, not many cases look like the one in the photo.

Ringworm may also be found on other parts of the body, such as the scalp (the area under the hair on the head) but it can also affect other skin areas.

Another fungal disease you may have heard of is thrush (candidiasis). Thrush can affect the mouth or the vagina. It is caused by a form of yeast called *Candida albicans* (not to be confused with the form of yeast used in bread-making or beer-making.)

The structure of fungi

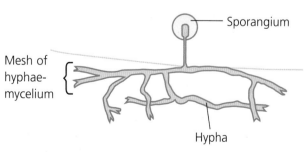

Mesh of hyphae-mycelium

Sporangium

Hypha

Most fungi have a thread-like structure (see Figure 16), although yeast consists of a single cell. The threads (hyphae) contain many cells that feed on the surface of our skin. There are reproductive parts (spores) sticking up from the hyphae that can be passed on to other people – via wet floors and puddles around swimming pools, for example. This is why most modern swimming pools make sure that people walk though an antiseptic footbath on their way to and from the pool. This helps reduce the spread of Athlete's foot.

Protozoan diseases

A protozoon is a single-celled organism. The most well-known disease caused by protozoa is malaria. Most people wrongly believe that malaria is *caused* by mosquitoes. This is wrong. A protozoon called *Plasmodium* causes the disease, but it is passed on from one person to another by mosquitoes. Malaria is probably the most common infectious disease in the world today, although there are not many cases in the UK. Sleeping sickness is another disease caused by a protozoon, *Trypanosoma*.

Transmission of diseases

We know that communicable diseases are caused by micro-organisms. So how do you catch a communicable disease? Have you ever been near someone who had a cold? Then a few days later, you also had a cold. You might say that you had not actually touched the person – in fact you had not even been near them.

Have you ever had food poisoning, or had an upset stomach? You might not have been near anyone else who had an upset stomach, yet you got one. In each case, the organism causing the disease got inside you. Think for a minute how that could happen.

Micro-organisms can infect a person in a number of ways:

- through the air
- in contaminated food
- in contaminated water
- by direct contact (including sexual contact)
- by **vectors**, such as insects.

Air-borne infection

There are many diseases that are transmitted through the air. Some of the common air-borne diseases are:

Viral diseases	Bacterial diseases
Cold	Pharyngitis (sore throat)
Influenza	Tuberculosis
Measles	Whooping cough

The micro-organisms pass through the air in tiny droplets of water, saliva or mucus, from the infected person to other people. If the infected person coughs or sneezes, this will speed up the transfer of these droplets.

Water-borne infection

Cholera and typhoid may be passed on by contaminated water. Remember John Snow and the outbreak of cholera in the nineteenth century. That was caused by contaminated water in a pump in the street. Fortunately, in this country nowadays, we have clean water that comes directly to our homes, and the incidence of cholera is very rare. This is not the case, however, in all parts of the world.

Food-borne infection

Salmonella food poisoning is transmitted when the *Salmonella* bacteria in someone's faeces contaminate food eaten by another person. Other types of food poisoning, such as that caused by certain strains of *E. coli* bacteria, are passed on in a similar way. Think how this could so easily be avoided. If only everyone would wash their hands after going to the toilet.

Cholera and typhoid may also be passed on in food, if the food is washed in water contaminated with the organisms that cause these diseases.

Direct-contact infection

If someone has micro-organisms on their skin, and we touch their skin, then some of the micro-organisms will be passed on to us. You can see why washing hands is very important. The fungus *Tinea*, which causes Athlete's foot, may be passed on through sharing towels – or simply by walking on the same damp areas barefoot as someone who has the disease. Diseases like chickenpox may be passed on by direct contact. At a certain time during the course of the disease, the spots will be infectious.

Some diseases can be passed on during sexual intercourse, if there is no physical protection, such as a condom. Examples of such diseases are AIDS, syphilis and vaginal thrush.

Sheila recently started work in a butcher's shop. One of her tasks is to clean out the areas where the meat is on display at the end of the day. Part of the display area holds cooked meat and the other part holds raw meat. Sheila noticed that sometimes there was blood from the raw meat in the area where the cooked meat had been. She mentioned this to the owner, Richard, who was unconcerned and told her 'We've always kept meat this way and there has never been a problem'. One day Sheila heard that several of the people who had been to the shop had taken ill with sickness and diarrhoea. Sheila knew that all the people had bought cooked meat and she wondered if there had been contamination from the blood of the raw meat. After visits from the environmental health inspector, her suspicions were confirmed. Richard's shop was closed and he had to put in completely separate storage areas for cooked and uncooked meat before the shop was allowed to reopen.

Infection through vectors

A vector is a living organism that carries a disease-causing organism from one person to another. One of the best known examples is the mosquito, which carries the malaria-causing **protozoon**, *Plasmodium*. Think of how the spread of malaria could be reduced. It could be reduced by killing the *Plasmodium* or by killing the mosquito.

Other vectors include ordinary flies – the kind you frequently see landing on food. Think what they are doing there, and what would happen if they had previously landed on some food that was infected.

Does age matter?

Are people more likely to 'catch' a disease if they are old or young? Having read the section on how communicable diseases are transmitted, what do you think? Whether disease-causing organisms get to your body will depend on whether you come into contact with people who are infected. This will depend on your lifestyle. In theory, it should not make any difference how old you are.

However, whether the presence of the disease-causing organisms results in you actually having the disease is a different matter. It will depend on how well your body 'fights' against the disease-causing organisms. In other words, it will depend on how well your immune system works. We shall hear more about this later. What we can say is that the immune system of the very young and the very old is not usually as efficient as that of people in other life stages.

Check your understanding

1 List the main points that all communicable diseases have in common.

2 List the four main categories of communicable disease, and give an example of each category.

3 Describe two differences between the structure of viruses and bacteria.

4 List the five main ways that diseases are transmitted. and for each one name a disease that is transmitted in this way.

extension**activities**

1 Find out more about two viral and two bacterial diseases mentioned in this topic. In particular which part of the body is affected, and how. You might like to work with a partner and summarise your findings to present to the rest of the class.

2 Carry out a small survey on communicable diseases and their transmission. Ask ten people what communicable diseases they can remember having, and how they think they caught them. See how well their answers match up with the information given in the topic.

Non-communicable diseases

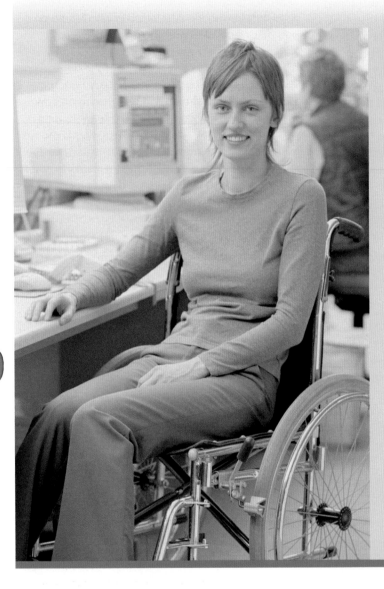

Getting you thinking

1 **What do you think might have caused the person in the picture to need the use of a wheelchair? Make a list of the different possibilities.**

2 **If the person had been older, do you think that the cause of them needing the use of a wheelchair might have been different? Explain your answer.**

KEY TERMS

Alzheimer's
A form of dementia.

Atheroma
Fatty plaques that form inside the lining of arteries.

Benign tumour
A discrete lump of cells that is harmless.

Coronary arteries
Blood vessels supplying the heart muscle with food and oxygen.

Dementia
A group of diseases where there is a progressive loss of brain function.

Malignant tumours
Lumps of cells that can travel around the body and grow in various organs, referred to as cancer.

Multiple sclerosis
A condition where the immune system attacks and destroys the nerves.

Myelin sheath
The insulating material that surrounds the nerves.
Osteoarthritis A degenerative disease affecting the cartilage of the joints, often occurring after injury.

Rheumatoid arthritis
A degenerative disease affecting the joints where the body's immune system attacks itself.

What do all non-communicable diseases have in common?

Non-communicable diseases cannot be 'caught' from someone else. They are not caused by micro-organisms and they are not transmitted from person to person in the conventional sense. They include a wide range of diseases such as degenerative diseases, deficiency diseases, inherited diseases and those associated with lifestyle or the environment. Different types of non-communicable diseases tend to affect us at particular life stages. Usually they require long-term support and treatment.

For your portfolio you need to compare a non-communicable disease with a communicable one. Communicable diseases were covered in Topic 3. In this topic you will be introduced to some non-communicable diseases. You will not be expected to learn everything about every non-communicable disease, but working through the topic will allow you to make an informed decision about which non-communicable disease you might choose to compare with the communicable disease you have chosen.

Before reading on, make a list of as many non-communicable diseases as you can. It might help to think of the four main categories:

- Degenerative diseases – ones that tend to get progressively worse

- Deficiency diseases – associated with something missing in the diet

- Inherited diseases – passed on from your parents

- Diseases associated with lifestyle or the environment.

Degenerative diseases

Degenerative diseases get progressively worse as time goes on. They tend to be associated mainly with later adulthood, although some may start much earlier in life. Can you think of an older person you know fairly well who has a condition that has got worse in the last few years? You may have thought about arthritis. Arthritis affects joints, and can make walking or movement difficult. You might know an older person who is increasingly becoming more and more confused. This person might have a form of dementia, such as Alzheimer's. You might know someone with multiple sclerosis. As well as affecting older people, multiple sclerosis can affect people in middle or young adulthood. Multiple sclerosis is a disease of the nervous system which may result in any movement

being difficult – with the person eventually unable to walk. Such diseases may be managed by drugs, and there are various types of support groups available.

Arthritis

Arthritis is a condition that affects our joints (see photo). There are different types of arthritis, the two most common being rheumatoid arthritis and osteoarthritis.

About 5 million people in the UK have **rheumatoid arthritis**. It usually starts around the age of 50, and three times as many woman are affected as men. It occurs when the body's immune system goes into action when there is no threat. In other words, the body starts attacking itself. Sometimes there is serious inflammation, known as 'flare up'. When this happens, the joints swell considerably, and the ligaments, holding the bones together, become stretched. It is important to seek treatment quickly because once joint damage has occurred, it can't be reversed.

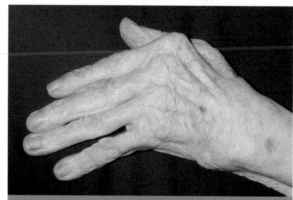

Arthritis can cause deformity of the joints, as in this person's hand.

About one million people in the UK have **osteoarthritis**, mostly in the hands, knees, hips and feet. It is more common in women over the age of 40, and in a joint where there has been an injury or operation. The smooth cartilage that takes the strain in a normal joint becomes rough, brittle and weak, and there is often inflammation (see Figure 18).

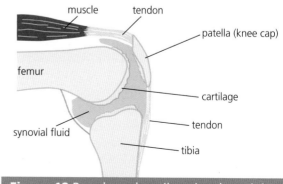

Figure 18 Roughened cartilage in a knee joint

To compensate for the impaired cartilage, the bone thickens and spreads out, forming knobbly outgrowths. The synovial membrane surrounding the joint thickens, and the fluid-filled space within it becomes smaller.

Alzheimer's disease

Alzheimer's disease is one of about a hundred different forms of **dementia**. Dementia is a term used to describe various types of brain disorders where there is a progressive loss of brain function. About 400,000 people in the UK have Alzheimer's. It affects about one in twenty people over the age of 65, and about one in five people over the age of 80. It is an illness that occurs in stages, with the person's ability to remember, communicate, understand and reason gradually declining.

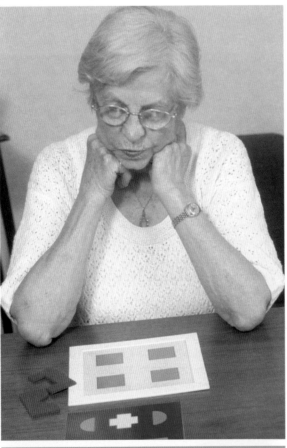

Alzheimer's disease affects thinking and memory skills.

In the early stages, there may only be minor changes in the person's abilities or behaviour. This means that diagnosis is not always easy – because there is usually a decline in memory and reasoning as people get older anyway. As Alzheimer's progresses, the changes become more marked. The person will need more support to manage their everyday lives.

Some people at this stage may become very frustrated or upset. In the later stages, the person with Alzheimer's will gradually become totally dependent on others for nursing care.

Multiple sclerosis

Multiple sclerosis is a condition that affects the central nervous system (the brain and spinal cord). Like rheumatoid arthritis, it is an 'autoimmune' disease, where the immune system starts to attack its own body. In particular, the insulating **myelin sheath** around the nerves starts to break down (see Figure 19). This myelin damage disrupts messages travelling along the nerve fibres. They can slow down, become distorted, pass from one nerve fibre to another (like wires short-circuiting), or not get through at all. As well as myelin loss, there can also be damage to the actual nerve fibres themselves. It is this nerve damage that causes the accumulation of disability that can occur over time.

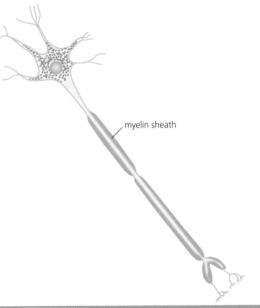

myelin sheath

Figure 19 A nerve, showing the myelin sheath

About 85, 000 people in the UK have multiple sclerosis. It is usually diagnosed between the ages of 20 and 40, and women are almost twice as likely to develop it as men. It is incurable at present, but treatments can help the symptoms to be managed.

Other degenerative diseases

Parkinson's disease was first described in 1817 by James Parkinson. It used to be known as the 'Shaking Palsy'. This is a very apt description of the characteristics of the condition – tremor, stiffness, or clumsiness, usually involving one side. The person can often have a blank, mask-like facial expression and may walk with a shuffling gait. The condition is caused by cell degeneration and the loss of some neurones in the midbrain. About 1–2% of people over the age of 50 are affected, although it can also occur in younger people.

Cataracts are the most common cause of blindness in the world today. The term cataract is used to describe any reduction in the clarity of the lens of the eye. This can mean anything from mild cloudiness to complete opacification. Most people over 50 have some haziness over the lens, but the situation only becomes a problem if the person's sight is being affected. The only method of treatment is to have the cataract removed surgically. This is a relatively minor procedure that can be done at a day clinic, using a local anaesthetic.

Deficiency diseases

One of the most famous examples of a deficiency disease is scurvy, which was common amongst sailors in the sixteenth century. They spent many months at sea at any one time, without any fresh fruit or vegetables. Scurvy resulted in gum disease and diseases of the skin. The disease was caused by a simple deficiency in the sailors' diet. What it lacked was Vitamin C – which we get mainly from fruit and vegetables. Fortunately, scurvy is very rare nowadays. Pellagra, however, a skin disease caused a lack of Vitamin B, is still found.

Today, deficiency diseases usually only occur in developing countries or the poorer developed countries. However, there is one deficiency disease that is relatively common all over the world – diabetes. There are two forms of diabetes, 'insulin-dependent diabetes' – caused by a lack of the hormone insulin, and 'non-insulin-dependent diabetes' – caused by the body's inability to use insulin. It is the first type, the insulin-dependent diabetes that may be classified as a deficiency disease.

Insulin-dependent diabetes

You may well know someone who has insulin-dependent diabetes. They will have regular injections of insulin to control the condition. This form of diabetes often starts in childhood or adolescence.

Pancreas releases insulin

Too much glucose detected by pancreas

Insulin changes excess glucose into glycogen which is stored in the liver

Normal concentration of glucose in the blood

Concentration of glucose in the blood returns to normal

Too little glucose detected by pancreas

Glucagon changes stored glycogen back into glucose

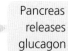

Pancreas releases glucagon

Figure 20 Regulation of diabetes

Two forms of diabetes

Babu is 50 years of age and overweight. Recently, he has been feeling very tired and very thirsty. He visited his doctor who tested his urine. This was found to contain glucose, a sign that he might have diabetes. Babu was referred to hospital for further tests. Blood tests revealed high levels of glucose, but normal levels of insulin. Babu was diagnosed with non-insulin-dependent diabetes. This means that his body produces insulin, but is unable to use it. He was advised to have small, regular meals to make sure his blood glucose did not fluctuate too much.

Babu has a son, Sunhil, who is 13. One day Sunhil collapsed and was taken to hospital. Tests found that he also had glucose in his urine and that his blood glucose was high. However, unlike his father, he was found to have very low levels of insulin in his blood. Sunhil was diagnosed with insulin-dependent diabetes and now has to have daily injections of insulin. Unlike his father, he can eat more or less the same as before.

If you have insulin-dependent diabetes it is important that the level of glucose in your blood is tightly controlled (fasting level around 4–7 mmol l^{-1}). If the value goes too high or too low, then you would go into a coma – and could die. You can see that if the level of blood glucose starts to rise, insulin is released and any excess glucose is joined together to form glycogen and stored in the liver. This would happen after you had eaten. What happens, then if the glucose level falls? You can see that another hormone, glucagon, breaks down the stored glycogen into glucose.

Insulin and glucagon are hormones that help maintain a near constant level of glucose in the blood. The maintenance of a constant level of blood glucose is an example of homeostasis (keeping things the same).

Inherited diseases

Inherited diseases are also known as genetic diseases, because the tendency to develop the disease is passed from parent to child in the genes. So when someone with a genetic disease has a child, that child may 'inherit' that possibility, and when they grow up, they may, in turn, pass it on to their children. As a result, these diseases tend to run in families.

About 20% of the UK population is affected by genetic diseases, including cystic fibrosis, haemophilia, phenylketonuria (PKU), Down syndrome and sickle-cell anaemia.

There is little anyone can do to affect the development of a genetic condition. However, the Human Genome Project is an international research programme to work out the DNA sequences of 50,000 –1,000, 000 genes in human chromosomes. The project aims to provide information for the possible treatment of genetic diseases. Already gene therapy has been developed for the treatment of cystic fibrosis.

Chromosomes, genes and DNA

Genetic diseases can be divided into two main groups – chromosome diseases and single gene diseases. But before we consider these two groups, we need to look at some cell biology.

There are chromosomes inside the nuclei of all our cells. We have 23 pairs of chromosomes, one set from our mother and one set from our father, making a total of 46. Each chromosome is composed of several genes, each one of which is coded for a particular characteristic, such as eye colour. DNA (deoxyribonucleic acid) is the chemical that makes up our genes and chromosomes. The relationship between chromosomes, genes and DNA is shown in Figure 21.

Figure 21 One pair of chromosomes

Each chromosome is made up of a molecule of DNA

This chromosome is from the male parent

This chromosome is from the female parent

A, B, C, etc. represent the position of genes for different features, such as eye colour

Chromosome diseases

Chromosome defects may involve changes in the chromosome number, the rearrangement of genes, or the duplication or loss of chromosome parts. Perhaps the best known chromosome defect condition is Down syndrome. This occurs when the individual is born with three chromosomes instead of the normal pair for one of the sets (chromosome 21). This triple chromosome condition is called 'trisomy', and it usually arises because chromosome 21 does not separate properly during the formation of the ovum. The ovum therefore has 24 chromosomes instead of the usual 23 (and the foetus would have a total of 47 instead of 46). The chance of this occurring increases as a woman gets older, which is why more Down syndrome babies are born to older mothers (see Figure 22).

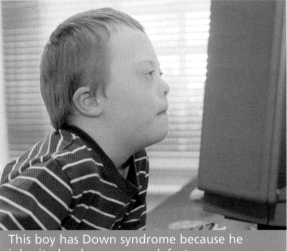

This boy has Down syndrome because he inherited a chromosome defect.

Figure 22 Age of mother and risk of trisomy of chromosome 21

Age of mother	Risk
20–29	1:1500
30–34	1:750
35–39	1:600
40–44	1:300
45+	1:60

Very few embryos with an abnormal number of chromosomes survive even until birth, apart from those with Down syndrome, and those involving the sex chromosomes. The absence of a sex chromosome or the presence of several sex chromosomes is less unusual and less life threatening (although in most cases it will cause fertility problems). The presence of the Y chromosome determines an embryo will be male, while its absence determines a female. For example, XY is normal male and XX normal female. If someone has only one X chromosome, (XO), this is known as Turner's syndrome and they will be female. An XXX female is known as a metafemale. If someone is XXY, they will have a condition known as Klinefelter's syndrome. They will be male because of the presence of the Y chromosome, but there may be some female characteristics.

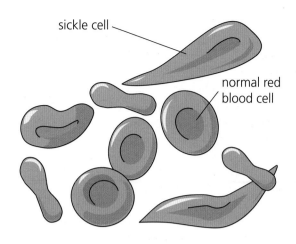

Figure 23 Blood cell shapes

people with cystic fibrosis producing abnormally large amounts of mucus from the lining of internal organs such as the lungs. This in turn leads to breathing problems and the inability to clear the airways of fluid, resulting in chest infections because micro-organisms get trapped in the lungs. Daily physiotherapy is needed to clear the lungs of mucus.

Down syndrome

Marie is 44 years of age and got married for the first time just two years ago. She and her husband were keen to start a family as soon as possible. As Marie said, 'I'm not going to get any younger, am I?' Marie became pregnant soon after the wedding. She was very excited, as this was to be her first child. Marie knew that there were risks in becoming a mother for the first time at her age, but she insisted that she did not want any tests during her pregnancy. 'If there is something wrong with the baby, I still want to have it' she would say to her doctor.

When Billy was born, it was clear he had Down syndrome. He had the characteristic wide-apart eyes and large tongue, yet Marie still declared 'He's beautiful!' Billy is not as quick as other babies to develop, but Marie and her husband are devoted parents and love him very much. Billy is a particularly affectionate baby and rewards his parents with a lovely smile.

Single gene disorders

Over 3000 single gene disorders have been identified, and around 1% of the population is affected. If a DNA sequence is altered in some way, then the resulting protein formed will be altered. This can have serious effects in some cases. For example, in sickle-cell anaemia, the protein haemoglobin which carries oxygen in the blood has a 'sickle' shape which in turn distorts the shape of the red blood cells. This means that they cannot pass easily along the capillaries.

In cystic fibrosis there is a change in one of the proteins on the cell membrane that regulates the transfer of chloride ions into cells. This results in

Diseases caused by lifestyle or by the environment

Diseases caused by lifestyle or the environment include cardiovascular diseases, respiratory diseases and cancers.

Cardiovascular diseases

We learned in Topic 2 that cardiovascular diseases have been the most common cause of death for the past 90 years in the UK. Cardiovascular disease include coronary heart disease and strokes. As we get older, fatty deposits called **atheroma** build up in the lining of our arteries. We cannot stop this happening, but we can control the rate at which it happens. Figure 24 (overleaf) shows the effect of the build-up of atheroma.

You can see that the space inside the artery (lumen) is reduced where there are atheroma present. You may also notice that the inner surface is rough. This may cause the body to think it is damaged and blood clots may form and block the flow of blood. If this happens in the coronary arteries supplying the heart muscle with blood, then a heart attack will occur, as the muscle cells cannot function without food and oxygen. If the blood flow is blocked to the brain or if a blood vessel bursts in part of the brain it will no longer have a supply of food and oxygen. Cells

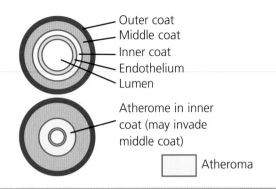

- Outer coat
- Middle coat
- Inner coat
- Endothelium
- Lumen

Atherome in inner coat (may invade middle coat)

☐ Atheroma

Figure 24 The effect of the build-up of atheroma

will then die and a stroke will occur. You may have noticed people who are paralysed down one side – this is likely to be the result of a stroke.

Respiratory diseases

Many respiratory diseases are associated with smoking, including lung cancer, emphysema and bronchitis. In emphysema, the walls of the alveoli (air sacs) of the lungs are broken down, so less surface area is available for the exchange of gases (see Figure 25). Think what the lack of oxygen getting into the body will mean.

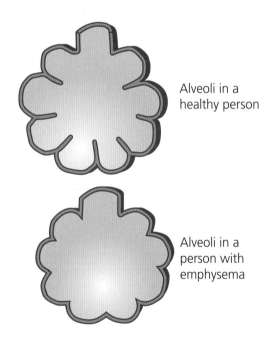

Alveoli in a healthy person

Alveoli in a person with emphysema

Figure 25 Emphysema and alveoli

A person is said to have chronic bronchitis if they have a cough where phlegm is coughed up, lasting for several months. Normally cilia in the bronchial tubes beat rhythmically to produce a constant upward flow of mucus from the bronchi to the back of the

throat where it is swallowed. The healthy mucus flow traps dust particles and micro-organisms so they do not reach the alveoli. Smoking stops these cilia from working properly so that the micro-organisms accumulate and cause infection. Smoking can also cause fibrous tissue to build up around the bronchioles, narrowing the air passages. Lung cancer usually develops in the lining of the bronchioles. It is often linked with emphysema and bronchitis. We shall learn more about cancers in the next section.

Smoking rates have declined across all age groups in the last 50 years, with the largest decrease amongst those aged 50 and over. Figure 26 shows that in 2002/03 people in their early twenties had the highest rates.

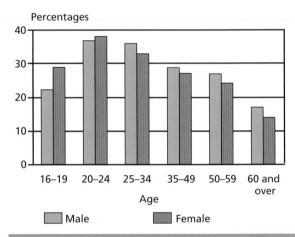

Percentages

Age

☐ Male ■ Female

Figure 26 Prevalence of cigarette smoking by age and sex in 2002/03 in the UK

Cancers

One in three people develop cancer during their lives. Figure 27 shows the number of people suffering from different cancers in 2002.

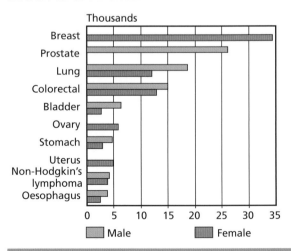

Thousands

Breast
Prostate
Lung
Colorectal
Bladder
Ovary
Stomach
Uterus
Non-Hodgkin's lymphoma
Oesophagus

☐ Male ■ Female

Figure 27 Incidence of the major cancers, by sex, in England in 2002

The four most common cancers – breast, lung, colorectal and prostate – accounted for just over half of the 223, 800 new cases of cancer. Cancer is predominantly a disease of the elderly – only 0.6 per cent of cases registered in 2002 were in children, and only 25 per cent were in people under the age of 60. Survival rates in England have improved for most cancers in both sexes over the last ten years.

Cancer is a range of diseases in which uncontrolled cell growth forms a **malignant tumour**. A tumour is a mass of cells which are undergoing repeated cell division, regardless of the body's need for new cells for growth and repair. (A **benign tumour** is one that forms a harmless lump. Most 'lumps' that are found in the body are benign tumours.) A malignant tumour is one whose cells are spread around the body by the blood and lymphatic systems to develop new tumours in other areas.

Check your understanding

1. List the features that non-communicable diseases have in common.

2. List three degenerative diseases. Choose one and describe why it is classed as degenerative.

3. Explain the difference between the two types of genetic diseases.

4. Explain how the build up of atheroma may lead to a heart attack.

5. Explain the difference between a benign tumour and a malignant one.

extension activities

1. Discuss the statement 'There are no cures for genetic diseases'.

2. Choose one communicable disease and one non-communicable disease. Summarise and compare the main points about the two diseases, under the following headings:
   - The effect that the disease has on the body
   - The possible ways the disease might have been contracted.

Getting you thinking

1 Can we always tell by looking at someone if they are ill?

2 How would we know the child shown in the picture is ill?

3 How can we find out exactly what is wrong with the child?

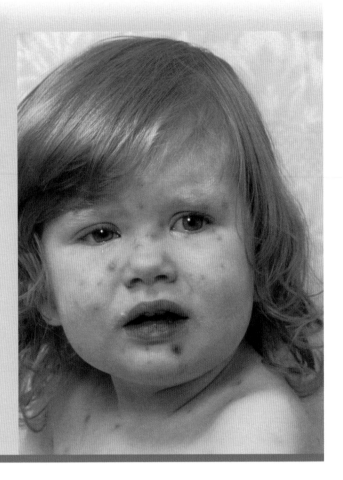

KEY TERMS

CAT scan
Computed axial tomography, a diagnostic technique which involves taking X-rays linked up to a computer.

Clinical features
Signs and symptoms of a disease.

Endoscope
A fibre-optic tube for seeing inside the body.

Monoclonal antibodies
'Magic bullets' designed to 'fight' disease-causing organisms within the body.

MRI scan
Magnetic resonance imaging, a diagnostic technique using magnetism which produces clear scans.

Non-invasive technique
Diagnosis or treatment method that does not involve piercing or cutting the body.

Nuclear imaging
Using a gamma camera and radionuclides to view abnormal function in the body, e.g. cancer cells.

PET scan
Positron emission tomography, a diagnostic technique similar to a CAT scan, useful for diagnosing brain tumours (but expensive).

Radionuclide
Low-level dose of a radioactive material.

Signs
Characteristics of a disease detectable by another person.

Symptoms
Characteristics of a disease felt by the person that have no visible physical manifestation.

Ultrasound
A diagnostic technique which uses high frequency sound to view soft tissues inside the body.

What does diagnosis mean?

The diagnosis of a disease is when it is formally identified. This identification is based on signs and symptoms, and may be backed up with laboratory tests and clinical investigations.

Signs and symptoms

If someone has a particular disease then they will show certain signs and symptoms. Think for a minute what this means. Someone with measles has characteristic spots and cannot stand bright light. Someone with arthritis in their hands will have painful joints and their hands may look deformed.

Signs are characteristics detectable by another person – such as a doctor. They include such things as the presence of a micro-organisms in the blood, a high temperature, swollen glands, or high blood pressure.

Symptoms are things which are felt by the patient which have no visible physical manifestation. They include headaches, pain, feeling tired or depressed.

Signs and symptoms are together known as the **clinical features** of a disease. Note that the term 'symptoms' is often used much more loosely, to include the signs as well.

Early diagnosis

The earlier a diagnosis is made, the more effective its treatment is likely to be. Early diagnosis is one of the main weapons we have against disease. It is particularly important in progressive diseases like cancer, where detection at an early stage can mean the difference between life and death. Screening programmes for cancer operate on this principle. (We shall discuss these later.)

Early diagnosis is also important in infectious diseases. For example, antibiotic treatment is very effective in stopping bacterial diseases from getting a strong hold on the body. Early detection of infectious diseases is important for other people, too, because their transmission could be reduced if infected people are quickly isolated.

A fairly new early diagnostic treatment is **monoclonal antibodies**. These 'magic bullets' can detect and even deliver drugs to specific foreign micro-organisms or diseased parts of the body.

General detection techniques

Faced with a patient complaining of a range of symptoms, a doctor's initial task is that of diagnosis. Diagnostic techniques often depend on being able to measure and monitor aspects of the patient's biochemistry, physiology and general internal state. **Non-invasive** methods, which avoid cutting or piercing the body in any way, are increasingly being used for diagnosis. The oldest of these methods is X-rays, but more and more procedures, involving ultrasound, radioisotopes and fibre optics, have appeared over recent years. Often the machinery to visualise what is going on internally can be linked to computers to enhance the quality of the picture or improve analysis of the data. Although many new instruments are costly, they may dramatically improve information and diagnosis.

Biochemical tests

Have you ever had to provide a urine sample or had a blood sample taken? If you have, then you will know that the sample is sent away for chemical analysis in a laboratory. There are many biochemical tests which can give valuable information about the internal state of the body. We shall look at some of the most common tests used.

One of the first signs of diabetes is the presence of sugar (glucose) in the urine. This is a simple test done at a local health practice with a clinistix – a strip of plastic impregnated with a chemical which indicates the presence of glucose. Try to get hold of some clinistix and test it on a solution of glucose. Your local pharmacy or health centre may be able to provide clinistix. There is also an automated method which gives a direct reading of glucose from either a urine sample or a blood sample.

Phenylketonuria, caused by the lack of a particular enzyme, may be detected by a build-up of an amino acid called phenylalanine in the blood. This is a relatively simple test that is carried out routinely at birth.

Biochemical methods are used to detect some micro-organisms. You may have had a throat swab taken for analysis. If bacteria were present in your sample they would have been detected by growing them on some nutrient agar (jelly).

Imaging techniques

X-rays

X-rays are used routinely for diagnosis in many branches of medicine. You may have had an X-ray yourself or know someone who has had one. But, have you ever wondered how X-rays work?

When a beam of X-rays passes through matter, such as body tissue, some of its energy is lost in the tissue, reducing the strength of the beam which reaches the 'plate' on the other side. The X-ray images recorded on the plate are, in effect, shadows of the objects placed in the beam. The X-ray image is clearest when there is the greatest difference in density of the materials. In the body, bones show up lightest, soft tissue not very well and air remains darkest of all. If the natural contrast produced in the tissue is not enough, it can be improved by introducing a contrast agent. For example, in investigations of the digestive system, which is all soft tissue, the patient is given a barium meal or a barium enema which places an X-ray-opaque barium compound in the tract. This shows up very clearly in the X-ray picture, particular if the rest of the digestive system is filled with air, which will stay dark (see Figure 28 below).

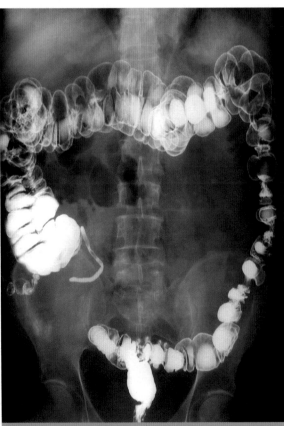

Figure 28 An X-ray of part of the digestive system of someone who has been given a barium meal

CAT scans

CAT stands for computed axial tomography. CAT scans involve an X-ray machine linked to a computer. The X-rays are used to take pictures at various levels of the body from many different angles, and the computer then analyses the data to give a series of cross-sectional pictures of, of example, the brain, spine or liver. The CAT scanner is a major improvement on conventional X-ray techniques because it allows soft body tissues as well as bones to be seen, enabling, for example, brain tumours to be identified.

Nuclear imaging

Nuclear medicine studies were first done in the 1950s using special 'gamma cameras'. The patient has a very low-level radioactive chemical called a **radionuclide** (radiotracer) introduced into the body. These radionuclides are absorbed temporarily by the specific part of the body to be studied. They emit faint gamma-ray signals which are measured by a gamma camera. An image of the part of the body is viewed on a computer screen.

Nuclear medicine imaging shows not only the structure of a part of the body, but its function as well. This information about its function can show if the organ is working properly. The amount of radiation that is taken up and then emitted by a specific part of the body is linked to how active the cells are. For example, cells which are dividing rapidly (like cancer tissue cells) may be seen as 'hot spots' of activity on a nuclear medicine image, since they absorb more of the radionuclide (see Figure 29 below).

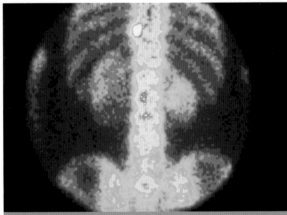

Figure 29 'Hot spots' on a nuclear medicine image

PET scanning

Positron emission tomography is a type of nuclear medicine scanning that involves taking pictures at various levels of the body from many different angles in the same way as CAT scans. It is particularly useful in diagnosing brain tumours, lung cancer and heart disorders. One of the disadvantages of PET is that it is very costly.

Magnetic resonance imaging

Magnetic resonance imaging (MRI) scans use magnetism to build up a picture of the inside of the body instead of X-rays. It is a much safer method, because radiation is not involved – and the pictures produced are very clear. MRI is used for viewing tumours in various parts of the body such as the brain, spinal cord and soft tissues. It is particularly good at showing how deeply tumours may have grown into body tissues.

Ultrasound

You will probably have heard of ultrasound scans in connection with pregnancy – they are used to show how well the foetus is developing. Ultrasound may also be used to diagnose problems with any soft tissue in the body, such as the heart, liver or kidneys. It can give information about how the organ works as well as it structure. For example, the flow of blood through the heart can be viewed, and problems such as a 'hole' in the heart diagnosed. Ultrasound is less costly than many of the other imaging techniques and offers a method of investigating inside the body without causing any damage.

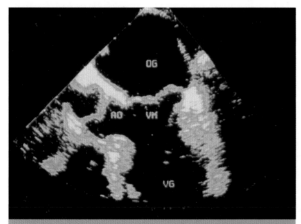

Figure 30 An ultrasound scan

Ultrasound works by emitting very high frequency sound waves into the body which bounce back, as a 'pulse echo', from the tissues they hit. The time lapse and intensity loss of the returning signals enables the nature and position of the organs and tissues to be calculated – and viewed on a computer screen. This technique is sometimes called **sonar** (sound navigation ranging). The principle was first developed in the Second World War to detect the echoes made by underwater objects – like submarines.

Fibre-optic endoscopy

You may have seen the principle of this method used in fibre-optic Christmas trees, where the central light source is transmitted through all the fibres to produce a tiny light at the end of each one. You can bend the fibre in any direction, but the light will always be there. An **endoscope** works on the same principle to see inside the body. It is a tube consisting of tiny light fibres inserted into the body through an orifice. Someone having this procedure may be seen in Figure 31.

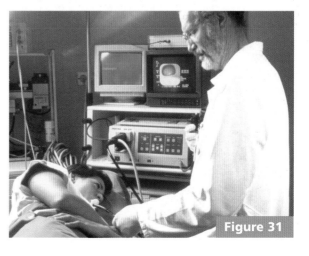

Figure 31

The viewing end of the endoscope contains the controls, an adjustable eyepiece and a connection to the light source and camera. A camera can be attached to the eyepiece of the image so that photographs may be taken. The images may also be displayed on a large screen. An endoscope is particularly useful for diagnosing problems of the digestive system. The information obtained may provide very clear evidence of, for example, bleeding ulcers, constrictions and tumours. Sometimes a small piece of tissue is taken (a biopsy) using the endoscope, for further examination of cells under the microscope. An example of this might be to check for cancer cells.

Tests for genetic conditions

Many genetic techniques are associated with pre-natal diagnosis of genetic conditions, such as Down's syndrome or cystic fibrosis. There are two main tests used – amniocentesis and chorionic villus sampling.

Amniocentesis

Amniocentesis involves sampling the amniotic fluid by inserting a long, thin, hollow needle through the wall of the abdomen into the uterus. A local anaesthetic is applied and it is usually accompanied by an ultrasound scan to confirm the position of the foetus so that it is not harmed. The amniotic fluid contains cells cast off from the amnion membrane surrounding the baby and from the baby's skin, and respiratory and digestive tracts. The cells are then cultured and their chromosomes examined.

Major chromosomal abnormalities, such as Down's syndrome, where the foetus shows 47 chromosomes instead of the normal 46, can be detected. The woman may then be offered an abortion. The amniotic fluid is also tested chemically for alpha-fetoprotein (AFP). A higher than normal level of this protein indicates spina bifida or other neural tube defects. Foetal cells can also be tested for the products of many other genetic diseases. Of the 600 genetic diseases now know, about one third can be detected in this way.

Amniocentesis is not offered to everyone, because there is a small chance of it causing miscarriage (0.5–1.0% risk). It is usually offered to older women since they have a higher risk of having a baby with Down's syndrome (see Topic 4).

Chorionic villus sampling

Chorionic villus sampling is an alternative to amniocentesis. It involves taking a small sample of the embryonic tissue from the chorion (developing placenta). The chorion has numerous projections called villi which contain many dividing cells. When cells are dividing, their chromosomes are visible,

so results of any chromosome abnormalities are known within a few days. It has the advantage of being able to be performed earlier than amniocentesis, as early as six weeks. However, it is a specialised technique and carries a slightly higher risk of causing miscarriage than amniocentesis.

Screening programmes

Screening programmes – designed to make early diagnoses of certain diseases – are becoming widely established in the UK. An example is screening for cervical cancer. About ten years ago, official statistics revealed an alarming increase in the number of deaths from the disease, with about 2,000 deaths per year. If detected early by a 'cervical smear' – a well-established screening technique in which a few cells scraped from the cervix are examined under the microscope – a complete cure can usually be effected very quickly.

There are now screening techniques for breast cancer. Breast cancer occurs in about 1 in 20 women. If diagnosed early, prospects for cure are good. If untreated, the disease is fatal. X-ray screening (mammography) is used for the early detection of lumps. If a lump is detected in this way, then ultrasound may be carried out to find out the nature of the lump. Sometimes some cells from the lump are taken for a biopsy.

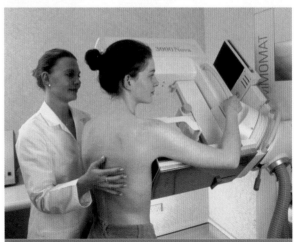

Figure 32 An example of a mammogram screening procedure

Screening for breast cancer – do we want to know?

Brenda is 53 years of age. She has received a letter inviting her to go for a mammogram in two weeks time. Brenda is apprehensive and does not want to keep the appointment. She tells her friend, Ruth, 'What if I find out I have cancer?' Ruth persuades Brenda to go and says the chances of finding any lump are not high. Even if a lump is found, it is unlikely that it will be cancerous. Brenda decides to have the mammogram. She finds the staff at the hospital very kind and sympathetic, and she met one of her neighbours there in the waiting area. They decided they had been called at the same time because they they their surnames both began with the letter 'T'. Brenda did not like the procedure very much. She tells Ruth it hurt a little having each breast squashed between two 'plates' to have the 'picture' taken.

Two weeks later Brenda received a letter from the hospital. She opened it very nervously, but was pleased to read that the mammogram was all clear and there was no sign of any abnormality. She told Ruth that she was glad she had kept the appointment and it was good to know that everything was OK.

Check your understanding

1. **Explain the difference between a sign and a symptom of a disease.**

2. **Explain the importance of the early diagnosis of a disease.**

3. **List the different imaging techniques, and for each one give a specific use.**

4. **Explain the difference between amniocentesis and chorionic villus sampling, giving an advantage and a disadvantage of each technique.**

extension activities

1. Choose two different diseases, one communicable and one non-communicable, and compare the different diagnostic techniques that could be used to detect each of them.

2. Choose an imaging technique. Research in as much detail as you can how the technique works. Present your findings to the rest of the class.

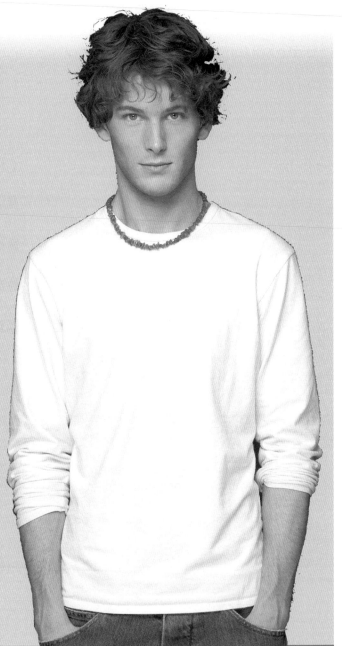

Getting you thinking

1 Who would treat this teenager if he had a headache, and where would he get the treatment from?

2 Who would remove stitches from a cut finger, and where is this likely to be done?

3 If this teenager needed an operation for a burst appendix, who would normally do this, and where?

KEY TERMS

Consultant
A care worker who specialises in a particular condition or disease or part of the body.

Informal carer
Someone (usually a relative, friend or neighbour) who looks after someone without payment.

Medication
Tablets or other forms of drugs given to aid recovery.

Ophthalmic
Relating to the eye and its diseases.

Prescription
An authorisation to obtain drugs, given by a GP.

Primary Health Care
Care provided by a care worker such as a GP, usually the first person to help a client.

Rheumatism
Painful muscles and joints.

What does treating a disease mean?

If we are ill, our first thought is usually, 'I feel bad'. Our second thought is, probably, 'What will make me better?' Once a diagnosis has been made, then steps can be taken to 'treat' a disease.

The Oxford dictionary defines 'treating' as 'dealing with'. So treating a disease means dealing with it. This can be done by a variety of approaches. We may take medicine, we may change our behaviour – or we may do both. Let's think of an example here. If you have influenza, you may take paracetamol to reduce any pain you have, and to reduce your temperature. You may also go to bed because you feel so tired and ache all over.

Some diseases may require that the individual needs additional support. That support may be practical or it may be emotional. We shall learn more about this shortly.

Who treats diseases and where are they treated?

Diseases may be treated by various people. Like diagnoses, treatment of diseases may be undertaken:

- by the individual themselves
- in a local health practice
- in a local hospital
- in a specialist national centre.

Treatment by the individual themselves

Throughout the ages, people have sought solutions and answers to medical problems through self-medication – that is, through treating themselves. Most self-treatment involves using over-the-counter medication. People choose self-treatment for many reasons, including:

- thinking that their condition is not serious enough to go to their GP about
- not wanting to bother anyone
- not having enough time to visit their GP
- to avoid contact with health care professionals
- a lack of satisfaction in or trust for the medical profession
- anxiety about what the GP may tell them
- fear of intimidation by the health care profession.

Think back to the last time you treated yourself when you were ill. Was it because of one of the reasons above?

Treatment at a local health practice

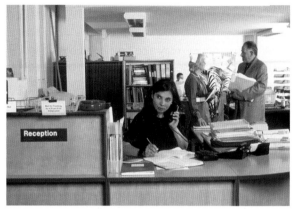

A local health practice is part of primary health care, and includes the basic, usually non-emergency, types of health care. Primary care services are delivered by a number of health care staff, working together as a team. A General Practitioner (family doctor) is often the leader or co-ordinator of the team. Other team members include practice nurses, district nurses, community psychiatric nurses and health visitors.

Some people need to use primary health care services regularly because they have a health problem or disability that requires continuing treatment or monitoring. An example would be someone with high blood pressure – can you think of others?

GPs may treat diseases by prescribing medicines (see Figure 33).

Rank	Generic drug name	What prescribed for
1	Acetaminophen; hydrocodone	Pain
2	Atorvastatin	High cholesterol
3	Levothyroxine	Thyroid problems
4	Atenolol	High blood pressure
5	Amoxicillin (antibiotic)	Bacterial infections
6	Lisinopril	High blood pressure
7	Hydrochlorothiazide	High blood pressure
8	Furosemide oral	High blood pressure
9	Albuterol aerosol	Asthma
10	Alprazolam	Anxiety disorder

Figure 33 *The top ten drugs prescribed in 2003 (by amount) and what they were prescribed for*

Take a moment to write down some observations about what the medicines were prescribed for. You might have noticed that pain was top of the list. You might also have noticed that four out of the drugs in the top ten were prescribed for high blood pressure. You might also have noticed that one of the drugs prescribed was for a mental disorder or that only one of the drugs was prescribed for a communicable disease.

Minor procedures may also be carried out at a local health practice. These will be carried out by the GP or the practice nurse. They include the removal of small cysts or fibrous lumps, or the removal of stitches. Can you think of any others?

Treatment at a local hospital

Treatment in a hospital, both local and specialist, is known as secondary care. This is because it is usually the second group of people who will see you. (Remember that the primary care is usually provided by your GP at your local health practice.)

People will be treated at a local hospital if their GP thinks that they need to see a consultant (a specialist in a particular area). This may involve attending an Outpatients Department where they receive treatment that does not involve a stay in hospital. They may require an operation or treatment that requires that they stay in hospital for a period of time. If someone has an accident that is fairly serious, they may also be treated at the hospital's Accident and Emergency Department. Can you think of when this might be? It could be after a road accident or if someone has had a heart attack. If a person's condition is very serious, they have be kept in an Intensive Care ward, where their condition will be very closely monitored (see below).

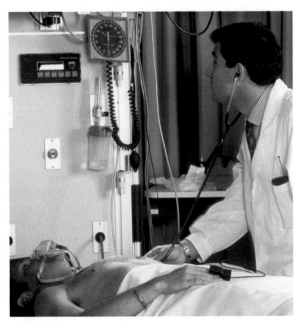

If you visit a hospital for treatment or an investigation, whether it be as an outpatient or for a longer stay, you will be looked after in a specific department (see table). The department usually depends on which part of the body you are having a problem with. You may well have noticed signs for different departments in a hospital (see Figure 34 below).

Figure 34 *Some of the different departments in a hospital and an example of what is treated in them*	
Department	**Example of what is treated**
Oral surgery	Removal of a wisdom tooth
Cardiology	Severe chest pains
Oncology	Cancer
Ophthalmology	Cataract
Radiology	Treatment for cancer
Podiatry	Ingrown toenails
Urology	Bladder infection
Orthopaedics	A broken leg
Ear, nose and throat	Deafness
Dermatology	Psoriasis
Rheumatology	Arthritis
Counselling	Bereavement
Psychology	Agoraphobia
Psychiatry	Mental illness
Gerontology	Senile dementia

Treatment at a specialist national centre

Specialist treatment and care often exists at many large hospitals. We have seen that hospitals can have many different departments. However, there are also some hospitals known as specialist national centres. Here particular diseases will be treated, and people may well come from a wide area. Perhaps you know of such a hospital in your area.

If you needed specialist care for heart disease in the North West of England, for example, you might be sent to the Cardiothoracic Centre in Liverpool. If you needed specialist eye care in the North East of England, you might be sent to the Yorkshire Eye Hospital in Bradford. Great Ormond Street Hospital for Sick Children and The Royal Homeopathic Hospital, both in London, are also specialist national centres.

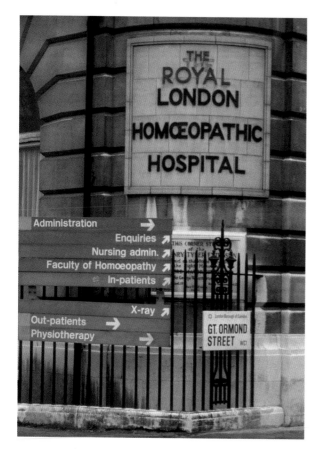

Facilities to support individuals with a disease

Once someone has had a disease diagnosed and treatment has begun, what happens then? Do they just wait to get better or are there other means of support? Imagine a child diagnosed with an eating disorder, or an older person who has just been diagnosed with Alzheimer's. Treatment has begun, but there are also other facilities providing support for the patient and their carers:

- Charities and support groups
- Clinics
- Domestic care.

Charities and support groups

Charities and support groups are organisations that are part of the voluntary care sector. Such organisations are not controlled by the government and do not have a legal duty to provide care. They provide care voluntarily, without making a profit. Examples include:

- British Heart Foundation
- Diabetes UK
- Epilepsy Research Foundation

- Institute of Cancer Research
- Multiple Sclerosis Society of Great Britain
- Muscular Dystrophy Association
- British Polio Trust
- Eating Disorders Association
- Alzheimer's Society
- Arthritis Research Campaign
- National Meningitis Trust
- MENCAP
- Stroke Association.

How can these organisations help people who have a particular disease? Think of a middle-aged woman living on her own, who has recently been diagnosed with Multiple Sclerosis. She is very frightened and wonders how she will cope in the future. The Multiple Sclerosis Society will be able to offer her advice and support. Their website offers many options (see below).

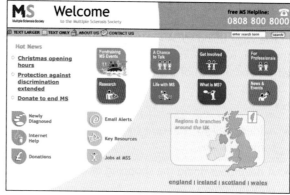

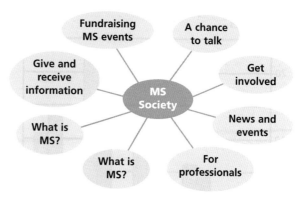

Clinics

There are clinics, often part of a local health practice, where people are treated for specific conditions. Usually, a particular clinic is held on a particular day of the week – blood pressure clinic on a Monday morning, for example, diabetes clinic on a Wednesday afternoon or asthma clinic on a Friday morning. As well as treatment, the clinic offers advice and support.

Topic 7 | Disease-prevention strategies

Getting you thinking

1 Look at the picture. Does it persuade you that smoking is unhealthy?

2 Why do some people continue to smoke after seeing pictures like this?

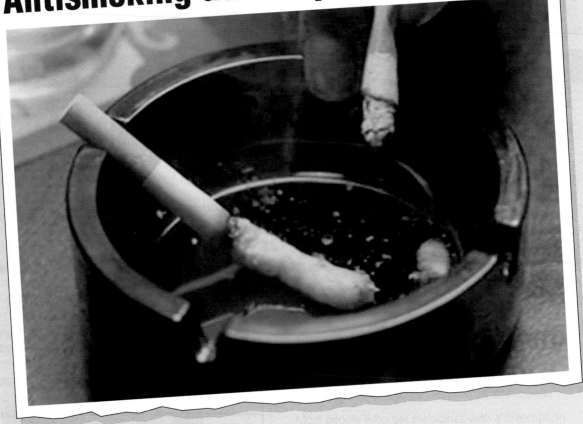

Antismoking ads help 1 million quit

KEY TERMS

Antibody
Protein formed by B lymphocytes, a type of white blood cell, in response to the presence of an antigen (on a disease-causing organism).

Antigen
Protein on the surface of a disease-causing organism that triggers the formation of antibodies.

Immune system
A system consisting of the lymphocytes (B lymphocytes and T lymphocytes) which produce a response to disease-causing organisms entering the body .

Lymphocyte
A type of white blood cell involved in the immune response (B lymphocyte and T lymphocyte).

Memory cells
A specific type of B lymphocyte that remains in the blood after the disease-causing organism has been destroyed, ready to make antibodies quickly, should the same organism enter the body again.

Pathogen
Disease-causing organism.

An overview of disease-prevention strategies

Prevention is better than cure. Rather than wait till we are ill, and then try to find a cure, it is much better to take steps to avoid getting ill in the first place –if we can. We shall see that there are many disease-prevention strategies. A very simple one is to encourage people to use handkerchiefs when they sneeze, especially if they have a cold or influenza.

Disease-prevention strategies may be at different levels. They may be:

- National strategies

- Local strategies

- Personal lifestyle choices.

Disease-prevention strategies will also depend on whether the diseases are communicable or non-communicable. Before we consider the different levels of disease-prevention strategies, we shall have a look at the way in which the body can protect itself.

Natural defences against infection

The body's natural defences are in two categories – non-specific defence mechanisms and the immune system.

The body has many non-specific defences against communicable diseases. An infection only occurs if an infecting micro-organism gets past the body's defences – or if the defences break down. The non-specific defence mechanisms of the body include:

- Harmless bacteria that live in or on the body competing with harmful micro-organisms for available nutrients.

- The skin, which offers a protective covering and is constantly being replaced

- The epithelial tissue, which lines tissues such as the respiratory passages (see Figure 36).

- Lysozyme, an enzyme present in tears and saliva, which kills bacteria.

- Blood clotting by platelets, when we cut ourselves.

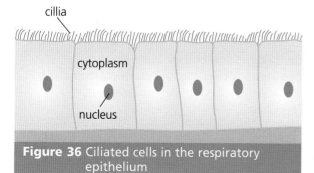

cillia

cytoplasm

nucleus

Figure 36 Ciliated cells in the respiratory epithelium

The immune system

Sometimes disease-causing organisms (pathogens) get past the body's natural defences listed above. What that happens, our immune system comes into action. The immune system provides a series of defensive responses to an invading pathogen. The body has two main types of white blood cell – phagocytes and lymphocytes. Phagocytes engulf foreign material such as pathogens. Lymphocytes, made in our lymph glands, provide a more directed attack.

Once inside the body, a pathogen is recognised as foreign material because of its **antigens** – specific proteins on its outer surface. These antigens are recognised by lymphocytes, some of which (the T cells) attach themselves to the antigens and destroy them. Phagocytes may then engulf and destroy the pathogen. Another type of lymphocyte (the B cells) multiply to produce large numbers of clones which release **antibodies**. These are proteins specific to a particular antigen, which bind it and destroy it.

Once the immune system has been activated, it usually destroys all of the pathogens that have entered the body. **Memory cells** – B cells specific to that particular pathogen – are then quickly produced, for a very important purpose. If the same pathogen gets into the body a second time, then the memory cells can help to make the appropriate antibodies immediately. This will ensure that the pathogens are destroyed long before they can cause the disease. This process, involving memory cells, explains why there are many diseases, such as measles, that we cannot catch twice.

But just think for a minute. Wouldn't it be wonderful if our bodies could have these memory cells without having to have the disease first. Well, they can – if we have a vaccination against the disease. We shall see that this is one the main national disease-prevention strategies.

National strategies

National strategies are broad plans that identify and explain the significance of public health issues. Many public health issues, such as the transmission of infectious diseases, are a *global* concern – BSE ('mad cow disease'), for instance and epidemics such as SARS or 'bird flu'. The National Health Service increasingly plays a role in preventative strategies. Examples of national strategies are:

- The NHS immunisation schedule

- The National Heart Forum's goals for prevention

- The government's anti-smoking campaigns.

Immunisation

Immunisation is artificial protection against infectious diseases. Most immunisation involves having a vaccination. A harmless part of a disease-causing organism is injected into the body, so that the body will make antibodies against it.

Figure 37 shows the NHS immunisation schedule. Notice that many different vaccinations may be given in one injection. Notice, too that it may require more than one injection for the person to be fully protected. This is because some of the memory cells may die and need replacing to be fully effective.

Figure 37 The NHS immunisation schedule

When to immunise	What is given	How it is given
2, 3 and 4 months old	Diphtheria, tetanus, pertussis (whooping cough), polio and Hib (DTaP/IPV/Hib)	One injection
	MenC	One injection
Around 13 months old	Measles, mumps and rubella (MMR)	One injection
3 years and 4 months to 5 years old	Diphtheria, tetanus, pertussis (whooping cough) and polio (dTaP/IPV or DTaP/IPV)	One injection
	Measles, mumps and rubella (MMR)	One injection
13 to 18 years old	Diphtheria, tetanus, polio (Td/IPV)	One injection

Goals against heart disease

The National Heart Forum (NHF) has helped to shape the public health policy agenda for about twenty-five years. It has argued for a strong policy focus on coronary heart disease prevention. As part of this process, the NHF contributed to the public consultation on the government public health strategy, *Saving Lives: Our Healthier Nation*. In 1999 the NHF released a major report reviewing the evidence on trends and prevention and setting out a prevention agenda for the twenty-first century, called 'Looking to the future: making coronary heart disease an epidemic of the past'. The NHF's seven policy goals are shown in Figure 38.

Note that the three established risk factors are poor diet, smoking and physical inactivity. These risk factors are also risk factors for strokes, diabetes and many forms of cancer. You can see why it is particularly important that there should be strategies for addressing these conditions, and that these strategies should be long term.

Figure 38 *NHF National Health Forum policy goals for the prevention of heart disease*

- A national coordinated and sustained strategy is needed to increase fruit and vegetable consumption to help people achieve the goal of at least five portions of fruit and vegetables a day.

- Schools and local authorities should support a whole-school approach to food, which promotes consistent healthy eating messages in the school dining room, in tuck shops and vending machines and in the classroom.

- Nutritional standards for school meals should be carefully monitored to ensure that meals meet established quantified nutritional recommendations and the standards should be strengthened as necessary.

- Emphasis should be placed on school nutrition education programmes including practical food skills for all children such as cooking and meal planning.

- In addition to the Department of Health, the Food Standards Agency should contribute to the formulation of a national nutrition policy, as well as dealing with food safety issues.

- Neighbourhood renewal strategies should: combat food deserts by attracting local shops into deprived areas through planning and business incentives; and promote healthy eating by encouraging discount schemes for the purchase of fruit and vegetables.

- Government should work with the food industry to make healthy changes to processed and pre-prepared foods by reducing levels of fat, sugar and salt.

The government's 'shock' anti-smoking campaign

The picture at the beginning of this topic shows one of the 'shock' pictures designed to put people off smoking. This campaign was created by advertising agencies, and it beat its targets. Other adverts showed children breathing out cigarette smoke to emphasise the effects of passive smoking. A study of the 'shock' advertising campaign claims that it has become so effective that it is now more powerful than GPs in persuading smokers to kick their habit. The study showed that this campaign prompted 32% of recent attempts to kick the habit, while GPs were responsible for 21%.

There have been many other government campaigns. Some of these were run by the Department of Health, others by a coalition of the NHS, Cancer Research and the British Heart Foundation.

Local strategies

What do we mean by a local strategy to reduce the risk of developing a disease? A local strategy is one organised by the local health authority or a local health practice or surgery. Local strategies include:

- Health information booklets.
- Well-women and well-men clinics.
- Exercise classes.

Health information booklets

Where would you go to get information on health? Many medical practices have leaflets available. You may have noticed that people sometimes pick them up and read them while they are waiting to see a GP or a nurse.

Camden and Islington have a Health Promotion Resources Service, where they give information about leaflets, posters and websites about difference aspects of health. The leaflets and posters may be ordered from the NHS website or there is a list at local GP practices and health centres.

Some medical practices have websites where there is information available or links to where people can get more information. The Goodwood Medical Centre in Hove has such a website (see extracts below).

> ### Stress see also The Complementary Therapy Centre
>
> Stress is thought to be responsible for a wide range of ailments ranging from migraine to heart attacks. Sometimes stress is caused by factors outside of your control but often it is not. To help reduce stress try taking regular breaks, doing more exercise, sleeping a full 8 hours (but no more), cutting down your intake of alcohol, cigarettes and coffee. Yoga and Meditation are also good stress relievers.

Well-women and well-men clinics

If your family owns a car that is over three years old, it will need an MOT. This is a series of relatively simple checks to make sure that the car is roadworthy. In a similar way, well-women and well-men clinics give people the opportunity to have simple checks taken, such as measurements of weight and blood pressure. Urine and blood samples are usually taken. This means checks are carried out for diabetes and high cholesterol. Women may be shown how to check for lumps in their breasts and men may be shown how to check for lumps in their testicles. Both these may be early indicators of cancer – although not every lump means cancer.

In most health practices, everyone is invited to attend such clinics, but it is up to the individual to decide whether they wish to attend or not. We shall see later that not everyone wishes to go.

Exercise classes

We shall see in the next section that exercise is important for a healthy lifestyle. Some people prefer to exercise with others, and taking part in organised classes increases their social well-being, as well. There are many different types of exercise classes available, yoga and step aerobics being two of the most popular ones.

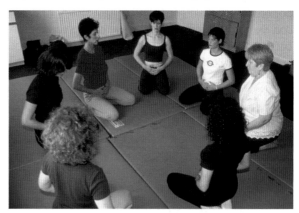

> ### Weight
> Weigh yourself – preferably without clothes ... Look at our Height Weight Chart to find out if you are in the correct weight range for your height.
>
> - If you are in the correct weight range, then try and maintain this by regular exercise and sensible eating of a mixed diet with vegetables, fruit and protein.
> - If you are underweight, then you can afford to eat a little more as there are other risks associated with insufficient body mass.
> - If you are overweight ... and this applies to the majority of people in the UK ... you should think about what you can do to lose some weight and
>
> become healthier in the process. This will mean increasing your exercise as well as decreasing the total amount of food that you eat. It is wise to avoid diets which work to produce a rapid weight loss as these do little to educate you into long-term healthy eating habits. Excessive weight puts a strain on your heart and causes a rise in your blood pressure and strain on the heart ... which leads to heart disease, heart attack and stroke.
>
> Come and talk to your doctor or nurse about how best you can lose weight, or for specialist advice make an appointment with our Nutritional Consultant.

Extracts taken from the 'Information Service' page on the *Goodwood Medical Centre* website

Getting you thinking

1 Why do you think young people drink too much alcohol?

2 Do you think that a paramedic might be able to change the behaviour of these young people?

3 What other factors might make young people drink less alcohol?

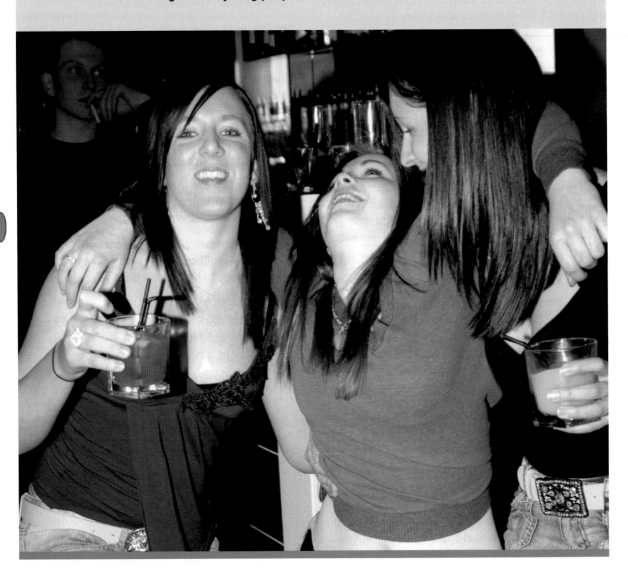

KEY TERMS

Compliance
The extent to which a patient's behaviour coincides with the medical or health advice given.

Concordance
Agreement between patient and doctor.

Why can't all diseases be prevented?

We learned, in Topic 7, about the large numbers of disease-prevention strategies that are being used. So why are there still high levels of disease today? You would think that, with a comprehensive immunisation programme, most infectious diseases would now be a thing of the past. This is not true – and we shall see why. You would also think that, with all the national and local strategies that are employed to reduce the risk of developing diseases, we should see significant decreases. That is sometimes the case, but not always.

There are many factors which interfere with the prevention of disease, and with the control of it spreading. These include:

- Public perception of risk

- Patient–doctor concordance

- Patient compliance

- Antibiotic resistance

- Funding available.

Public perception of risk

In Topic 7 we learned about risk behaviour, such as smoking, taking drugs and unsafe sex practice. Why do people put themselves at risk by continuing to practise these unhealthy behaviours?

Janine smokes twenty cigarettes a day. She says, 'I'll be OK. My grandfather is 90 years old and he has always smoked more cigarettes a day than I do. I'm more likely to die from crossing the road, than from smoking.' One of the reasons Janine continues to justify her smoking is because she has an inaccurate perception of risk and susceptibility.

Many people have an unrealistic optimism when it comes to their chances of contracting a serious illness, compared to other people the same age as them. They think that it will never happen to them. You could test this by asking people you know. Why are most people unrealistically optimistic? Factors that contribute to this include:

- Lack of personal experience of the problem.

- The belief that the problem is preventable by individual action.

- The belief that if the problem has not yet appeared, it will not appear in the future.

- The belief that the problem does not occur very often.

These factors suggest that our perception of own risk is not always a rational process.

The media can affect our perception of risk. We are made aware of health risks in the news and in documentaries. Examples include serious outbreaks of food poisoning or legionnaire's disease. We are also made aware of health risks in TV dramas, such as *Casualty* and *Holby City*. Being aware of health risks may make us more careful in our behaviour. However, over-dramatisation of health risks may scare us so much that we don't even want to think about them.

Charities such as the Imperial Cancer Research Fund and Health Watch also heighten our awareness of risk. Again, people's perceptions of risk will differ. Some people will take the advice to examine for lumps in the breast as reducing the risk of dying from cancer, whilst others may prefer not to know if there is a problem. An article on breast screening, published by Health Watch says, 'As for cancer, if the result of a smear or mammogram is doubtful (as is quite common) intense anxiety may be caused. Further tests will need to be done and distressing doubt may continue for weeks or even months.' The article also says, ' Many of those given a complete medical check up will now be labelled as unhealthy in some way. If no cure is available this may sometimes adversely affect the peace of mind and quality of life of people who previously thought of themselves as healthy.'

Patient–doctor concordance

Ask most people and they will say that, in health matters, 'the doctor knows best'. Is this always the case? Do all people believe that the doctor knows best?

Doctors are usually perceived as those knowing most about health and disease. However, Arksey (1994) showed how patients suffering from repetitive strain injury (RSI) can inform doctors about health issues. RSI is a general term for a number of neck, shoulder, wrist and elbow disorders occurring in both manual and non-manual workers. Arksey carried out a study of doctors' and patients' perspectives on the diagnosis of RSI. At the beginning of the study one GP was quoted as saying, 'I'm not really into this RSI thing, I think it's a load of nonsense.' However, at the end of the study, after talking to many patients, the GP admitted that he had 'learned a hell of a lot from the experience of talking to the patients and that he now recognises RSI as a problem, quite a major problem at that'. This study showed that medical knowledge cannot be taken for granted as the truth.

Patients can also resist the knowledge imparted to them by their doctors and they can challenge it. Some patients are able to evaluate the advice of their doctors. They might believe some of the advice, but not necessarily all of it. Calnan and Williams (1992) carried out a survey using self-completed

questionnaires with a random sample of the
population aged 18 and over (see Figure 41 below).

Figure 41 *Patients' evaluation of medical knowledge (percentage of sample)*

Doctors' recommendation	Accept without question	Accept with explanation	Not accept readily / not at all
Antibiotics	54	41	5
Hernia operation	30	63	7
Bowel cancer op.	29	60	12
Tranquillisers	8	29	63
Hip replacement	25	62	13
Hysterectomy	20	65	16
Faith in doctors	**Lot of faith**	**Quite a lot**	**Not very much**
	31	56	13

Source: M. Calnan and S. Williams, 'Images of scientific medicine', *Sociology of Health and Illness*, vol.14, no. 2, 1992

Notice that when antibiotics were recommended
the majority of people accepted this and did so
without question. However, when tranquillisers were
recommended few people accepted this readily and
even fewer did so without question. It is interesting to
note that most people accepted the doctors'
recommendation to have an operation, but most only
did so after an explanation.

Patient compliance

Have you always followed the advice given by your
doctor? Have you ever stopped taking medicine
before you were supposed to?

Compliance may be defined as 'the extent to which
the patient's behaviour (in terms of taking medications,
following diets or other lifestyle changes) coincides
with medical or health advice' (Haynes *et al.*).

Compliance is regarded as important – because
following the recommendations of health
professionals is considered essential to patient
recovery. However, studies estimate that about half of
the patients with chronic illnesses, such as diabetes
and hypertension, are non-compliant with their
medication regimes, and that even compliance for a
behaviour as apparently simple as using an inhaler for
asthma is poor (Dekker *et al.*).

Ley (1989) claimed that compliance may be
predicted by a combination of patient satisfaction
with the consultation, understanding of the
information given and recall of this information (see
Figure 42).

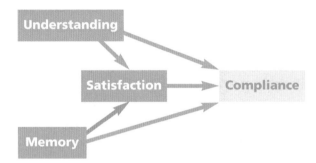

Figure 42 Ley's model of compliance

Researchers have examined how well patients recall
the information given to them during the consultation
with their doctor. In one study, Bain (1977) found that
37 per cent could not recall the name of the drug, 23
per cent could not recall the frequency of the dose,
and 25 per cent could not recall the duration of the
treatment. Recalling information after the consultation
may well be related to compliance.

In addition, if the doctor gives advice to a patient
or suggests that they follow a particular programme
of treatment and the patient does not understand the
causes of their illness, the correct location of the
relevant organ or the processes involved in the
treatment, then this lack of understanding is likely to
affect their compliance with the advice.

Compliance will only work if a patient wants it to.
But doctors could help to increase it by improving
their communication, in several ways:

- Tell the patient the most important piece of
  information first.

- Stress the importance of compliance.

Unit 9 Investigating Disease

- Simplify the information.

- Use repetition.

- Be specific.

- Follow up the information with additional interviews.

Bert thinks he knows best

Bert was feeling unwell. For days, he had been feeling tired and listless, but what worried him most was the fact that he got breathless every time he walked uphill. He decided to visit his doctor. The doctor told Bert that he was overweight and had high blood pressure. He was given medication for the high blood pressure, told he should eat less and that he should give up smoking. The doctor said that he was a high risk for having a heart attack. Bert was shocked to hear this and agreed that he would following the doctor's advice. He stopped smoking and started to eat more salads, but he found he was always hungry – and he felt 'on edge' all the time. After three weeks, his wife told him she was fed up with him being bad tempered, and if that was how he was going to behave, he should start smoking again! Bert was not happy with the medication for his high blood pressure. He said it was giving him a tickly cough and he was stopping taking it. After a few days, his wife said he ought to go back to the doctor. Bert said he did not think that was necessary as he was feeling better.

Antibiotic resistance

Antibiotics are prescribed for bacterial infections. However, there has been a move recently to reduce their usage (see table below). You might well wonder

Figure 43 *The number of antibiotic prescriptions dispensed in England*

Year	Prescription items (millions)
1991	43.7
1992	43.4
1993	47.7
1994	45.8
1995	49.4
1996	46.6
1997	46.4
1998	42.6
1999	38.6
2000	36.9

why, if they are effective in preventing bacteria from multiplying. The problem is that for as long as antibiotics have been used to treat bacterial infections, the bacteria have been fighting back. Not all bacteria are susceptible to all antibiotics. For example, penicillin does not work against a group of bacteria called Gram negative bacteria. There has also been a development of resistant strains among bacterial species that were generally susceptible to particular antibiotics.

It is important to remember that resistant bacteria are not *caused* by antibiotics. Bacteria that become antibiotic-resistant do so by a mutation (spontaneous change) in their genes. An antibiotic-resistant bacterium develops and is able to grow and reproduce successfully despite the presence of the antibiotic. Imagine that in a population of bacteria most are susceptible to a particular antibiotic, but there are some that are resistant. Which ones will be killed and which ones will be able to go on a reproduce? The ones that are susceptible will be killed and the few that are resistant will go on and reproduce. Over time, the percentage of bacteria that are resistant in the population will vastly increase. What will happen to the effectiveness of the antibiotic then? It will decrease. In fact, it will be pointless giving a patient that antibiotic to treat that particular infection.

Funding available

There is no getting away from the fact that the prevention and control of disease cost a lot of money. Where does this money come from? Is there always enough money available?

The modern welfare state in the UK was created just after the end of the Second World War. Its instigator was Sir William Beveridge. He described disease as one of the five main evils in society. He proposed that there should be a National Health Service which everyone was entitled to use, regardless of their ability to pay. The idea was that as the health of the British people improved, less money would need to be paid out for sickness and disability, thus saving the country money in the long run. At first the costs of the welfare state were almost all paid for by the government out of taxation and the New National Insurance scheme. But the NHS quickly ran into financial difficulties, and the government had to make some hard choices. In 1952 selective charges were first introduced for:

- Dental treatment

- Prescriptions

- The costs of glasses.

It could be argued that some people do not visit the

dentist or the optician for checkups because of these charges. They may prefer to wait until they have a problem and need treatment, rather than take preventative measures. Likewise, some people may not wish to collect medicine and pay the prescription charges.

In the 1980s the Conservative government split parts of the NHS into separate purchasers and providers of health care. District health authorities and GP fundholders became purchasers, and self-governing health care trusts – such as hospitals – become providers. Health care purchasers shopped around for the best value health care of their patients from a range of competing providers. The government then believed that such a market-like mechanism was the best way of delivering public services because it created competition between providers, created choice for purchasers, cut costs as providers tried to win contracts and reduced inefficiency and saved money.

In 1997, the new Labour government introduced reforms to the NHS internal market. One of those was to abolish fundholding GPs and to create primary care groups in their place. The new NHS has been designed to reduce competition and encourage co-operation and integration within the NHS.

The Department of Health, like all government departments, gets its money from the Treasury, which is the central government department responsible for balancing the country's finances. Every year, the Department of Health competes for money with all the other central government departments, such as education, defence, environment, and the Home Office. It never gets as much money as it wants, so one of its functions is to set priorities. Prevention and control of disease has to compete with all the rest of the Department of Health's priorities, which is why the funding available is one of the main factors affecting disease prevention.

Figure 44 shows how funds were allocated for three years from 2003 to 2006. The aim of changes in the proportion of funds allocated to different services has been to produce a fairer means of allocating resources. A key criterion of the new funding has been to contribute to the reduction of avoidable health inequalities. Notice the increased amount given to statutory bodies such as the Health Protection Agency. This can only be good news for the prevention and control of disease.

Figure 44 *Central Health and Miscellaneous Services (CHMS), 2003–04 to 2005–06 (£000s)*

Budgets	2003–04	2004–05	200–06
Improving services and outcomes in:			
Cancer	39,000	43,692	58,000
Mental health	1,000	4,000	4,000
Children	525	487	450
Reducing health inequalities	47,101	46,744	51,061
Contributing to the reduction in drug misuse	3,331	3,308	3,331
Other CHMS budgets:			
Central payments made on behalf of DH (e.g. EEA Medical costs)	334,893	353,726	375,893
Public health (e.g. Welfare Foods)	127,915	127,839	127,887
Statutory Bodies (e.g. Health Protection Agency)	94,451	97,501	101,311
R&D	37,794	37,529	37,794
Residual CHMS budgets (e.g. communications, grants to voluntary organisations)	61,758	62,306	63,579
Non-cash CHMS budgets (including Capital Charges, Provisions, etc)	27,713	29,611	31,359
Total	**775,481**	**806,743**	**854,665**

Alison has always been particular about looking after her teeth. She goes to the dentist every six months for a check-up. Her dentist works for the National Health Service. This means that, although Alison pays for her dental treatment, she pays less than if she went privately. Recently, Alison moved to another part of the country. She asked a neighbour for the name of good dentist. Her neighbour said that there were lots of good dentists, but that there was only one dentist, Mr Chang, working for the National Health Service, who was prepared to taken on any new patients. Alison rang Mr Chang's receptionist who said that 'his books' were now full, and if she wanted treatment she would have to go to a dentist who was in private practice. Alison decided not to bother signing up with a dentist in private practice, as check-ups and treatment would be too expensive. Anyway, she told her husband, 'it's not as if I am having any bother'. Her husband said that he thought she might suffer in the long run as not having her teeth checked might mean having to have more treatment in the future.

Check your understanding

1 List the factors which might interfere with the prevention and control of disease. For each factor, identify a particular disease that may be especially affected.

2 Explain which doctors' recommendations people agreed with most, and which they disagreed with most.

3 Give three reasons why patients may not comply with their doctors' recommendations.

4 Explain why there is an ever-increasing number of antibiotic-resistant bacteria present today, compared with several years ago.

5 Explain why the Health Service does not always have the same amount of money to spend each year.

extension activities

1 Imagine you are in charge of allocating money to different areas in the NHS. Put forward a case for giving a larger sum of money to disease prevention than before. (Think carefully of the consequences of doing this, first.)

2 'Compliance will only work if a patient wants it to.' Explain why this may be so, despite the patient having a complete understanding of the advice being offered to them.

Topic 9 Putting it all together: case studies

Getting you thinking

1 **What might be wrong with each of these people?**

2 **Who might each of them be waiting to see?**

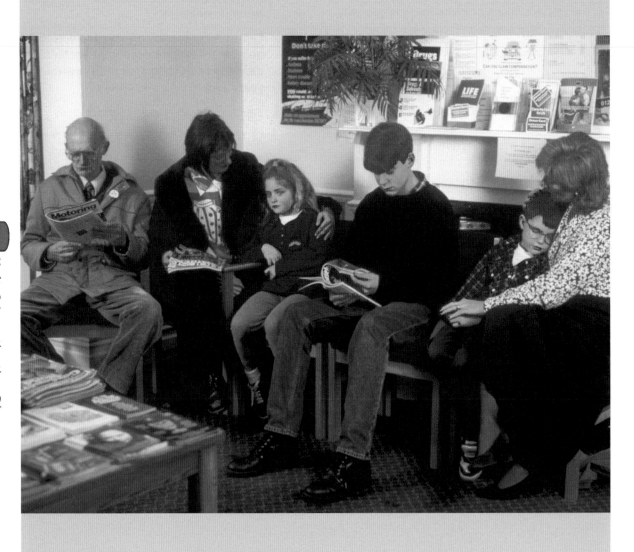

Preparing for your portfolio

Now that you have studied Topics 1 to 8 in this unit, you are in a good position to decide which communicable and which non-communicable diseases to compare. The following case studies will cover a variety of diseases. We shall use them to make comparisons between diseases based on the following aspects:

- The biological basis of disease
- The body's response to disease
- The cause and distribution of disease
- The availability of support for disease
- Factors that may affect treatment of a disease
- Strategies for the prevention of disease
- Factors that may affect the prevention of disease.

Meet John, the GP

John is one of six GPs in a busy health practice. The health practice is in a small industrial town where a large number of the population work at a local engineering factory. The town has a high number of families receiving income support, and the secondary school has a high proportion of its pupils receiving free school meals. Recently, there has been an outbreak of food poisoning amongst young children. The town has a higher population of people over the age of retirement than nationally.

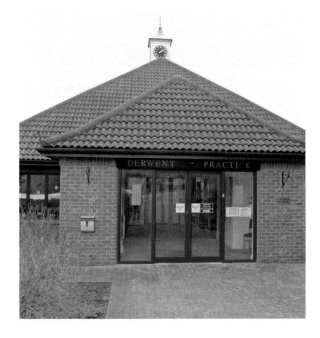

It is Monday morning, and John notices that the waiting room seems fuller than normal. He calls for his first patient.

Four-year-old Amir and his mother

Amir is brought in by his mother, Fatima. Amir is looking very tired – and Fatima is looking very stressed. They both look underweight. John asks how he may help them. Fatima tells him that Amir has been vomiting and has diarrhoea. She also says that this is the final straw, and she just doesn't know how she is going to cope, because she is a single parent with three other children to look after. John asks how long Amir has been unwell. Fatima says that Amir started being sick yesterday evening and this continued all night. She says he has not eaten breakfast, but neither of them ever does.

John thinks that both Amir and Fatima need help. He will deal with Amir first, because he suspects that, like many other children locally, he may have food poisoning. He takes Amir's temperature, because a raised temperature is a sign that he might have an infection. Remember that food poisoning is caused by a bacterium, usually *Salmonella* or *E.coli*. This may be confirmed by taking a faeces sample and sending it off to the microbiology laboratory at the hospital for analysis. Amir may be prescribed antibiotics if the food poisoning does not clear up, but John knows the importance of not prescribing antibiotics too readily. John asks Fatima if he can take her blood pressure. He suspects that she may be stressed and he wants to check for hypertension. If her blood pressure is too high, he will ask her if she is happy to have a visit from the health visitor to discuss how she might lower her blood pressure. John is not sure that Fatima will agree to this, but he hopes that Fatima will accept this offer of help.

Comparing food poisoning and hypertension

Let's now compare what we have learned about the two diseases in this case study. The communicable disease is food poisoning and the non-communicable disease is hypertension.

We have not considered fully the factors affecting the treatment and support of the diseases, apart from Fatima agreeing to having a visit from a health visitor and John's hesitation in prescribing antibiotics. Other factors might include the waiting time for Amir's diagnosis to be confirmed, funding available to pay for the health visitor's visit and Fatima's perception of the long-term risk of having high blood pressure.

Figure 45 Comparing Food Poisoning and Hypertension

	Food poisoning	*Hypertension*
Biological basis of disease	Bacterium, usually *Salmonella or E.coli*	Narrowing of the arteries or a very fast heart beat
Transmission	Infected food, usually caused by the person preparing the food not washing their hands after going to the toilet	Not applicable, but related to lifestyle
Signs	Vomiting and diarrhoea	Both systolic and diastolic blood pressure being significantly above normal for age
Symptoms	Dehydration, tired	Feeling stressed
Further confirmation of diagnosis	Microbiological analysis of faeces to check for the presence of the specific bacteria	Angiogram (scan of blood vessels) of the brain to check on how much the blood vessels have narrowed. This will only be done if it is thought that the hypertension is a significant risk to future health.
Treatment	Antibiotics	Prescribing medication to reduce blood pressure. Change in lifestyle, to include healthier diet and exercise. Steps taken to help reduce stress.

78-year-old Matt and his son

Matt is John's next patient. He has been brought to the surgery by his 43-year-old son Luke. Matt has difficulty in walking and is very breathless. Luke helps Matt by giving his arm to lean on.

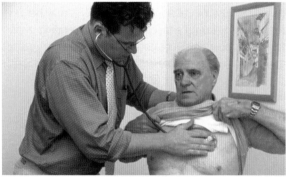

Matt tried to tell John that he is feeling very tired and can't catch his breath. Luke has to help his father explain what's wrong. John asks how long Matt has had these symptoms, and if he smokes. Luke says that Matt has been like this for about a year, but that he hasn't wanted to see a doctor until now. He also says that Matt smokes about thirty cigarettes a day. Matt nods in agreement. John can see that Matt can't breathe properly and he listens to his breathing, using a stethoscope. He finds it irregular and laboured. John tells Matt that he would like to send him for an X-ray. He says Matt may need to wait for a while, but he will do his best to get it done as quickly as possible. Matt is not keen to have an X-ray, but John explains to him about emphysema and what might have happened in his lungs. He says that if this is confirmed, then he will recommend that Matt has an oxygen cylinder in his house to help him breathe more easily. He also tells Matt that smoking will continue to make his condition worse. Matt is not so sure about this. Just as they as about to leave, Luke asks John if he will have a quick look at his foot. He thinks that he might have Athlete's foot. John says that although he is busy he will do this. John notices that Luke has broken and flaky skin between his toes. Luke asks if he can have a prescription for some medication. John says that a prescription is not necessary, as the medication may be bought cheaply over the counter without prescription.

Athlete's foot and Emphysema

Let's now compare what we have learned about the two diseases in this case study. The communicable disease is Athlete's foot and the non-communicable disease is emphysema.

Figure 46 Comparing Athlete's foot and Emphysema

	Athlete's foot	*Emphysema*
Biological basis of disease	Fungus, *Tinea*	Breakdown of the walls of alveoli in the lungs
Transmission	Contact with someone who has had the disease, such as using the same towel or walking barefoot	Not applicable, but related to lifestyle, particularly smoking
Signs	Flaky or broken skin between the toes	Laboured breathing
Symptoms	Itchiness between the toes	Tiredness, inability to 'catch' breath
Further confirmation of diagnosis	Not usually necessary	X-ray of the lungs to check the condition of the alveoli
Treatment	Fungicidal cream	No cure, but symptoms may be alleviated by breathing pure oxygen or oxygen-enriched air

Some of the factors affecting the treatment and support of the diseases have been mentioned. Matt was reluctant in coming to see the doctor in the first place and he is also reluctant to go for an X-ray. An earlier diagnosis might have prevented the emphysema from being as serious as it is now. Matt has to want to have the diagnosis confirmed. Another problem that will affect the treatment of the disease is that Matt does not fully agree with John about the importance of not smoking.

Meet Abeni, the practice nurse

Abeni runs several clinics at the health practice. Some are aimed at disease prevention and others are for routine procedures, such as immunisation or the removal of stitches. She runs a well-women clinic two afternoons per week and a well-men clinic one afternoon per week. She finds that many men are reluctant to have their health checked. This is the afternoon of the well-men clinic, and Abeni calls for her first patient.

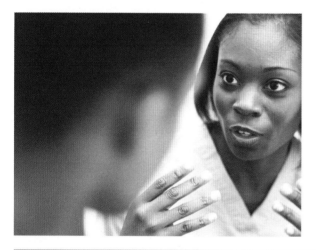

48-year-old Clive

Clive has been asked to bring a urine sample with him. Abeni checks this for the presence of glucose, which might indicate that Clive has diabetes. She notes that there is no glucose present in the urine. She measures Clive's weight and sees that it is within the normal range for his height. She also checks Clive's blood pressure which is normal and takes a blood sample to be sent away for analysis. Clive has asked if his blood could be checked for the presence of the HIV virus as he has had sexual contact with someone he thinks might be HIV-positive. He mentions to Abeni that a lump has developed in one of his testicles and that he is worried that it might be a sign that he has testicular cancer. Abeni asks one of the doctors on duty to examine Clive there and then. The doctor says that this should be investigated further and says he will arrange for Clive to be referred to the oncology department of the local hospital.

AIDS and cancer

Let's now compare what we have learned about two of the diseases in this case study. The communicable disease is AIDS and the non-communicable disease is prostate cancer.

Clive has attempted to diagnose his own diseases, but he has taken the opportunity to mention the problems on his visit to the well-men clinic. Not all men would have acted in the way that Clive did. Peter Jenkins in a magazine called *Achilles' Heel* (1991) explored the strained relationship between men and their health. He concluded that the culture-borne technique of denying injury and disease explained the abnormally low uptake of health care amongst men. He finds this strange because, apart from the complications of childbirth and the drop in hormones associated with the menopause, women are no more prone to illness than men.

Figure 47 Comparing AIDS and Testicular cancer

	AIDS	Testicular cancer
Biological basis of disease	Human Immunodeficiency (HIV) virus that acts on the immune system	A malignant tumour in one of the testicles, part of the male reproductive system
Transmission	Sexual contact with someone who is HIV-positive. By infected blood or sharing syringes.	Not applicable
Signs and symptoms	A flu-like illness initially. Later on the person might contract a form of skin cancer or pneumonia.	First detected by a lump in one of the testicles.
Further confirmation of diagnosis	Blood test to look for the presence of the HIV virus	Ultrasound, biopsy to check for cancerous cells.
Treatment	Very little at present. Anti-viral drugs.	Surgery, chemotherapy or radiotherapy or a combination of all three.

18-month-old Damien

Abeni meets Damien at the immunisation clinic. Damien has been brought in by his father to have an MMR injection. MMR stands for measles, mumps and Rubella (German measles). Damien's father is worried because he has heard that this triple injection may be linked with autism. Damien's father does not want to run the risk of Damien developing autism, but equally he does not want him to develop measles, mumps or German measles. Abeni tells Damien's father that he will need to make the decision whether Damien is immunised and she gives him some leaflets to take away and read.

Let's now compare some of the features of one of the communicable diseases of the MMR – Rubella – with autism.

prioritise them for treatment, according to the severity of their condition. Those who have minor ailments may have to wait a long time, depending on who else arrives.

17-year-old Tom

Tom is brought into A&E by his mother and father one Friday evening. He has had a fever for a few days, and now has a severe headache and a very sore stiff neck. He knows that he has been in contact with someone who has developed viral meningitis. Charles examines Tom and decides to do a lumbar puncture to get a sample of his cerebral spinal fluid. A sample of this fluid will be sent to the microbiology laboratory to determine whether Tom has viral meningitis or the more serious bacterial form of the disease. Charles knows that the laboratory is short-staffed and that it

Figure 48 Comparing Rubella and Autism

	Rubella (German measles)	Autism
Biological basis of disease	A rubivirus. Can cause deafness and other congenital abnormalities in the foetus if present in the mother.	Not completely known. A connection between the lack of a particular enzyme in the gut and autistic brain dysfunction has been claimed by some researchers. This connection is disputed by others.
Transmission	Droplet infection or direct contact with an infected person.	N/A
Signs and symptoms	Initial period of high temperature, then the appearance of a pink rash with small spots.	Withdrawn, limited imagination.
Treatment	Increased fluid intake, rest	Management of the person's environment to minimise change.

Note that the prevention of German measles depends very much on whether there is a high percentage of the population immunised. The public perception of risk of German measles weighed against the perceived risks of the side effects of the immunisation is important in determining the extent to which German measles is prevented.

Meet Charles, a consultant – and Nazy, a triage nurse

Charles and Nazy both work in the Accident and Emergency department of a large city hospital. They never know from day to day who will arrive or what will be wrong with them. When people arrive at A&E, they are seen by a triage nurse, such as Nazy, who will

will be difficult for him to get a result of the test for several days. Charles decides to admit Tom and to give him antibiotics intravenously. The hospital is short of beds and Charles may have to put Tom in a side ward off one of the main medical wards. This is not ideal because Tom might be very infectious at this stage.

53-year-old Angus

Angus is brought into A&E by ambulance, accompanied by his wife.. He has collapsed and has severe chest pains. Nazy is in no doubt that Angus needs to be seen immediately as his condition is life-threatening. Charles performs an ECG on Angus and confirms that his heart muscle has been damaged. He is taken to the intensive care ward where he can be closely monitored. Charles noticed that Angus was very overweight. His wife told Charles that Angus smokes heavily and has a stressful job as a headteacher.

A comparison of the factors affecting the diagnosis, treatment and prevention of Tom and Angus's diseases

Angus's diagnosis of a heart attack was confirmed very quickly, whereas Tom's diagnosis of meningitis (including the type) will take several days. Tom's diagnosis is also affected by the short-staffing in the laboratory.

Angus's treatment is started immediately by sending him to the intensive care laboratory. Tom's treatment is also started immediately by giving him antibiotics. This is a precaution in case he has the more serious bacterial form of meningitis.

Angus might have prevented his heart attack had he reduced the risk factors of not smoking, reducing his weight and not having such a stressful job. Tom may not have been able to prevent himself being in contact with someone who had meningitis. Meningitis can be immunised against, but it is not routinely carried out unless there is thought to be a high risk.

Check your understanding

1 List the communicable diseases and the non-communicable diseases in this topic. Choose two diseases that have not already been compared in a table and write a comparison between the two.

2 Write a comparative table for meningitis and a heart attack under the following headings:
- **Biological basis of the disease**
- **Transmission of the disease**
- **Signs of the disease**
- **Symptoms of the disease**
- **Diagnosis**
- **Treatment.**

3 Write a short paragraph comparing the ways in which food poisoning and hypertension may be prevented.

extension activities

1 Find out about groups which support emphysema, heart disease or autism. Give a short Powerpoint presentation to the rest of the group on your findings.

2 Choose two diseases not mentioned in the case studies, and write a comparative table, similar to the ones presented here. One disease should be communicable and the other non-communicable.

THIS UNIT IS ABOUT THE ROLE OF RESEARCH IN HEALTH AND SOCIAL CARE. It will develop your understanding of how research can contribute to best practice and policy in health and social care by showing you how experimental research, survey investigations and epidemiological and census data can contribute to effective care. It will also help you to understand why the evaluation of current measures and the trying out of new interventions are so important.

Because this unit requires you to conduct a research project on a health and/or social care issue, we also examine and weigh up some key research techniques – questionnaires, interviews, observation and experiments. Additionally, you will gain knowledge of – and (we hope) commitment to – the dignity, rights, safety and well-being of the people whom researchers study. We consider other ethical issues too, such as the informed consent of participants.

Finally, the unit will show you how to plan and conduct your own small-scale research project and how to write a research report. Carrying out an investigation into an aspect of health and/or social care that interests you will help you to gain a practical understanding of the link between research and care issues.

Although some writers distinguish between 'practice' and 'policy', unless otherwise indicated, we sometimes use 'practice' to denote both terms. The need for good practice applies as much to those responsible for health and social policy as it does to frontline care practitioners.

Understanding Research in Health and Social Care

Key questions

By the end of the unit you should be able to use the knowledge and understanding that you develop to answer the following questions:

1 What contribution can health and social care research make to evidence-based care practice and policy?
2 What are the more common research methods that are used in the health and social care field?
3 How should ethics play a role in care research?
4 How can you undertake a small-scale research project on a health and/or social care topic?

Introducing health and social care research

Getting you thinking

1 Suggest how research findings might help a care practitioner to provide high-quality health advice and care services for the person in the photograph.

2 Explain how research has shown that obesity is linked to unhealthy lifestyle choices.

3 What ethical considerations should a researcher take into account when interviewing a sample of overweight or obese people for research purposes?

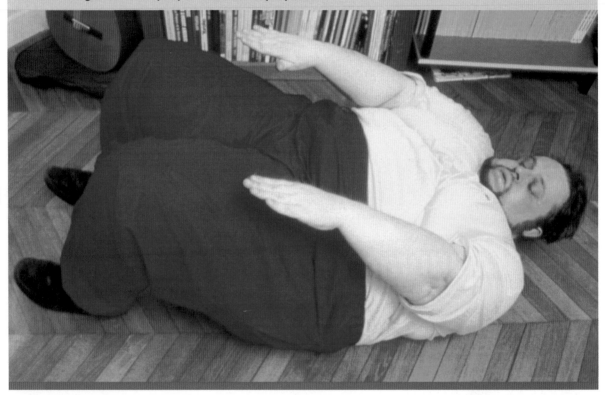

KEY TERMS

Research-based evidence
Findings that are based on data collected through systematic investigation.

Empirical evidence
Evidence based on direct observation and collection of data

Evidence-based practice
Practice that applies the best available evidence, some of it available from research studies, some of it gained from practical experience.

Governance of research
The process of applying and monitoring approved research 'rules' and procedures.

Qualitative data
Non-numerical data – usually presented as 'talk' or 'text' though it can also include images and objects – that provide some form of information.

Quantitative data
Information presented in numerical form. Typically, this involves some form of quantifiable measure.

Secondary data
Existing data that has been collected and analysed by a previous researcher but which can be reanalysed and reused in a subsequent research study.

The significance of health and social care research

Many of the advances in health and social care over the last century have depended on the work of researchers. At times, their contributions have helped to move the field of practice and policy from guesswork to science. Today high-quality **research-based evidence** is used in many specialist areas of health and social care. Research-based evidence is produced through careful research studies and is made available through printed and online journals as well as through specialist books. Computer terminals in some care settings can give health care professionals electronic access to research-based evidence on a variety of topics, almost instantaneously.

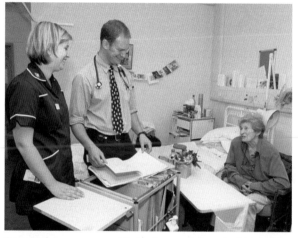

Care workers can now get hold of research-based evidence fast.

Research is generally seen as a good thing by health and social care practitioners. However, there have also been occasions when research procedures have failed to meet the high standards that the public expect and deserve. This is why strong **governance of research** is crucial. This point has been forcibly stated by the Department of Health (2001, p. 3) who say:

'The public has a right to expect high scientific, ethical and financial standards, transparent decision-making processes, clear allocation of responsibilities and robust monitoring arrangements.'

In this unit, we will focus on research that aims to produce real health and social care benefits for the individual and the community. Often the aim of this research is to provide a clear evidence-base for care practice. This is not to say that a 'gut feeling' or practice based on practical learning and experience is necessarily wrong. But what makes 'good practice' right is not the strength of the feeling associated with it or the length of time that people have been doing it, but rather the collection of supporting evidence that verifies it. Research plays a key role here, but so too does sound professional experience. Health and

social care research is (or should be) based on solid data, and one of the best ways of obtaining such data is to conduct systematic research.

The nature of scientific research

When I was a sociology student in the 1970s, I spent countless hours studying statistics. Statistics uses quantitative data (that is, data expressed in numbers) to obtain scientific insights and to draw reliable conclusions. This kind of data can help us to tackle major health and social care issues. For example, what percentage of the UK population is poor? What is the relationship between being poor and being ill? These are the kinds of question that statistics helped me to answer. I could have made some guesses, but being a social scientist, I had to look at the evidence. Science helped me determine the truth or falsehood of an idea. It let me arrive at a conclusion independently of who said what or who thinks she or he knows best.

While statistical analysis is a very important tool in scientific research, so too is the analysis of **qualitative data** (that is, data mainly expressed in words). Using the example of poverty and illness again, scientists need both numerical and non-numerical data. By non-numerical data, we mean the views of the people who are being studied. The focus here is on how they interpret their circumstances in their own terms. For example, a poor person whose health is affected by an inadequate diet might produce very useful qualitative data by recording her experiences in a research diary or by telling an interviewer about it in her own words.

The word 'science' comes from the Latin verb scire, meaning 'to know'. In the English language, science often conjures up images of white-coated experimenters. However, in some languages, the term also applies to knowing about the social world. While we can know things in lots of different ways, scientific knowledge is based on objective evidence. In ideal terms, this means that one scientist's truth is another scientist's truth, not because of what they believe but because of how they arrive at their beliefs. To prove something scientifically, scientists have to provide **empirical evidence** that can be checked and confirmed by other scientists. The result is a collectively agreed body of 'facts' that can be scrutinised and tested. Scientific researchers argue that this kind of evidence provides a much better basis for care practice than 'common sense' or ad hoc guesswork.

When people are ill, seeking forms of treatment that have scientifically proven benefits makes good sense. Similarly, it is wise to implement social policies that research has found to be effective. We can only know what works well – and the best ways of using

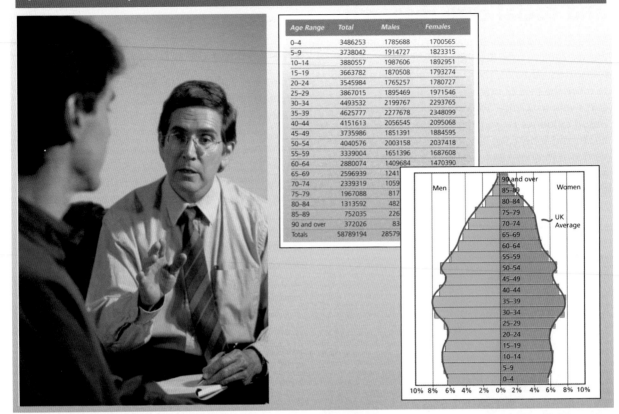

Age Range	Total	Males	Females
0–4	3486253	1785688	1700565
5–9	3738042	1914727	1823315
10–14	3880557	1987606	1892951
15–19	3663782	1870508	1793274
20–24	3545984	1765257	1780727
25–29	3867015	1895469	1971546
30–34	4493532	2199767	2293765
35–39	4625777	2277678	2348099
40–44	4151613	2056545	2095068
45–49	3735986	1851391	1884595
50–54	4040576	2003158	2037418
55–59	3339004	1651396	1687608
60–64	2880074	1409684	1470390
65–69	2596939	1241	
70–74	2339319	1059	
75–79	1967088	817	
80–84	1313592	482	
85–89	752035	226	
90 and over	372026	83	
Totals	58789194	28579	

Figure 1 Used together, quantitative and qualitative data give a fuller picture

these effective approaches or treatments – by carrying out research into 'good practice'. In addition, health and social care researchers are also interested in the discovery of new and better treatments and care policies. This is why researchers need to find out:

- What is already known about an issue
- What gaps there are in existing knowledge.

Investigating existing practice

In order to avoid 'reinventing the wheel' in the care field, researchers can consult 'systematic reviews' of previous research on a particular topic. These reviews rigorously sift through and assess the research evidence on the effectiveness of specific health and social care practices throughout the world. They provide an analysis of existing research in order to find out if lots of studies support current practice and procedures. Two of the most prominent organisations that conduct and publish systematic reviews are the Cochrane Collaboration, which assesses health interventions, and the Campbell Collaboration, which assesses social interventions.

When systematic reviews bring to light shortcomings in current knowledge, the challenge for

science is to discover new and better ways of doing things. If, for example, a systematic review reveals (and this is entirely hypothetical) that public anti-smoking campaigns are not having the desired effect, this finding invites further exploration. Perhaps the health message needs to be repackaged, perhaps more preventative work needs to be done in schools, perhaps additional restrictions should be placed on advertising, and so on.

On the subject of smoking (and this time for real), systematic reviews have discovered that simple, one-off advice from a doctor during a routine consultation increases the proportion of smokers quitting smoking and not relapsing for at least one year.

Another way of investigating current practice in health and social care is to use data that are available centrally, such as national statistics on births, mortality, morbidity, life expectancy, poverty, education and pensions. Sometimes inspections of existing, that is secondary, data confirm existing conclusions. At other times, unanswered gaps in knowledge come to light, prompting further study.

Among the reviewers of **secondary data**, are scientists who are interested in finding out which diseases are increasing or decreasing in incidence and how such trends are linked to particular policies and practices. This field of investigation forms part of what is known as epidemiology, the study of the incidence, distribution and causes of disease.

Breaking new ground

Once a new care delivery or treatment approach is seen as promising, it is time to investigate its potential. The gold standard for doing this is the experiment, which is used to measure the effectiveness of an intervention. Effectiveness is measured by exposing one group to an intervention – for example, a new surgical technique – and comparing the outcome with a group that has not been exposed to the intervention. Each of these groups should be randomly selected beforehand. If there are different outcomes, then this is taken as evidence that the intervention has had an effect. This type of research might show, for example, that a less invasive surgical technique produces quicker recovery rates than more aggressive surgery.

Although the experiment is often the first method to be considered, there are many other ways of obtaining new knowledge about health and social care. This is partly because different kinds of question require different kinds of evidence. Thus, for example, while experiments can help clinical psychologists to identify the most effective way to treat depression, in-depth interviews with depressed patients can throw new light on what it feels like to be depressed.

Irrespective of the methods used, all investigations should be carried out not just using rigorous scientific principles, but also following faultless ethics.

Research ethics

Research ethics are principles that offer researchers guidance on how they should value and treat the people who participate in their research studies. Many of the ethical principles focus on respecting and protecting the rights of participants.

Arguably, the most important ethical duty in care research is to protect the dignity, safety and well-being of participants. Researchers should also obtain informed consent from participants and, if appropriate, from their relatives. Other ethical principles include: confidentiality of personal information, active involvement of participants whenever possible in the research process, and, if the research involves an element of risk to participants, explaining this to them and keeping it to an absolute minimum.

Participants should also be told that they are free to withdraw at any time from a research project. Furthermore, researchers are under a moral obligation to answer honestly and fully any questions that participants might have about the study.

As far as honesty is concerned, there are differing views. Is it, for example, permissible for a researcher to use a bit of deception in order to get at the truth, or is complete openness essential? Putting these questions into a concrete context, is it, for example, wrong for me to secretly observe you going about your care work on the grounds that if you knew you were being watched, you might act 'unnaturally'? Or should I tell you that I am observing you as part of my research study?

Epidemiological and census data

In an earlier section, we briefly considered systematic reviews of existing data. Among the most comprehensive sources here, are epidemiological and census data.

> ### Hurricane Katrina: an epidemiological challenge for New Orleans
>
> Hurricane Katrina hit the city of New Orleans in 2005, with devastating consequences. Epidemiologists are investigating the short- and long-term health effects of this disaster. Among the issues that they are seeking answers to are these:
>
> - the effect of exposure to mould in healthy and vulnerable populations within the city
>
> - the physical and emotional impact on first responders and health care providers to the devastation caused by the hurricane
>
> - the experiences of people who evacuated and those who stayed.
>
> The hope is that epidemiological research will help policy-makers in New Orleans to avoid the mistakes of the past during the process of rebuilding the city.

Epidemiology is the study of the distribution and determinants of disease within a given population, such as the residents of a town or, on a much larger scale, the citizens of a nation. Some epidemiologists conduct their own medical studies and produce their own data, but many look for undiscovered patterns in existing data. The sources of contemporary information include relevant published studies in medical journals and government statistics.

The most complete store of official (government) statistical information that we have in the UK is the

Census. The most recent Census was carried out on Sunday, 29 April 2001. The Census is a national headcount of people and households, and since 1801 this count has been made every 10 years. The information that the Census contains helps health and social care authorities to prioritise and plan their services for years to come.

What we can learn from care research

There are many lessons to be learned from health and social care research. The main focus here is on using proven good practice more widely. If, for example, we know from research findings, as indeed we do, that many buildings cannot be easily accessed by wheelchair users, then policy-makers need to approve only the construction of buildings that are accessible for everyone.

Doing your own research

During your course, you will complete a research project on a health and social care topic. At this stage, you will not be expected to produce an action plan, but there is nothing to stop you from jotting down a few possible ideas. One way of adding weight to your proposals is to find support for them in background literature and other information sources relevant to your chosen topic. You might, for example, refer to research highlighting problems of access for wheelchair users and then produce further evidence supporting this finding from your own study.

Irrespective of what you find out when you conduct your own research, you will gain a better understanding of the research process by doing a 'hands-on' project. And that in itself is a worthwhile endeavour.

Wheelchair users are the real experts in disability research

Midshire Local Authority is keen to provide support for disabled people living in its local authority area. Following a consultation with disabled people, it has agreed to develop and fund a project aimed at improving indoor mobility for wheelchair users living at home. It has therefore asked Tariq, who has cerebral palsy and is an experienced wheelchair user, to help them out.

Tariq will work as a consultant to the Disability Support section of the social services department. His role will be to provide advice and guidance on possible strategies and to review any project plans.

His personal experience and insights into disability and wheelchair use are seen as vital to the success of the project.

Tariq feels that the project team needs some basic information before they begin suggesting ways of modifying disabled people's homes. For example, he has arranged a demonstration of several different types of wheelchair. The aim of this is to show the team how the turning circle of a wheelchair affects a person's ability to turn his or her wheelchair around within a room.

Figure 2 Doing your own research: preliminary preparation

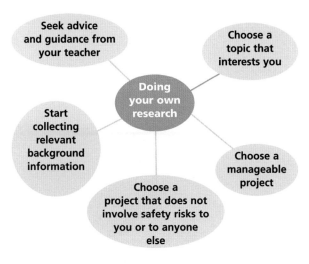

Figure 2 Doing your own research: preliminary preparation

Check your understanding

1 What is research-based evidence?

2 Explain why it is important to apply research-based evidence in care practice whenever this is possible.

3 Identify one example of quantitative data and one example of qualitative data and explain how they can provide important insights into health and social care.

4 Why is it important for scientists to check their research findings with each other?

5 What are systematic reviews and how can they help researchers from having to 'reinvent the wheel'?

extension **activities**

1 In the USA, where medical care is very costly, some poor people who are sick are encouraged to enter free clinical trials of experimental drugs or experimental approaches to treatment that might help them to get better. Identify and discuss the ethical issues that you think arise in this kind of situation.

2 Imagine that you are a care researcher addressing an audience of care professionals. You can specify what they do – for example, social work, nursing. How could you persuade your audience that evidence-based practice might help them to do their job even better? Produce an outline for a 15-minute talk.

Getting you thinking

1 What role do you think medical laboratory researchers play in the development of health care practices?

2 What comes to mind when you hear the word 'science'?

3 Is there a difference between science and opinion? Explain what you think this might be.

4 Is it possible to be scientific and caring at the same time?

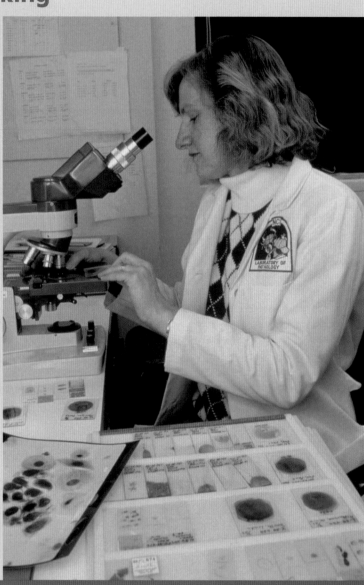

KEY TERMS

Empirical evidence
Things that we can verify with our senses, such as by observing and listening.

Hypotheses
Intelligent but untested propositions.

Reliable results
Findings that can be confirmed by other scientists.

Science
A way of knowing, based upon testing the truthfulness of ideas against empirical evidence.

Valid results
Findings that are based on the most appropriate research instruments.

The value of scientific research

The word 'science' often conjures up images of people in white coats, surrounded by brightly coloured chemicals bubbling away in test tubes. Yet this is an example of **science** rather than a comprehensive definition. Science is a way of knowing, based upon testing the truthfulness of ideas against **empirical evidence**. In turn, empirical evidence refers to what we can verify with our senses, such as by observing and listening. The scope of scientific research is wide, and includes the study of human behaviour as well as the properties of chemicals in a laboratory.

Scientific research provides care professionals with objective knowledge about good and bad effects. If, for example, research shows – as it does – that increasing the minimum wage helps the children of low-paid, recent immigrants, here is evidence of a good effect. If, on the other hand, research shows – and again, it does – that smoking increases the risk of the smoker dying from lung cancer, here is proof of a bad effect.

In general, health research achieves a higher degree of scientific precision than social care research. This has nothing to do with the quality of researchers in the respective fields, but everything to do with complexity. It is easier, for example, to produce stronger statistics on the effect of a new drug treatment than the effects of a scheme to combat racism at work. Even so, social care research is definitely able to estimate the outcome of various measures. And the findings of care researchers can help care professionals – nurses, social workers, etc. – to do a better job.

In defence of science

Science enables care researchers to distinguish between opinion-based practice and verifiable knowledge. We are reluctant to use the word 'fact' here because the vast majority of scientific conclusions are statements of probability based on overwhelming evidence. In that sense, even the best scientific argument on how to treat diabetes or how to reduce unemployment is only to be trusted for the time being – for as long as there are no alternative positions that stand up to tough scrutiny. It is precisely this rigour that helps to make a scientific assertion much more convincing than an opinion, a guess or a whim.

What characterises science is that it sets out the conditions that must be fulfilled before an assertion can be trusted. It is not enough to tell you that I know the best way to tackle the problem of obesity. I must also convince you that my claim is based on sound evidence. To do this, I need to persuade you that my findings are both reliable (other scientists would arrive at the same or very similar conclusions) and valid (I have used the most appropriate research instruments for the task at hand).

This doesn't mean that 'common sense' opinions may not be helpful. Opinions are often the starting point for scientific thinking, especially when they are stated as **hypotheses**, that is, as intelligent but untested propositions. They can then be tested to determine how well they are supported by evidence. This is particularly important when judging different claims to truth, such as 'This surgical procedure is better than that one', or 'This social work initiative is more promising than the other one.'

When to state a hypothesis

In general, a research hypothesis should be stated before collecting any data. An exception would be an exploratory study. For example, if you were investigating the possible reasons for high levels of satisfaction among social work clients, you might not already have a specific hypothesis in mind.

Which of these research questions do you think could helpfully be investigated using a hypothesis?

- The effect of walking to and from work for a year on the fitness of 10 employees.

- The effect of attending a healthy living conference on the behaviour of a group of obese patients during the following month.

- The effect of a power-driven wheelchair compared to a manual wheelchair on mobility at home among two groups of wheelchair users.

Explain your reasoning.

In being able to judge such assertions, scientists can only arrive at a consensus after repeated experiments and other rigorous testing procedures. Even then, however, science cannot afford to rest on its laurels. However well a scientific claim is supported by compelling evidence, such as the assertion that about 90 per cent of the most common lung cancer cases are caused by years of smoking or inhaling second-hand smoke, scientific propositions can only survive as long as they are not contradicted by other credible evidence. This is why medicines undergo (or should undergo) years of testing before being licensed for public use.

Getting you thinking

1 What are the advantages in care research of identifying and assessing existing clinical and social care practice?

2 If care researchers find that a current care practice is highly beneficial, what advice should they give to care practitioners?

3 If care researchers find that a current care practice is not up to scratch, what advice should they give to care practitioners?

4 Is it possible to retain best practice while simultaneously seeking to improve practice in the field of health and social care?

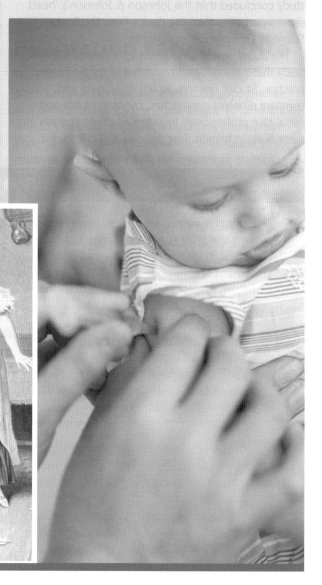

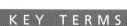

KEY TERMS

Audit
This refers to the monitoring of current practice or policy and its evaluation against predefined standards.

Meta-analysis
A quantitative systematic review.

Synthesised
Distilled and fused into a digest or detailed summary

Systematic review
A systematic analysis of other analyses.

Investigating existing ways and breaking new ground

In care practice and policy, if a measure or approach to care is working well, there is no immediate need to change it. Why, for example, replace an effective treatment for managing wounds if a current technique works well? On the other hand, when the evaluation of contemporary approaches to care practice indicates that they are inadequate, inappropriate or, in some cases, even damaging, then it is time to break new ground. If, say, a policy for helping more working-class students to study medicine fails to achieve its goal, a fresh approach is called for.

Some of the methods that researchers use when they investigate current practice and when they try out new approaches are similar or even the same, so there is some overlap. For example, an experiment can help to determine if an existing surgical procedure is better than a new technique that is being tested. On the other hand, some methods work better with a particular kind of study. For example, a **systematic review** (see below) is more likely to be used when studying existing practice or policy than in testing new procedures.

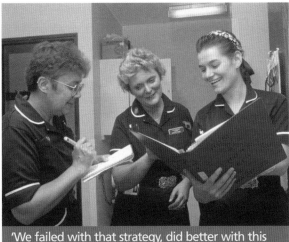

'We failed with that strategy, did better with this one, and can do even better with a new approach.'

Current practice

The main instrument for checking if current treatments and social care arrangements are effective, is called a systematic review. This is an objective investigation of numerous research findings in the same field. Put simply, a systematic review is an analysis of many existing research studies. Among the numerous studies that are reviewed some or all may support the effectiveness of an existing practice or policy. If, however, the results are inconclusive or indicate that present-day arrangements are poor, then it makes

sense to look for new solutions. This turns the systematic review into a 'win–win' research instrument. Either way, care practice and policy benefits.

The systematic review

The systematic review is justifiably regarded as the best method for summarising the key findings of existing and relevant studies in a particular field. High-quality systematic reviews weed out all relevant research studies (both published and unpublished) and then put each one through a rigorous reassessment. The goal is to identify the effectiveness of clinical and social interventions, and often tens, even hundreds, of clinical trials and other measures are examined closely.

Systematic reviews bring together the relevant research findings on a particular care topic, synthesise this evidence and then present it in a structured way.

Figure 3 Main steps in a systematic review

3 Rigorously reassess each relevant study

1 Identify all relevant research studies in a specific care field

Main steps in a systematic review

2 Summarise the key findings of the top studies

Some of the selected studies may well contradict each other. This is the challenge for the systematic reviewer: to summarise the current state of knowledge while including all the studies that meet the selection criteria. The same (or even a more demanding) level of rigour must be applied in the selection process as was originally used in the best studies being examined. Then, the findings from the top studies are **synthesised** (distilled and fused) into a 'bottom line' report.

In some cases, particularly in social care studies, the synthesis is qualitative. But more often, especially in clinical research, the systematic review is presented in quantitative terms. For example, it might be concluded that 90% of the relevant studies indicate that a specific clot-busting medication demonstrated beneficial effects for heart attack survivors. A quantitative systematic review is known as a **meta-analysis**.

The sources that are used to locate relevant studies for systematic review are many, but electronic databases are usually the most important starting point. Journals are also used, as are reference lists and conference papers. It is important to identify key search terms, such as 'child poverty', 'postoperative complications', 'depression', 'random controlled trials', 'NHS best treatments' and 'disability initiatives'. Researchers can also consult databases that already contain systematic reviews – such as the Cochrane Database of Systematic Reviews (CDSR) and the Database of Abstracts of Reviews of Effectiveness (DARE).

Current practice in health and social care can also be evaluated using an **audit**. This is the methodical monitoring of current practice or policy and its evaluation against predefined standards.

Audits can be planned for future checks as well, as in, for example, the regular UK audits of child poverty. In 1999, the Prime Minister, Mr Blair (picture below), set the social policy auditors an historic task: the elimination of child poverty within 20 years. The government subsequently produced targets for reducing child poverty by at least a quarter by 2004/05, halving it by 2010/11, and eliminating it by 2020.

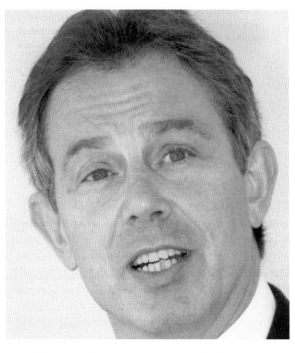

Audits often involve a range of methods – document checks (e.g. review of social work case notes), checking outcomes against pre-defined targets (e.g. monitoring the aim of reducing hospital waiting lists) and focus-group interviews (e.g. obtaining the views of a group of disabled people on the accessibility of local public transport).

Another way of measuring the effectiveness of a health or social care measure is the experiment, a method that we will discuss in more detail in Topic 5. Experiments are more commonly used in new research and we will therefore briefly consider their use below.

Breaking new ground

Innovative (new) research seeks to generate new knowledge by using scientific methods – usually experiments – to test hypotheses. The technical procedure is essentially the same as when researchers use experiments to investigate the effectiveness of existing practice, but the aim now is to test new suggestions.

There are different kinds of experiment, but at its most basic, an experiment is used to measure the effects of an intervention. It typically begins with a 'pre-test' (e.g. patients' anxiety levels before therapy), followed by an intervention (e.g. 20 hours of therapy with a clinical psychologist), and, after that, a 'post-test' to measure the effect of the intervention (e.g. a reduction in anxiety). In more sophisticated experiments, researchers expose one group of participants to the intervention and another group to a different intervention or even none at all. The object is to compare results between the two groups in order to see if there are different outcomes. But there are ethical issues to consider. Is it ethically justifiable, for example, to offer a promising treatment to one group

A new (and hopefully a better) treatment for John

John is 54 years old and is suffering from cancer. The standard current treatment helps about 70% of patients with this cancer to survive at least 5 years (and probably much longer) after treatment begins. A new but untested treatment might increase the predicted survival rate by 20 percentage points that is, to 90%. John's surgeon has asked him if he would like to participate in a clinical trial whose aim is to find out if the new treatment will work better than the standard treatment, or otherwise. The doctor has explained to John that, if he agrees to take part in an experiment, he will be randomly assigned to one of two treatment groups: one to receive the standard intervention, the other to be treated with the new intervention. Afterwards, the survival rates of both groups will be compared over a period of 5 years in order to find out if the new treatment is more effective. Beforehand, the doctor has explained to John that the 'roll of a dice' will determine if he receives the standard treatment or the new treatment, and, if the latter, there is no guarantee that John's survival prospects will improve. Indeed, it is possible though probably unlikely, that John's condition might worsen as a result of the new regime.

of patients but not to another group in order to find out if the treatment really works?

In practice, it is really quite difficult to conduct proper experiments in non-clinical settings. For this reason, social care researchers sometimes use a less controlled form of experimental investigation when they want to try out new measures. For example, they might compare the effect of introducing free school breakfasts on pupils' learning by comparing two different schools in similar neighbourhoods, the only difference being that one school adopts this measure and the other school does not. Moreover, the two schools will probably have made their own decisions without any prompting from the researcher. This, in itself, could reduce the value of the experiment by making it less likely that the two schools have identical characteristics.

The most common form of experimental research in the care sector is the clinical trial, which we will look at in more detail in Topic 5. Clinical trials are at the cutting edge of health care research because they help care researchers to decide which is the best treatment.

In the example opposite, a new cancer treatment will be tried out on John. Studies like this might improve care for cancer sufferers. On the other hand, there is the risk that the new treatment will not be as effective as the standard treatment.

The best of both worlds

As we have emphasised in this topic, effective practice and policy in the field of health and social care must be based on finding and keeping the best of current measures, as well as continually looking for even better answers. That way, care researchers will avoid having to spend valuable time and resources on constantly having to 'reinvent the wheel', while at the same time identifying and filling important gaps in existing knowledge.

Check your understanding

1 What is the difference between a 'systematic review' and an 'audit'?

2 What is a 'meta-analysis', and when might this research instrument be helpful in care research?

3 Give some examples of care research where the clinical trial might be an appropriate method, and justify your argument.

extension activities

1 In groups, discuss the case of John (above). Think about the risk factors and the ethical considerations involved. In addition to summarising the risks and ethics of the proposed clinical trial, try to make a decision about what you would do if you were in John's position. Present your conclusions to the rest of the class, either in writing or orally.

2 Using the internet and other helpful sources, see what you can find out about an evaluation of an existing social measure and a new medical intervention that are about to be, or have recently been, trialled.

Getting you thinking

1 Identify three principles or types of behaviour that you think should be part of an 'ethical' approach to research ('being honest' is an example).

2 Can you think of any circumstances in which it is acceptable for a researcher to harm the people whom they study, provided that this brings benefits to society at large?

3 Why is it important that strict ethical guidelines govern the conduct of research?

4 What kind of ethical safeguards would you expect to be in place before you agreed to participate in a care-related research study?

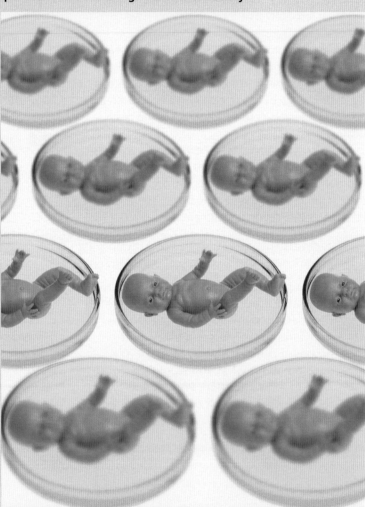

KEY TERMS

Beneficence
Acts of charity or generosity that go beyond what people are normally expected to do.

Distributive justice
This refers to the fair distribution of goods and services according to need.

Ethics
A code of behaviour based on moral principles.

Morality
This refers to ideas about 'goodness' and 'badness'.

Research ethics

In order to ensure that the public can have confidence in and benefit from care research, it is essential that high standards of science and **ethics** are put in place. The term ethics refers to the values and standards of behaviour that a person adopts in relation to others. For example, a care researcher has an ethical duty to seek to help those whom she studies.

The overriding ethical duty of care researchers is to protect those whom they study. This principle is stated in the Department of Health's Research Governance Framework for Health and Social Care (2005, Second Edition), which sets out standards for improving ethical and scientific quality and preventing misconduct and poor performance. In this document, the Department of Health provides a concise checklist of ethical principles (see below) that, according to the Department, can contribute towards a quality research culture in health and social care:

Researchers must respect the rights of human participants in research settings, just as they would do in other circumstances. In short, there is no special permission to ignore ethical principles when conducting research, even if the research findings will be later used in a good cause.

The need for ethics in care research

Research clearly contributes much to good practice in health and social care. But there are times when researchers have failed to protect the safety of those whom they study. For example, during the nineteenth and early twentieth centuries, the risks associated with being a research subject often fell upon poor patients, while the benefits of medical research generally flowed to well-off patients.

The worst abuses of human participants in experiments have concerned unwilling prisoners, especially concentration camp prisoners during the Second World War. John Cornwell's (2003) book, *Hitler's Scientists: Science, War and the Devil's Pact*, is a chilling tale of scientific practice that was conducted with no regard to the rights and dignity of humans. The poison gas scientists who served Hitler used chemical science to terrible effect, including the murder of Jews and other 'lives not worth living'. As well as being profoundly unethical, much of what passed as Nazi science was also factually flawed – the so-called 'scientists' who exploited Jews as human 'guinea pigs' making nonsensical assumptions about genetics.

In many respects, science has moved on, both ethically and factually, since the era of the Third Reich, but there are some notable exceptions. Arms dealers, new merchants of poison gas and drug barons still openly ply their terrible trade in some parts of the world, and they need (and get) scientists to make this possible.

Another cause for ethical concern involves drug

By way of illustration, the writer of this unit was recently involved as a participant in a clinical trial which was testing a new medication for the treatment of heartburn (see below for relevant details). While he hopes that his own modest contribution as a 'guinea pig' may result in benefits to other sufferers, his interest in the project was initially motivated by a desire to improve his own health.

Social justice

Although the principles of respect for persons need to be set out in rules and regulations, it is also important when conducting care research to cultivate the practice of **beneficence**. This term refers to acts of kindness and charity that go beyond mere formal obligation and which constitute a commitment to social justice. For example, the Scottish Centre for Research on Social Justice describes its mission as one of promoting better understanding of, and more informed debate about, the nature of social justice in Scotland, particularly with regard to public policy. The Centre argues, for example, that to improve social justice, housing policies should pay particular attention to the housing needs of the poorest people, through **distributive justice** (fair distribution).

This belief in 'ethical social research' considers that if research can help us to make society a fairer place, then we should use it to do just that – and tackle social suffering, using the best scientific evidence. Policy-makers can then be more confident that their efforts to improve the health and well-being of those in society who are socially disadvantaged are based on sure scientific and ethical foundations.

A clinical trial

As he writes this unit, the author is recording his stomach problems on an electronic patient diary supplied by a clinic that is conducting a clinical trial on the effects of a new medication for heartburn (reflux of stomach acid into the oesophagus).

The clinic asked for and obtained the author's consent. Each morning, he takes two tablets, which is one of four randomly selected possible treatments. The researchers will later seek to determine which one of the four treatments offers the best result.

Before going to bed and when he gets up, the patient switches on an electronic diary and answers some closed questions about his condition, such as 'During the night how would you rate your heartburn symptoms on this scale?' Because he completes two daily reports, it is not too difficult for him to remember his symptoms. He knows too that regular checks are made on his reports because the clinic downloads data at regular intervals. This keeps the patient on his toes and he always completes the electronic diary, as required.

But what's in it for him? Quite a lot, actually. The doctor has checked his stomach before, during and after the clinical trial, and has confirmed that things have improved. The patient has also reported that he feels a lot better. Yes, there are some risks, and he hopes that they do not come to anything. He also hopes that he has contributed towards helping other patients with similar symptoms. That really would be a wonderful outcome!

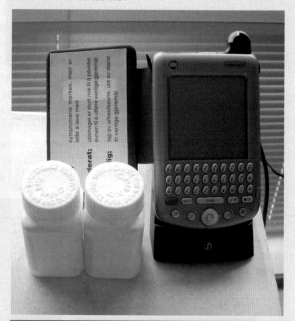

The author's electronic diary and two boxes of tablets

John Dee is a local authority councillor in Midshire. He is passionate about reducing poverty in Midshire. He believes that the local authority could do much more to tackle poverty experienced by older people and children in particular. John has approached both the population planning and the social services teams at the council to consider his ideas for a series of projects to tackle poverty in the local area.

At the first meeting John pointed out to his colleagues that tackling poverty is a government priority. He quoted from a speech given to the Labour Party Annual Conference in 2004 by Gordon Brown, the Chancellor of the Exchequer, who said:

'We have lifted one million children and more than one million pensioners out of poverty. But we must do more.'

John Dee is keen to do more. However, whilst his colleagues agree with this sentiment they told John that research into the numbers of people in poverty in Midshire and the possible causes of this would be required before any work could be done on tackling this social justice issue.

Check your understanding

1 Identify three examples of ethical principles used in research.

2 Explain why high ethical standards are an essential part of any care research study.

3 Is it ever ethically justifiable to deceive research participants when conducting research?

4 What is 'distributive justice' and how can it be applied to ethical social policies?

177

Topic 4 Ethics in care research

extension**activities**

1 In groups, use the internet and other sources to find a Research Ethics Guidelines document. Read it carefully and extract and critique the main points in the form of a concise report. Present your report to the rest of the class and invite critical discussion.

2 After you have completed the first assignment, and still in groups, construct your own Research Guidelines in Care Research document.

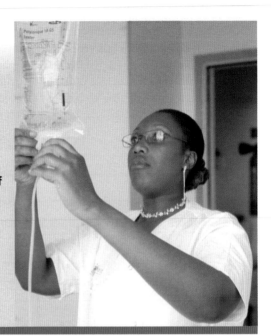

Getting you thinking

1 **What kind of quantitative (or statistical) data might be present in the photograph?**

2 **How could a researcher obtain quantitative data if they wanted to do a piece of research about the use of drips in hospital care?**

3 **How might care practices like that pictured be improved on if research evidence about it was available to care practitioners?**

4 **Can you think of any limitations to research that only uses quantitative data to draw conclusions about care practice?**

KEY TERMS

Clinical trial
An experiment that tries out a potentially helpful procedure on human volunteers in order to find out how well the procedure may or may not work. A clinical trial also attempts to discover and assess risks that may occur during and/or after the procedure.

Control group
A group that is not exposed to a new drug or intervention during a clinical trial but which is compared to a group that is.

Convenience sample
A sample of individuals that is selected for reasons of convenience. That is, the individuals are chosen because they fit the researcher's selection criteria but are not chosen randomly.

Data
Facts that might consist of observations, measurements or other information.

Data analysis
The procedures that scientists use to make sense of the data that they collect.

Descriptive statistics
Statistics that enable researchers to describe what the data are, without drawing conclusions about why this is so.

Double-blind assignment
Assignment of people to experimental and control groups such that neither the researcher nor the participants know who is in which group while the research study is being carried out.

Experiment
A research procedure that exposes one of two samples to an intervention (e.g. a new medical treatment) in order to see if the intervention has an effect.

Experimental group
A group that is exposed to an intervention.

Hawthorne effect
The tendency of participants to behave differently when they know they are being studied.

Inferential statistics
Statistics that enable researchers to make inferences from their data to more general conditions.

Matching
A procedure that helps to ensure that any 'extreme' characteristic in an experimental group (someone with an eating disorder, for example) has a match (counterpart) in the control group.

Placebo
An inactive substance or procedure that resembles the experimental intervention being studied.

Placebo effect
The tendency of some participants to think they have been affected by a research intervention even though they haven't been. This occurs because they know about the aim of the research in which they are involved and are suggestible.

Population
The total of all persons who possess a common characteristic that that is being studied (e.g. all poor children in Birmingham).

Quasi-experiment
A research study that is based on, or mimics, the experimental method but which doesn't fulfil all of the criteria required in closely controlled experimental research.

Random sample
A sample of individuals selected from a population where all have an equal chance of being chosen.

Sample
A portion of some people in a population.

Survey
A method for obtaining information from a sample of a population.

Research methods

Getting to the right conclusion in scientific care research requires choosing the right tools for the job. In broad terms, there are two ways of achieving this:

1 Using quantitative methods

2 Using qualitative methods.

Quantitative methods

In this topic, we will examine some of the more commonly used methods in quantitative research. It is important, however, to emphasise that some of these methods (with certain variations) are also used in qualitative studies. For example, questionnaires containing closed questions (such as 'Tick one of the boxes') produce quantitative data, whereas those with open questions (such as 'Tell me in your own words') yield qualitative data. It is, of course, entirely possible – and often very useful – to construct questionnaires that are made up of a mixture of closed and open questions.

Quantitative research seeks answers to questions about quantity, such as:

- How many disabled people find it hard to use public transport?

- Does being male predict a higher risk of suicide?

- How might this surgical procedure help to cure more patients?

The numbers, words and other factual information that researchers collect are called data, and by carefully examining these data, researchers can draw scientific conclusions. Such conclusions can, in turn, help care professionals to make sound evidence-based decisions.

Data analysis in quantitative research

Data analysis describes the procedures that researchers use to make sense of the information that they collect. In this topic, we will look at data that are expressed in numbers. In Topic 6, we will turn our attention to data in the form of words.

Quantitative research puts data into numbers. It addresses questions such as: How many people in the UK are in poor health, as a percentage of all people? This is an example of **descriptive statistics**. These statistics let the numbers speak for themselves. They simply describe what the data are, without drawing conclusions about why this is so. Examples of descriptive statistics include total numbers, percentages and averages.

If we want to make inferences from our data apply to more general conditions, **inferential statistics** will help us to do this. Statistics of this kind tell us more than the data at hand. They help us to infer, for example, if the risk of poor health in the UK is related to social class, ethnicity, place of residence, and so forth. Inferential statistics enable researchers to go beyond a description of what is happening because they enable them to offer explanations about why something is happening. For example, inferential statistics would be needed to explain why there are differences in health outcomes between different areas of the UK.

When using inferential statistics, it is important to distinguish between a **population** and a **sample**. A population describes the total of all persons who possess a common characteristic that is being studied. This might be a national population (e.g. all British citizens), but more often it will be a smaller group, such as all poor children in Birmingham. Because populations are large and often difficult and expensive to study, researchers usually conduct a **survey** of a sample of the total population. A survey is a data-collecting method that typically obtains information from a sample – a portion of some people in a population.

Another important research procedure, the **experiment**, also makes use of samples. Unlike the survey, however, which does not attempt to influence the sample of individuals that it studies, an experiment does just that. Essentially, an experiment exposes one of two samples to an intervention (e.g. a new medical treatment) in order to see if the intervention has an effect. Surveys and experiments are widely used in quantitative care research, and we will examine both in this topic.

If a researcher wants to infer a finding from a sample that is likely to be the same (or very similar) in the population that the sample represents, then it is best to use a **random sample**. In a random sample, all individuals in a given population have an equal chance of being chosen for the sample. This ensures that a randomly selected sample is a representative cross-section of the population.

A simple way of understanding a representative cross-section is to think of a big apple pie. I can get a good idea of what the whole pie tastes like just by eating a slice of it. Similarly, if I interview a representative sample of one-parent mothers in Glasgow, I can get a good idea of what the rest of the one-parent mothers in the city think .

A common instrument for collecting information from a representative (and, sometimes, a non-representative) sample of individuals is the survey. There is no hard and fast rule for sample size that can be used for all surveys. Even so, researchers often find that a moderate sample size is sufficient for statistical purposes. For example, some national polls use samples of about 1,000 people to obtain representative information about national attitudes and opinions (e.g. the general public's view on nurses' pay).

Although random samples are best for survey research, not all surveys use random selection. Sometimes, a sample is chosen for reasons of convenience – e.g. people near at hand and easy to recruit – a convenience sample. A sample of this kind is non-random and therefore, cannot be considered as representative of a wider population.

The survey

The survey is commonly used in care research and it enables researchers to collect data from small, medium or large populations. Most surveys collect information using questionnaires. Typically, the researcher selects a sample of respondents from a population and supplies a questionnaire, either for the person being surveyed to complete or to be completed by the interviewer in a face-to-face or telephone interview. While paper and pencil can do the job, today field researchers often use Computer Assisted Personal Interviewing (CAPI).

When UK policymakers want accurate information about the state of the nation's health and well-being, they usually consult the government's social research organisation: the Social Survey Division of the Office for National Statistics. The Social Survey Division (or just Social Survey, as it is also called) mainly uses interviews, either face-to-face or by telephone, when it collects information. Social Survey typically employs random sampling methods and often selects respondents from the Post Office's list of addresses throughout the country.

Questionnaires/interviews in survey research

In quantitative research, questionnaires and interviews often use a closed-question design – using questions of the 'circle one' (single-coded) kind, such as:

Figure 7 Single-coded question design

How many pints of beer did you drink yesterday? (circle one)

| none | 1 | 2 | 3 | 4 | 5 | 6 or more |

If you were asked to complete questions like this yourself, the research method would be defined as a 'self-completed' questionnaire. If an interviewer did the circling for you, then the method would be termed an 'interviewer-completed' questionnaire. For simplicity's sake, we have used the term 'circle one' to

denote a closed-question design. In practice, however, this design can also incorporate so-called 'multi-coded' questions that let respondents select a number of responses to one question, such as:

Figure 8 Multi-coded question design

Which of these qualities do you value in a GP? (circle one or more)

Sound clinical skills

Kind disposition

Matter-of-fact manner

None of the above.

For research purposes, a closed-question design has the advantage of obtaining greater uniformity of measurement and of being more easily coded (and therefore quantified). A disadvantage, however, is of forcing respondents to make what they think are inappropriate or insufficient choices from a predefined

A survey to assess patient satisfaction

The Rand Corporation is a US-based, non-profit Think Tank that has produced many practical surveys for improving quality of care. Here is a concise description of a Rand health survey.

Dialysis Patient Satisfaction Survey
The aim of this survey is to assess renal patients' satisfaction with their health care. This includes satisfaction with their specialist kidney doctor, the nurses they see at the dialysis clinic, other staff at the dialysis clinic and at their primary kidney doctor's office, the physical environment at the clinic, and their health plan.

The survey is designed to be self-administered by mail, but it could easily be adapted to be interviewer-administered. Average interview time during the pretest was 13 minutes. The questionnaire contains 40 closed questions, and the respondent checks off one or more responses for each question. There is also one open-ended question at the end of the questionnaire for respondent comments.

Question 4 of the questionnaire asks respondents to rate the kidney doctor they saw most often in the last six months on a scale from 0 to 10, where 0 is the worst kidney doctor possible, and 10 is the best kidney doctor possible.

How might this kind of patient rating scale help healthcare professionals to assess their own performance?

list of possible options. Moreover, a circle or a tick does not permit a deeper, more accurate response.

The decision to use a self-completed questionnaire or to have an interviewer pose questions directly rests with the researcher. Each technique has its strengths and limitations, but overall the interview arguably has the edge. Survey respondents are usually more willing to answer questions in a face-to-face situation than to fill out a questionnaire and send it back. So response rates for face-to-face interviews tend to be relatively high. Moreover, the presence of an interviewer makes it easier to clarify questions that may be confusing – and to include respondents who have various disabilities, such as visual impairment.

Figure 9 *Advantages and disadvantages of mail (postal or electronic) questionnaires*

Advantages

- They enable researchers to reach a widely dispersed audience relatively easily and quickly.

- In general, mail questionnaires are cost-effective with regard to distribution and return.

- The risk of the respondent being biased by the presence of an interviewer is eliminated.

Disadvantages

- The response rate for questionnaires is often notoriously low (e.g. because of general indifference or, in the case of internet questionnaires, inability to handle electronic data).

- Low response rates reduce the likelihood that a sample is representative, not just because too few people reply, but also because those who do might be untypical (e.g. they may have strong views on a particular issue).

- It is often difficult for the respondent to seek clarification if she or he does not understand a question or an instruction.

The experiment

The true experiment is the backbone of evidence-based medical practice, forming the basis of **clinical trial**s. In social care research, it is much more common to use what is called a '**quasi-experiment**'. Either way, the essential feature of all experiments is to test if a specific intervention (e.g. a new drug therapy or a new wheelchair design) has an independent effect (e.g. a higher cure rate or improved mobility).

At its most basic level, the true experiment requires the random assignment of participants to one of two groups: an **experimental group**, which is exposed to an intervention, and a **control group**, which is not exposed. Ideally, the random assignment should be double blind, meaning that neither the researcher nor the participants know who's in what group. This precaution helps guard against the **Hawthorne Effect** and the **Placebo Effect**.

The Hawthorne Effect refers to the tendency of participants to behave differently when they know they are being studied, especially if they think they have been singled out for some experimental intervention. The Placebo Effect refers to the tendency of some participants to think they have been affected by a research intervention even though they haven't been. This occurs because they know about the aim of the research in which they are involved and are suggestible.

From the outset, the persons in the experimental and control groups should have broadly similar pre-test characteristics: e.g. Diabetes 1 patients, heroin users, overweight persons, and so on. Randomisation will take care of some of this, but the procedure known as **matching** (which is more often associated with quasi-experiments) will also help. Matching helps to ensure that any 'extreme' characteristic in one group (someone with an eating disorder, for instance)

Figure 10 *Advantages and disadvantages of face-to-face interviews*

Advantages

- Once an interview is underway, the response rate is guaranteed and immediate.

- They enable the interviewer to clarify anything that the interviewee might not understand.

- It is easier for the interviewer to use relevant prompts, such as pictures.

Disadvantages

- Interviews can be expensive (e.g. owing to travel and salary costs).

- Interviews are often very time-consuming.

- Some interviewees are likely to give biased responses when face-to-face with a researcher (e.g., because they give the answer that they think the researcher wants to hear).

has a match (counterpart) in the other group.

Examples of experimental interventions include medications, combinations of medications, vaccines, devices and lifestyle changes. In clinical trials, the participants in the control group are usually given a placebo, which is an inactive substance or procedure that resembles the experimental intervention being studied. Care researchers can then compare notes between the two groups. If there are statistically significant outcomes here – e.g. people in the experimental group are in markedly better health compared to people in the control group – then it can be inferred that the intervention has had an independent effect – in this case, a beneficial one. The true experiment can also be used to compare one care intervention with another intervention, and both to a control group, in which case there would be two experimental groups and one control group.

True experiments are the first choice of medical researchers. However, social researchers, who have to deal with many more factors than their medical colleagues, are more likely to use quasi-experiments. The word 'quasi' means 'almost', so our second type of experiment, the quasi-experiment, can be defined as 'almost a true experiment'. A quasi-experiment, unlike a true experiment, does not randomly assign participants to experimental and control groups. For example, someone measuring the effects of a new social work strategy in a town might try to find a similar town in the same region where the new initiative is not in use.

This other town would need to have demographic characteristics (e.g., size, ethnic variation, etc) that are broadly similar to the experimental town. Strictly speaking, the non-experimental town is not a 'control' group, but a 'comparison' group. That said, the aim of a quasi-experiment, as with a true experiment, is to find out if an intervention has had an independent effect.

Figure 11 *Advantages and disadvantages of experiments*

Advantages

- The experiment is probably the best research method for identifying and measuring cause and effect – particularly important, for example, in clinical trials.

- Experiments, particularly when used in medical research, give researchers a lot of control over the variables that they are investigating.

- Because experiments employ standardised procedures and measures, tests can be repeated over and over again in order to find out if the same results are obtained.

Disadvantages

- Some experimental designs create rather artificial settings by 'over-controlling' what in normal circumstances would be a more 'fuzzy' reality.

- Related to the first point, it is not always possible, especially in social care research, to take account of all the possible (often hidden) influences that form part of a complex social world.

- It can be difficult to obtain representative samples when conducting experiments.

Clinical trials

In health care research, researchers often use experiments to test new procedures in the laboratory and on non-human animals. Afterwards, the experimental procedures with the most promising results are then tested in clinical trials. A clinical trial tries out a potentially helpful procedure on human volunteers in order to find out how well the procedure may or may not work. A trial also attempts to discover and assess risks that may occur during and/or after the procedure. The clinical trial is one of the most important applications of experimental investigation in care research. In very broad terms, there are three types of clinical trials (see below).

Clinical trials raise numerous ethical questions, not least the risk that the procedure being trialled might do more harm than (any) good. That said, the clinical trial is a very effective way to find treatments that work in people.

Figure 12 *Types of clinical trial*

- Treatment trials, which test new treatments, such as new drugs and surgical techniques which may lead to a cure or more effective palliation (reduction of pain or other discomfort).

- Prevention trials, which test new approaches, such as new medicines and lifestyle choices which may lower the risk of a disease occurring in the first place or its re-occurrence after successful treatment.

- Screening trials, which test new ways of detecting and diagnosing illness, especially in its early stages, so that effective interventions can be made.

Check your understanding

1 What are the essential characteristics of quantitative data?

2 How can quantitative data help care researchers to assess the effects of care interventions?

3 What are the advantages of using closed questions in survey research?

4 What are the essential similarities and differences between 'true experiments' and 'quasi-experiments'?

extension**activities**

1 Identify a health or social care issue that could be investigated through an experiment or clinical trial. Describe how the experiment could be carried out, who the participants would be and what the investigation would be hoping to find out. You should also consider whether the proposed research raises any ethical issues.

2 Imagine that you are going to interview a health professional on ways to improve mental health services for children and young people. Construct a short questionnaire using closed questions that would help you obtain relevant information from this respondent during the interview.

Topic 5 Quantitative research

Qualitative research

Getting you thinking

1 What can researchers learn by getting respondents to tell 'their story' in their own words?

2 How do you think a conversation between friends might be different to an interview for research purposes?

3 How might the detailed observation of a care practice, such as a ward round, help researchers to offer care professionals valuable advice?

4 Can you think of any limitations to research that only uses qualitative data to draw conclusions about care practice?

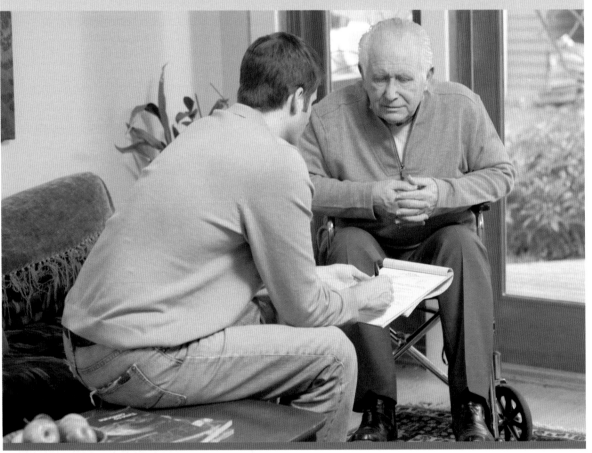

KEY TERMS

Interview guide
A basic checklist of themes that guides an interviewer on the particular issues that they should explore.

Observation
In qualitative research, this procedure usually refers to watching people in their natural settings.

Open-ended interview
An informal interview in which the sequence and wording of the questions are not decided in advance.

Qualitative methods

In the last topic, we looked at data that are expressed in numbers. In order to obtain a broader view of care issues, we also need to consider data that are expressed in words. For this purpose, we can use qualitative methods. Suppose, for example, researchers are investigating the debilitating psychological effects of poverty. Numbers are important (e.g. percentage of poor people who have psychological disorders), but so too are direct quotations about what it feels like to be poor. In this particular setting, researchers need to know about the real-life experiences of poverty that the statistics have concealed. By using qualitative methods they can research further, and obtain rich data – in the form of direct quotation and careful description of observed behaviours.

Qualitative research usually seeks to answer questions about what individuals express in their own words, such as:

1 What do disabled people have to say about public transport?

2 How do men who have suicidal dispositions describe their mental state?

3 What do surgeons think about trying out new surgical procedures?

Data analysis in qualitative research

Qualitative researchers obtain data that contain much personal opinion, story and feelings. The aim is to reconstruct, as far as is possible, the experiences of the participants in their own words, keeping faith with their perceptions. The analysis is their analysis, or as close to this as is achievable.

A large amount of data analysis in qualitative research involves presenting excerpts from transcripts of interviews, thereby capturing the participant's 'voice'. These dialogues are then 'clarified' by the researcher by being sorted into major themes. One way of doing this is by drawing up a list of categories and 'cutting and pasting' each segment of transcribed interview data into one of these categories. This can be done either manually or by using computer software. The different interviewees' remarks on a particular theme can then be compared with one another, and more sophisticated comparisons can be made, like: 'Did individuals who held opinion X also tend to express opinion Y?' From a scientific point of view, it also helps if qualitative researchers constantly check with each other and/or the participants to see if they agree about what segments fit into which categories.

In order to explore the goal of capturing the participants' voice a little further, let us have a look at a qualitative study carried out by Professor Stein Erik Ohna (2004) in Norway. Ohna wanted to find out how deaf people relate to each other and to hearing persons. In order to do this, he had 'guided conversations' (in the form of **open-ended interview**s) with 22 deaf people, using sign language. The interviews were video-recorded, and the text was translated from sign language into standard text. All of the respondents received a copy of the translation in order to check that the interviewer's interpretation corresponded with theirs.

Here is an excerpt from one of the interviews, where Gro (20 years old) tells how she, as a 12-year-old girl, discovered that not everyone understands sign language:

Interviewer: When did you discover you were deaf?

Gro: … when I was 12 years old. When I was supposed to be an 'adult' and should act as an adult. Before, well, I knew I was deaf, but I didn't understand what it meant to be deaf. I just went straight up to a man I didn't know, and then I said. 'Hi, I am deaf; you must use sign language with me'. Even when he didn't know my language, I said this. I took it for granted that everybody knew sign language because I am deaf. So my mother explained to me then.

These are fragments of a dialogue, presented as the literal words of the respondent. Next, comes the researcher's 'clarification', his 'reading between the lines', his interpretation:

Now she relates her discovery of what it means to be deaf to the moment when she, as a teenager, should behave as an 'adult'. She says that she always knew she was deaf, but previously did not understand what it meant to be deaf.

Based on these and other words in the interview transcript, Ohna begins to draw out central categories that emerge from the data. For example, he thinks that Gro's sense of deafness changes when she sees a connection between her hearing loss and her relationships with hearing persons. Being deaf starts to mean that something is wrong and makes her feel abnormal. Ohna uses the category (or concept) of 'alienation' (in this case, being cut off from hearing persons) to capture Gro's unease. Referring to another remark from Gro – 'I can only be myself with other deaf persons' – Ohna sees this as an indication of her sense of fitting in with her 'own kind'. In other words, Gro can be herself among people like her.

Census and epidemiological data

Getting you thinking

1 How could you find out how many people live in your local area and what their health and social care needs are?

2 What sources of data are available to care professionals who are involved in planning health and social care services in your area?

3 Identify three examples of diseases or viruses that could pose a major threat to the health of the UK population.

4 How might detailed data on past epidemics of infectious disease help care practitioners and planners to prevent or minimise the impact of future epidemics?

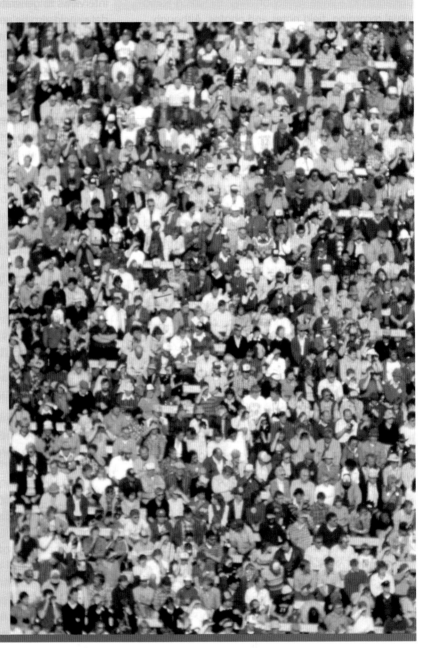

KEY TERMS

Census
A national headcount of people and households.

Epidemiology
The scientific study of patterns of disease in human and other populations.

Hypertensive
Having persistent high blood pressure.

Statistics used to support care practice and policy

Data from the **Census** and epidemiological studies help care practitioners and policymakers to plan, implement and evaluate health and social care services. Both sources provide statistics on the state of the nation: the Census on a wide range of issues, **epidemiology** on the specific area of patterns of disease.

The Census

The Census is a survey of all people and households in the nation. It provides vital information from national to local level for policymakers and care professionals. The most recent Census was in 2001, and the next one will be taken in 2011. The 2001 Census offers a goldmine of health and care data. Here are a few examples that apply to England and Wales:

- Nearly 9.5 million people (18.2%) say they have a long-term illness, health problem or disability that limits their daily activities or the work they could do. Of these, 4.3 million are of working age (16–64 for men; 16–59 for women), which is more than 1 in 8 of the age group.

- The proportion of people with a limiting long-term illness has gone up since 1991, when 13.3% of the population of England and Wales were recorded as having a long-term illness. In the same period, there has been a 3.4% increase in the number of affected people aged 65 and over.

- There are 5.2 million people providing unpaid care, which is one in ten of the population. Carers are people looking after or giving help to family, friends, neighbours or others, because of long-term physical or psychological ill-health or disability, or problems related to old age.

The main results of the 2001 Census are available free on the Office for National Statistics (ONS) website, so go online and have a look. (Do consult a range of issues – but you should really pay particular attention to health and social care data.)

The Census data that have been released so far indicate a number of key changes in the nation's population profile over the last ten years. For example, the proportion of households containing a married couple – essentially the norm for past generations – is now about 45% of all households, compared with 55% in 1991, and 64% in 1981. The overall proportion of one-person households has also increased, up from 26% in 1991 to 30%. People are living longer, but are spending more of that time alone.

Such data have clear social policy implications. Living longer, particularly doing so alone, places new demands on health and social services. Age brings with it a higher risk of diseases such as cancer, osteoporosis and dementia. It also requires society to develop more extensive and different care arrangements. There are, of course, opportunities to seize when a society increases its overall longevity. Older people are working longer (not always willingly), thereby bringing depth of experience to the workforce and boosting the nation's economy. It is also good to know that, due largely to the implementation of evidence-based policies and practices, we can look forward to more time with our grandchildren, friends and neighbours and, in most cases, to an extended period of leisure.

Epidemiological studies

As already indicated, the Census covers a wide range of issues. So, in order to sharpen the focus on care (and more specifically, health) issues, researchers also carry out and consult epidemiological studies. Unlike the Census, which takes account of the entire national population, epidemiological research is based on samples. Provided that these samples are properly selected, statistical tests will make it possible to infer more general patterns.

'Europe's high blood pressure crisis is spinning out of control', reported *Time* (front cover) on 13 December 2004. Epidemiological research findings indicate that in 2003 (before the entry of ten new member states), 50 million people in the then European Union – 16.5% of those 15 and older – were **hypertensive** (that is, suffering from persistent high blood pressure). Unless we take steps to change the way we live (more exercise and healthy eating) perhaps as many of half of us will die from either heart disease or stroke – hypertension's all too common final consequences.

Epidemiology – the study of patterns of disease in populations – is concerned with causes and effects. No wonder then that epidemiologists are finding statistical links between bad lifestyle choices (not forgetting that for the poor, such choices are often 'forced' upon them) and increasing risks of hypertension. Too many Europeans smoke, drink heavily, eat fast and processed food and, crucially, take too little exercise.

To tackle the European (and global) problem of hypertension, epidemiologists are having to deal with many factors – especially people's diet and lifestyle. Countries such as Finland and Poland, where diets are high in unhealthy fat and low in fruit and vegetables, will need to change their ways. So too must the most

Hypertension: a stealth killer

In a special report on hypertension, which it defines as a stealth killer, *Time* magazine notes that the sinister thing about the condition is that most of the creeping harm it does occurs without the patient knowing it. People with less severe hypertension may notice nothing at all until disaster strikes. One of the more common of such alarming pressure-related events is a heart attack. The brain can take a tragic 'hit' too in the form of a stroke.

Doctors have now identified a category of risk called prehypertension, which defines a borderline blood pressure now considered a warning sign of trouble to come. Worryingly, it is not just middle-aged and older people who are turning up at the doctor's surgery. So are children. It is therefore important for everyone to consider how their lifestyle choices might help to reduce their risk of developing hypertension.

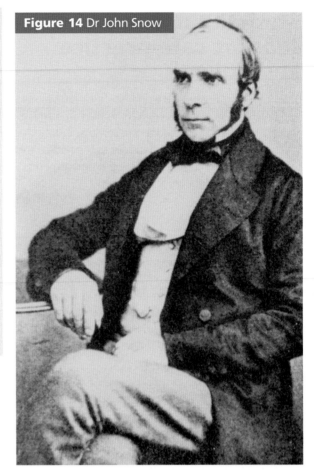

Figure 14 Dr John Snow

at-risk population – children. It is now recommended that taking blood pressure becomes a routine part of any visit to the paediatrician. Reducing weight (especially abdominal fat) and quitting smoking are also vital steps, as is cutting down on drinking. Exercise is crucial because as little as 30 minutes of brisk walking three or four (or preferably seven) days a week lowers overall blood pressure.

The above issue – high blood pressure – illustrates the important contribution that epidemiology makes with regard to identifying the distribution of health problems. Such data provide other researchers, practitioners and policymakers with better opportunities to tackle many diseases that have reached epidemic levels.

As a discipline, epidemiology owes much to the pioneering work of John Snow (1813–1858), an unassuming London physician who came to prominence during the 1830s and 1840s, when severe cholera epidemics threatened the city. In 1849, Dr Snow published a pamphlet, *On the Mode of Communication of Cholera*, in which he proposed that cholera was a contagious disease caused by a poison that reproduces in the body and is found in the vomitus and stools of infected patients. He believed that the main mode of transmission was contaminated water.

In 1854, the good doctor proved his theory was right when another serious cholera epidemic hit London. Through painstaking scientific research, Dr Snow found that cholera occurred much more frequently among customers of one water company, the Southwark and Vauxhall. This company drew its water from the lower Thames River, where it had been contaminated with London sewage. A memorable incident deserves special mention. In one neighbourhood, the crossroads of Cambridge Street and Broad Street, there were so many cholera cases that Dr Snow concluded that the cause was centred around the Broad Street pump. On his advice, the pump handle was removed so that the pump could not be used and, subsequently, the epidemic was contained.

The pump handle remains to this day a symbol of effective epidemiology, as does the memory of Dr Snow, whose evidence-based intervention is a good example for scientists involved in disease prevention and control. Like, and inspired by, Dr Snow's pioneering research, they are able to use epidemiological information to prevent and manage diseases that have already started.

Crucial to epidemiology is the measurement of disease in populations that have some characteristics in common – which could be geographical (e.g. all inhabitants of Dublin), age-specific (e.g. all children in the UK aged 5–11), occupational (e.g. all steelworkers in Wales), or diagnostic (e.g. all persons in Glasgow who had diagnosed hypertension in 2006). Within such broad categories, other variables such as social class, sex and ethnicity are often added.

From the 'study population', it is common to select a study sample, preferably a random sample. Thus, for example, if epidemiologists were studying the incidence of headaches in a study population from ten English counties, they might select, say, a 20% sample of all patients aged 16–64 who presented with this symptom during visits to their GPs in 2006. With this design, further extrapolation to the study population might be possible, provided proper statistical procedures were followed. For example, it might be found that headaches are more commonly reported in industrial than in rural communities, among women compared to men, and so forth. These findings would produce other leads to follow up.

Whether using Census or epidemiological data, researchers are able to help care professionals and policy-makers to make informed decisions. Both sources provide the statistics that scientists use when they alert us to the risks that we face from smoking, drug misuse and other threats. There is also good news to be recorded – such as the benefits of regular exercise and healthy eating.

Check your understanding

1 What are the similarities and differences between data from the Census and data from epidemiological studies?

2 Why is Dr John Snow considered to be a pioneer of epidemiology?

3 How might Census and epidemiological data help policy-makers to make informed decisions about healthy school dinners?

4 Why are the data from the Census and epidemiological studies mainly of the quantitative kind?

extension activities

1 The 2001 Census discovered that 5.2 million people in England and Wales (one in ten of the population) provided unpaid care to family, friends, neighbours or others, because of long-term physical or psychological ill-health or disability, or problems related to old age. In groups, write a letter to a local MP or a local notable (such as Head of Social Services) bringing this information to her or his attention and suggesting what resources and policies might helpfully make life better for unpaid carers and the people they care for.

2 Data from the last Census reveal that we are living longer. What health and social care challenges and opportunities does this bring to care policy and practice?

Care research and public policy

Getting you thinking

1 Do you think that independent living is likely to have a positive or a negative effect on a disabled person's development?

2 What kinds of research methods could be used to find out whether independent living has a positive effect on the development and wellbeing of the person pictured?

3 How might research into the availability of independent living help the government to develop its policy on supporting disabled people?

4 If you were the Prime Minister, what areas of care research would you prioritise and why?

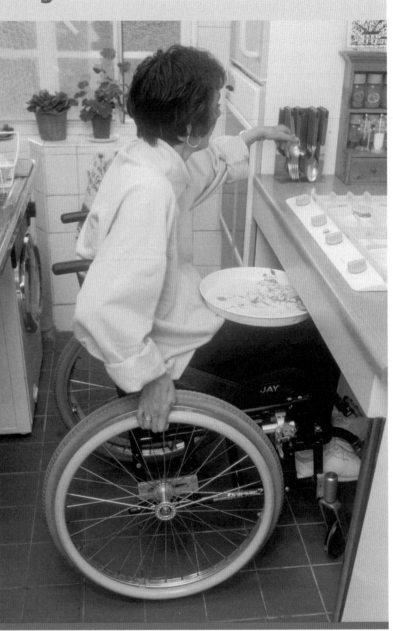

KEY TERMS

Independent living

A philosophy which holds that disabled persons have the right to live with dignity and with appropriate support in their own homes, to participate fully in their communities, and to have control over their lives.

Inclusive design (or Universal design)

The design of products and environments for use by all people, to the greatest extent possible, without the need for adaptation or specialised design.

Evidence-based care policy

It is a government priority that decisions in health and social care policy are based (and can be seen to be based) on evidence. So politicians regularly consult academic experts for research data on the feasibility and impact of national and local policies, and, of course, for new ideas. Scientific research that aims to support health and social care has a long history in the UK. For example, the well-being of British citizens today owes much to the pioneering work of scholars such as:

- Seebohm Rowntree, who, in the early twentieth century, devised a scale to measure the minimum necessities for 'physical efficiency'.

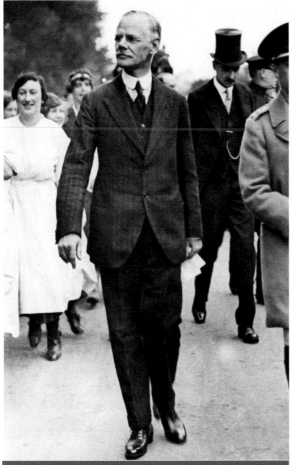

Figure 15 Seebohm Rowntree

- Sidney Webb who, in the same period, drafted the Labour Party's first policy statement, *Labour and the New Social Order* (1918).

- Peter Townsend, who from the late 1940s to this day, combines science and ethics to help in the struggle against the root causes of poverty and inequality.

There has long been a steady flow of data and recommendations into UK policy-making. Researchers from key Think Tanks exert substantial influence here through regular meetings with Cabinet (and Shadow Cabinet) members and via close contacts with civil servants. One such body, the Centre for Evidence-Based Social Services (set up in 1997 and funded by a consortium of Social Services Departments in England) aims to ensure that decisions taken at all levels in Social Services take account of research findings. Another Think Tank, the National Centre for Social Research (NatCen), conducts research that has been guiding health and social policy debates for more than 30 years. Findings from its largest survey, the annual *Health Survey for England*, are used to improve the targeting of national health policies.

'Who could be against evidence-based policy? Who would wish to advocate superstition-based practice?', asks Harry Torrance (2004, p. 187). Imagine a social policy-maker who arrives at decisions on the basis of a crystal ball, or a doctor who prescribes pills according to her patients' favourite colours. The case for applying best evidence to policy and practice decisions is often seen as obvious. But politics is a complex business, and it would be naïve to suppose that policy-makers always act on the best empirical evidence.

Policy settings

Policy decisions involve many more (and less easily controlled) variables than those normally found in care settings, such as hospital wards and social work offices. Deciding, for example, to invest public money in another psychiatric centre in a region or to move two neurosurgical units to one hospital is a complex process. It can involve hospital managers, health professionals, local user groups, the media and politicians. Decisions may be affected by heated emotions rather than by evidence and sober thought. For this reason, it is hard to apply the same degree of rigour in evidence-based policy as it is when using research findings to improve clinical and social practice.

Despite this, the goal of improving services and care practice is always worth pursuing and can lead to important improvements. For example, evidence shows that the incidence and severity of disability in a population can be reduced by:

1 Developing and supporting the daily living skills of disabled people.

2 Making changes to the social and physical environments in which disabled people live.

Acting on such knowledge makes good scientific (and ethical) sense. In this topic we are going to use the disability issue to show how policy-makers can make better use of research findings.

Disability in the UK: what the research shows

The government says that it is committed to improving the life chances of disabled people in the UK. At the same time, it recognises that there is more to do in terms of using research to find ways of, for example, tackling the barriers in attitudes, building design and policies.

In that spirit, the Strategy Unit of the government, which provides strategic evidence-based advice on major policy issues, was asked by Mr Blair to carry out a project that would:

1 Assess the extent to which disabled people were doing less well than non-disabled people, socially and economically.

2 Identify why this is occurring, and what its implications are.

3 Assess what could be done to improve the situation, in particular, by making better use of existing resources.

By systematically sifting the evidence and venturing into the field, researchers at the Strategy Unit found that disabled people are, for example, more likely to have problems with employment, income and education. They are also more likely to face discrimination and prejudice, and they frequently have difficulties with housing and transport.

Such problems are both a cause and a result of disability. Low incomes, non-employment and limited education all independently increase the probability of a person becoming disabled. Moreover, the onset of ill-health or impairment often worsens pre-existing difficulties. The disadvantages that disabled people face, place heavy economic, social and personal costs not only on themselves, but also on their families and friends, on the wider community and on the economy. Instead of being empowered to participate and to be included, many disabled people are forced to depend on welfare benefits and other forms of government support.

Government researchers think that a better and a more just society can be achieved by ensuring that future policies are inclusive, effective and informed. In more concrete terms, the Strategy Unit concludes that:

1 Disabled people's needs should be actively included early on – alongside those of other citizens – within all mainstream policies.

2 Disabled people should receive effective personalised responses to their specific needs, to a high standard, when they need them and for as long as they need them, so that they are empowered as consumers and citizens.

3 Policy design and implementation should be informed by disabled people themselves, by their preferences.

Each of the strategies above is linked to a series of interventions, including the inclusive design of products, services and environments, so that people of all abilities and ages are able to use them in their everyday lives. Examples include 'accessibility audits' of buildings to improve mobility for everyone from wheelchair users to parents pushing prams, and a big-button phone selling as a mainstream product – irrespective of visual impairment.

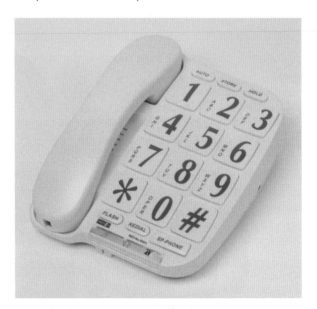

Inclusive design: an example of good practice and policy

Inclusive design (or universal design, as it is often called) refers to the design of products and environments for use by all people, without the need for adaptation or specialised design. It requires designers and manufacturers to actively consider the widest possible audience for their products and services. Take buildings, for example. One way – an inadequate one – is to comply with accessibility standards after the fact – adding a ramp, for example, to 'solve' the problem of inaccessible hospital entrances. With inclusive design, however, an inclusive approach to the total needs of all possible users is an integral part of the original plan, right from the start.

Why, for example, fit door knobs in a social services building when we know that not everyone can use them? We know that lever handles, because of their shape, are usable by nearly everyone. Better still, everyone can use power doors with automatic sensors. Adjustability is another important detail to consider. For example, public buildings, such as hospitals and nursing homes, can be fitted with adjustable sinks at fairly low cost. Just press the button and set the sink to the desired height of the user – high for tall people, low for shorter or seated people.

Inclusive design is a proven cost-effective method for helping all sorts of people, including older persons and those who are disabled, to have a more profitable and productive role in society. Inclusive design allows disabled people 'to boldly go where everyone else has gone before'.

Independent living

The philosophical foundations of inclusive design is to be found in the '**Independent Living** Movement', a lobby group that came out of the disabled people's struggle for civil rights. Independent living is the view that disabled people have the right to live with dignity and with appropriate support in their own homes, to participate fully in their communities, and to control and make decisions about their lives. For independent living to be more than just rhetoric, however, the policy-makers must redesign our built environment so that housing and the transport systems, for example, are made more accessible for disabled (and non-disabled) people.

This is broadly recognised by government policy-makers, who accept the fact that, historically, the tendency has been to see disabled people as dependent and in need of 'care', rather than being recognised as full citizens. At the same time, the Strategy Unit has found that the support that is made available to disabled people today is generally not fitted to the person. Instead, disabled people are expected to fit into the services – which does little to help them realise their rights or voice their needs.

The promise of evidence-based care policy

Unfortunately, there is no guarantee that good research will be put to effective use. Indeed one of the most important studies of health inequalities in the UK, the Black Report of 1980, just sat on library bookshelves instead of provoking the action that was needed to put things right. This is why heath and care professionals and policy-makers should not only examine evidence but also, crucially, look to evidence as a means of improving practice.

Check your understanding

1 Define the terms, 'inclusive design' and 'independent living'.

2 Referring to examples, indicate how research findings have influenced UK social policy in the past.

3 How can emotion get in the way of rational thinking in policy-making circles?

4 What is the relationship between inclusive design and independent living?

extension**activities**

1 According to Walsh *et al.* (2000, p. 352), in a perfect world, 'social policy would be the application of social scientific knowledge in the pursuit of human social needs.' In groups, critically discuss this claim, citing one or more concrete policies along the way. Each group should present their findings and deliberations to the whole class.

2 How do you respond to Harry Torrance's (2004, p. 187) rhetorical question, 'Who could be against evidence-based policy?'

Getting you thinking

1 If you were to conduct a small-scale research project on school or college students' attitudes towards smoking, what method (or methods) would you use to collect the data, and why?

2 Referring to Question 1 above, construct a short questionnaire (about 10 questions) that contains both open and closed questions.

3 How would you find scientific information on the effects of smoking on physical health?

4 What ethical matters would you consider if you were to undertake this research project into smoking in your school or college?

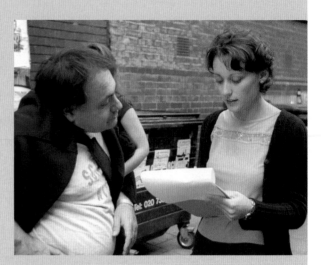

KEY TERMS

Exploratory question
A question that requires an open enquiry.

Doing care research

One of your tasks as an A Level Health & Social Care student is to conduct and write up a small-scale research project. And it really must be 'small-scale'. No one is expecting you to solve the problems of the National Health Service or to eliminate poverty in one stroke!

Here are a few of the main things to take into account:

- Relevance is a key priority. You must make sure that the research issue is linked to the A Level course, so do consult the specification and talk to your tutor before you start any serious work.

- Your own curiosity in an issue will help, because it is very motivating to investigate something that intrigues you.

- Practicality is a must. It is vital to make your project a 'doable' venture, so define clear limits – and keep to them.

- Ethical and safe research is central. Is there a risk that your proposed project might harm you or the people you are studying? If the answer is 'yes' – or even 'possibly' – then you must not proceed.

Choosing a topic to research

A Level teachers often exchange notes at conferences on research projects that students want to carry out, including the obvious unsuitability of some proposals. Two of the boxes on the opposite page show a few examples of unsuitable topics and procedures. But, you may ask, what constitutes a suitable topic or method? The first expert to consult is your teacher. Otherwise, a few suggestions are given in the bottom box on the opposite page.

'I think' or 'Let's see'

Once you have settled on a topic to investigate, it is time to consider your general approach. In broad terms, you need to decide if you are going to test an 'I think' hunch or carry out a 'Let's see' exploration. For the former, you would propose a hypothesis, that is to say, an 'intelligent prediction' and then test it against empirical evidence. For the latter, you would raise an **exploratory question**, which is an open enquiry, and then analyse the empirical evidence that arises.

These two examples illustrate the two approaches:

- Hypothesis: Young people from working-class backgrounds are more likely to smoke than those from middle-class backgrounds.

- Exploratory question: What do teachers think should be done to reduce or remove child poverty in the UK?

Figure 16 *Unsuitable research topics*

- Undertaking field research into criminal and other doubtful behaviours. The only safe way to study these issues is to review, for background purposes, a relevant text or a radio or television broadcast.
- Investigating areas where privacy might be compromised. For example, interviewing people on their sex life is definitely not a good idea. Nor should you breach patients' or social clients' confidentiality rights.
- Adopting overly ambitious aims. To study the lifestyle habits of a representative sample of 16-year-old people in West Yorkshire is better left to the National Office for Statistics. Thinking small with regard to sample size is the right approach.

Figure 17 *Suggested research topics (with examples of suitable research methods)*

- Students' or teachers' actual lifestyle choices, particularly with regard to health matters (questionnaire; interview; diary)

- Students' or teachers' attitudes on a range of lifestyle choices – e.g. smoking in general, smoking during pregnancy, drink–driving, healthy eating, vegetarianism, extreme sports (questionnaire; interview)

- A disabled person's reflections on her or his challenges and successes in life (interview, particularly an unstructured interview). The disabled person should be known to you or to your teacher

- A health or social care professional's views on what constitutes good professional–patient/client relationships (interview, particularly an unstructured interview). The health or social care professional should be known to you or to your teacher

- A 'modest' systematic review of a clinical or social intervention – e.g. a cancer treatment or an inclusive design initiative (internet search engines).

Figure 18 *Unsuitable research procedures*

- Interviewing or observing strangers (e.g. knocking on people's doors). Only interview or observe people whom you know or whom you are sure can be trusted (e.g. your GP, family friends, students at your school or college, etc.)

- Hurting people (including their feelings) and deceiving them. The literature is full of cases of unethical research. Do not follow bad examples.

- Following on from the last point, do not ask respondents to take, reduce or stop prescription medications. Leave such things to qualified health professionals.

Choosing a method

The next thing is to choose a method for carrying out the study – or possibly two methods. More than two methods is inadvisable in a small-scale project.

In order to obtain reliable and valid evidence in the field of health and social care, researchers must ensure that they use the best data-gathering methods. The first step in a good research project is to fit the methods to the study. If, for example, you wanted to find out what the residents of a particular nursing home think about the quality of care they receive, it would be advisable to use a questionnaire or an interview in order to obtain the information. If you do not know the residents, use the teacher as a go-between.

Previously in this unit, you will have read about various methods that care researchers use. For present purposes, we think that you should restrict yourself to just a few methods:

- Systematic reviews (of the modest kind)

- Questionnaires (closed or open questions, or a mixture of both)

- Interviews (closed or open questions, or a mixture of both)

- Observation (qualitative or quantitative).

Combinations of the above methods (e.g. a basic systematic review accompanied by a short questionnaire) would work well, or you might decide that one method is sufficient and appropriate.

Real experiments are not a serious option because they involve complex statistics and very controlled settings. For similar reasons, quasi-experiments are best avoided. Observational methods might be possible, but only if you can gain access to safe relevant settings. If this is feasible, appropriate confidentiality standards should be strictly followed.

Systematic reviews

A trimmed-down version of this method is suitable, either in the introduction, or for the whole project. Let's say, for example, that you want to do a systematic review of the *British Medical Journal's* (BMJ) guidance on the best forms of treatment for Obsessive Compulsive Disorder (OCD), a psychological disorder characterised by persistent worries (e.g. exaggerated fears of contamination) and repetitive behaviours (e.g. excessive hand-washing).

You could, of course, look up the BMJ's own systematic review of interventions. But that would be a case of looking at a systematic review rather than doing your own. It would be much better to enter OCD into a BMJ search engine, and then review the relevant studies that appear over, say, the last 12 months. If you find that the medical terminology is too difficult (actually, compared to other medical journals, many BMJ articles are quite readable), you could consult a different journal. Either way, it is sensible to read fairly widely. Articles, quality newspapers and reports from public bodies are good sources, so use the library and go online.

At this level, the examiners will not expect you to evaluate the reliability and validity of your sources. But do be 'critical' if some of your sources are of the tabloid kind. Otherwise, it is enough that you report and, as appropriate, briefly comment on the relevant findings.

Questionnaires and interviews

First, decide on the degree of structure: structured or unstructured or a combination. A structured questionnaire, whether self-administered or interviewer-administered consists of closed questions. For example, respondents might be asked, 'Do you think that smoking should be banned in all UK pubs and restaurants?': definitely; probably; probably not; definitely not. This type of question is suitable in quantitative research.

At the other end of the spectrum, are unstructured questionnaires and interviews, both of which employ open or semi-structured questions. As indicated earlier, the challenge with unstructured research methods is to give respondents flexibility, whilst not drifting too far from the issue at hand. Also, during the course of an unstructured interview, the researcher may pose further questions in order to pursue interesting leads.

Here are a few examples of unstructured questions:

- Think of a problem you had to deal with affecting your mobility as a wheelchair user. Tell me exactly what happened and how you handled it.

- Think of a day when you had many things to do on a busy ward, and describe how you scheduled your time.

- Describe a time when you had to tell some unpleasant news to a patient. What happened?

Whether or not you use a structured or unstructured (or in-between) format, here are some important points to bear in mind when you construct a questionnaire or interview schedule:

- Ask clear questions, using easily understandable and appropriate language.

- Do not use leading questions, such as, 'Do you agree that the best way to tackle poverty is to get the poor into work?'

- Ask one question at a time, and keep each question short.

- As appropriate, use follow-up questions to obtain more depth and detail. For example, you could follow 'How do you rate the care you receive?: excellent; good; not so good; poor' with: 'Please add comments in your own words.'

- When interviewing, either listen carefully and make notes or, better still (with the respondent's permission) use an audio recorder.

- When interviewing, show respect for the interviewee. She or he is doing you a big favour, so make it clear that you value this.

- When interviewing, try not to sound like an NYPD cop conducting an interrogation. Establish neutrality and a sense of personal rapport.

Observation

As with questionnaires and interviews, the degree of structure is important. If you are going to use quantitative observation, you will need to decide beforehand what you are going to count. Suppose you want to count the number of times a health professional offers advice on not smoking during a 'healthy living' lecture to an audience of college students. Each time such advice is offered, you would count this as one incident. You might go further, and time the duration of each incident.

Should you decide to conduct qualitative observation, you will still have a focus, but, this time, the emphasis will be on watching things unfold as they happen, rather than measuring a predefined set of incidents. The result will be rich description rather than precise counting. In the example of the 'healthy living' lecture, you could write down what you see and hear, thereby providing a running description of activities and settings. Try though to separate important detail from the trivia. We advise you to use non-participant observation because being a participant involves more complex access issues and can also take a lot more time to carry out.

Writing up

Care researchers often use a fairly standard style when they write up their findings in articles or reports. The style is straightforward, so we think it would work well for you as well. As far as writing style is concerned, keep it simple and direct.

Start with an Introduction. This should set out the issue that you are studying, indicating why you have chosen it. For example:

- Reducing child poverty is high on the government's agenda, which is why it deserves my attention in this research project.

- I want to be the kind of nurse/social worker/ local councillor who makes practice/policy decisions on the basis of scientific evidence. This why I am going to interview my GP to find out what she thinks about the relevance of research in her professional work.

- Being ethically committed to the goal of making the built environment more accessible for disabled people, I want to interview a disabled friend in order to record and analyse his 'story'.

Your Introduction should also contain a brief literature review (why not make it a short systematic review?) that highlights a few relevant studies in the field, and, if appropriate, identifies a few gaps that you intend to (partly) fill.

Next, comes the Methods section, in which you should briefly outline the method(s) that you are using for data collection, and say why you have chosen them. In the example of the disabled participant, you might explain your choice of an unstructured interview by saying that it is appropriate because it takes the point of view of the participant.

Then, write up your Results, which should be more factual than analytical. For example, if you were using a structured interview to obtain quantifiable data from local councillors on how they propose to tackle child poverty in your area, you could present the findings in simple tables.

Last, but definitely not least, is the Discussion. This is the 'exciting' part of your report, in which you should tell the reader how you make sense of the data that you have obtained and, as appropriate, how the data might be useful when developing good practice and policy. Be modest here. It is also customary in the Discussion to state any limitations that might affect the validity and reliability of your results and conclusions. Do not be too hard on yourself here.

There are two final sections: the References, which list your sources (consult your teacher on an appropriate standard style) and, if this is applicable, an Appendix containing for example your interview schedule, questionnaire or observation checklist. When you seek advice on a suitable reference style, ask the teacher to brief you on how to cite sources in the main text of your report.

Now you are all set, so get out there and do a good job – and good luck!

Check your understanding

1. Why are ethical and safe procedures vital when you conduct your own research?

2. What is the difference between research that involves a hypothesis and research that is exploratory?

3. Identify a potential small-scale research project in which it would be suitable for you to use a modest systematic review and a questionnaire. Justify your answer.

4. What should the Discussion part of a research report contain, and why?

extension activities

1. Identify a local or national example of a situation where a user of care services has received poor quality care. Investigate the reasons for this, and the response of the care organisation. Suggest ways in which the organisation could improve the quality of services that they offer to ensure that a similar situation doesn't occur again.

2. Use the Department of Health website to research the government's approach to improving the quality of care services. Find and review the main points of the policy titled *A First Class Service: Quality in the New NHS* and any other recent additions to the government's quality-focused policies.

THIS UNIT IS ABOUT SOCIAL ISSUES AND WELFARE NEEDS. It will help you to develop your knowledge and understanding of the perceived social issues and welfare needs in our society. Some of these issues have been with us since records began – and probably before that. Others are new areas of concern and, arguably, a product of more recent social and economic changes. This unit will provide you with the background knowledge that you will need to complete Unit 11 of the Edexcel GCE Health and Social Care award. You will learn about:

• The origins of issues that are of social concern.
• How changes in the size and structure of the population can present new issues and influence welfare provision.
• How social and welfare issues are linked with the political, social and economic circumstances of the society.
• How governments have responded to the identified areas of welfare need.

Social Issues and Welfare Needs

Key questions

By the end of this unit you will be able to use the knowledge and understanding that you develop to answer the following questions:

1 How are social issues linked with the wider social and political culture of the society?

2 How do changes in the population affect the welfare needs of the society?

3 What are the perceived key issues and welfare needs that exist in our society?

4 How have government and other influential groups responded to identified welfare social needs?

Getting you thinking

1 **Should the family look after frail older relatives, or should the state provide residential care?**

2 **Should people put money aside for a 'rainy day' – periods of ill health or unemployment, for example – or should the state help?**

3 **Should the state help only the poor – and others should pay for their care?**

4 **Do social security benefits lead to people becoming scroungers?**

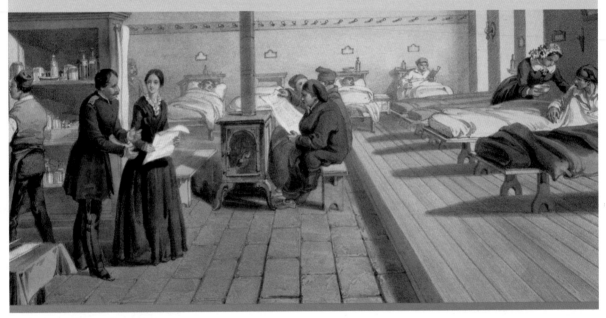

KEY TERMS

Dependency culture
The view that a welfare state will create a society where people rely on state benefits and services rather than working, planning for the future and taking responsibility for their own lives.

Industrialisation
The move towards basing an economy on the production of goods in factories, mills and mines rather than on agriculture and other cottage industries.

Laissez-faire
A view that the government should not interfere in the workings of the economy or in the provision of welfare services. The government should 'leave well alone'.

Post-industrial society
A society whose economy is no longer dependent on the production of goods but is now based on services and office-based occupations.

The New Right
A political viewpoint committed to minimal state provision of welfare services. Taxes should be low and people should decide how they spend their money – making their own provision for health and welfare needs.

The Third Way
An approach to welfare that tries to combine individual freedom and responsibility with state provision for those most in need.

Urban living
Living and working in towns and cities, rather than living and working off the land in agricultural communities.

Welfare state
A term, first used during the 1940s, referring to a system in which government took a primary responsibility for the health and welfare of the nation through the provision or monitoring of services. The services, developed following the Second World War, included the National Health Service, Family Allowance, secondary education for all, and social security benefits and pensions.

Who cares for the vulnerable?

In all societies there are groups of people who are potentially vulnerable. These include children, older people, people with disabilities and the poor, for example. Whether they are supported and how they are supported, however, varies from society to society and at different times in history.

In some societies, the care of the vulnerable is seen as the responsibility of the family or the village. In others, it is principally the responsibility of the state, through community provision. In Israeli kibbutzim, for example, the care of children is seen as the responsibility of the whole community, and not principally the concern of the birth parents. In other societies the care of children is the prime responsibility of their parents, and in some it is the responsibility of the extended family. Attitudes to the vulnerable vary. Those on benefits may be seen as 'lazy scroungers', or their situation may be seen as the result of poor parenting or the inevitable consequence of economic changes. The response to their need will vary according to the dominant attitudes in the society, the views and priorities of government, the wealth of the nation, and how that wealth is distributed and managed.

The state, the church and the family

In England, the state has had some involvement in providing for the poor since Elizabethan times. The 1601 Poor Law allowed officials to collect money from each household in their parish and to distribute it to the needy. There were two kinds of poor law relief – 'outdoor relief' and 'indoor relief'. Outdoor relief was the financial help given to people who were living in their homes but regarded as destitute. In order to receive indoor relief people had to live in an institution, normally called the workhouse. State support, however, was minimal, and personal care was considered to be largely the responsibility of the individual and their family. The poor, it was thought, had only themselves to blame. If people worked hard, saved for 'rainy days' and understood the value of family life they would not be needing relief. Depending on 'poor law relief' was seen as shameful and unnecessary.

The political approach at the time – **laissez faire** – was informed by a view that the government should not interfere in the workings of the economy or in the provision of welfare services. The church and other voluntary groups provided charitable support, but the state 'left well alone'. Not until the opening years of the twentieth century did the state begin to take a proactive role in the care and welfare of its citizens.

The Liberal reforms

The growth of **industrialisation**, **urban living** and the associated poverty, homelessness, ill-health and high mortality rates led social reformers and politicians to the view that the state would have to play a bigger role in the provision of welfare services. The Poor Law provisions were not meeting the needs of the individual or the economy. Employers needed a healthy, educated and reliable workforce. The Liberal government of the early twentieth century played a key role in increasing state involvement in personal health and care services and, some would argue, laid the foundations of the **welfare state** (see below). There was a gradual move away from the laissez-faire economic liberalism of earlier years to a more supportive welfarism by government.

Welfare reforms introduced by the Liberal government (1905–1915)

1906
- The Education (Provision of School Meals) Act
- Providing school dinners for poor children

1907
- The Old Age Pensions Act
- The Labour Exchange Act
- School medical inspections
- The introduction of juvenile courts

1911
- The National Insurance Act

Figure 1 Reasons for state intervention

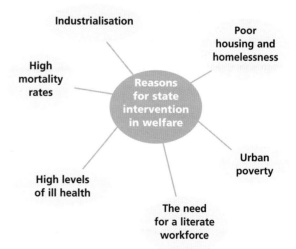

Mrs Brothers is 85 years old and lives quite independently in a small and comfortable flat in the north of England. She has three adult children, one in Australia and the others, both married who live in London. Her GP's surgery is nearby. She has meals-on-wheels delivered three days a week and a home care assistant visits her once a week to help with household chores. This is very different from her childhood memories. Her grandparents lived in the countryside. There were no pensions, they had to pay to see the doctor, they had to find the rent for their house and there was certainly no meals-on-wheels. While her grandfather was working they had managed to pay their bills. They had saved a bit of money too but this money ran out and in the end they were forced to go and live in the workhouse to survive.

The birth of the 'welfare state'

The 1940s saw the development of legislation that reflected an agreement across the main political parties that the state should take an increased responsibility for the funding and provision of welfare services. The specific measures taken were based on the proposals of Sir William Beveridge (1879–1963) and published in his *Report on Social Insurance and Allied Services* (1942), more commonly known as the Beveridge Report. Beveridge based his recommendations on his concern to defeat five 'giant evils' that, despite the measures of the early twentieth century, were still hindering social and economic progress in Britain. The five evils identified were:

• Want (poverty)

• Disease (ill-health and high mortality rates)

• Ignorance (inadequate education)

• Squalor (poor housing and homelessness)

• Idleness (unemployment).

The existence of poverty in Britain was the underlying reason for commissioning the report, but legislation was passed and services introduced that addressed each of the 'five giants'. These measures, together, represented a radical approach to welfare services, building on the initiatives of the Liberals at the turn of the century but representing an agreement that the state had a central role in ensuring basic standards of care and support for all.

The development of what came to be known as the 'welfare state' was a sea change in the approach to welfare. There was a new focus on the role of government, government policy and state intervention in welfare. A brief consideration of the key services – which largely remained in place until the 1970s, and some we would still recognise today – provides a clear picture of how the new system would provide care and support 'from the cradle to the grave'.

Want (poverty)

• Family Allowance Act 1945 introduced a financial payment for children under 15. This did not apply for the first child but applied for all subsequent children.

• The National Insurance Act 1946 allowed for the payment of unemployment benefit, sickness benefit and retirement pension, maternity benefit and widow's pension for all who, when in work, paid weekly from their wages into the national insurance scheme.

• The National Assistance Act 1948 provided a 'safety net' – a minimum income for people who did not pay into the national insurance scheme and were, therefore, not eligible for those benefits.

Disease (ill-health and early mortality)

• The National Health Service Act 1948. Before the introduction of the National Health Service (NHS), if people needed to see a doctor or have hospital treatment they normally had to pay. A national service was central to the post-war welfare reforms and was based on three principles:

1. That health services should be free to all at the point of delivery (when they are actually used).

2. That the service would be truly national, covering the whole population in all parts of the country.

3. That access to services would be based on clinical need (not on the ability to pay).

Idleness (unemployment)

In the post-war period, rather than 'letting well alone' the government intervened in the running of the economy, using the approach of John Maynard Keynes (1883–1946) to support a policy of full employment, which was recommended and necessary for the success of the Beveridge reforms. It was through full employment that his reforms would be financed.

Ignorance (inadequate opportunities for education)

- The 1944 Education Act provided free secondary education for all. Up until this change, most young people in secondary schools paid for their education. Only a minority had free scholarship places. The school leaving age was raised to 15, and grants were made available for people studying at university.

Squalor (poor housing and homelessness)

- The New Towns Act 1946 provided for new towns to be built or developed to address housing shortages, e.g. Stevenage, Welwyn Garden City and Cumbernauld.

- The Town and Country Planning Act 1947 required local authorities to agree building plans for their local area that would benefit the community as a whole.

Welfare and the 'New Right'

The services which arose after the Second World War established a framework for provision and a range of services that remained in place for the generation that followed – and many are still in place today. These were not significantly challenged until the Conservative victory at the 1979 election. The view of this government – led by the first woman prime minister, Margaret Thatcher – was, once again, that the government should interfere as little as possible in the running of the economy and the provision of welfare. The view of her government was that care and welfare should be the responsibility of individuals,

their families or charities. The welfare state, it was argued, supported a **dependency culture**. The **'New Right'** was concerned to see a 'rolling back' of the welfare state.

The 'Third Way'

The Third Way is an approach to welfare associated with 'New Labour' and the Blair governments. Its aim is to steer a line – some would say shape a compromise – between the welfare state's full involvement of government in welfare and the **New Right's** reluctance to intervene in welfare at all. The proponents of the Third Way aim to foster personal and family responsibility for welfare and the quality of community life but, at the same time, provide support to avoid the extremes of deprivation. They are trying to develop a spirit of community in which people accept responsibility for themselves but also for the most vulnerable in society. People would therefore be maintaining a balance between their individual freedom and their responsibilities towards society as a whole.

205

Check your understanding

1. What is meant by the term 'laissez faire'?
2. What is meant by the term 'welfare state'?
3. What were the five 'giant evils' addressed in the Beveridge Report?
4. Why may a welfare state produce a dependency culture?
5. Briefly describe the approach of the new right.

extension activities

1 Using the local library, find out if there was a workhouse in the area where you live. When did it close? What provision was then made for the vulnerable elderly who were not able to live in the community?

2 What provision is in place in your area now for the vulnerable elderly? Would you say that it reflected the provision of a welfare state, the new right or the third way?

Topic 1 Social factors and areas of welfare need

Getting you thinking

Think about all the television adverts that portray 'families'.

1 How is the family typically portrayed in these adverts?

2 Do you think this is a typical family in modern Britain? Give reasons for your answer.

3 Are there often older people in these adverts? If not, why not?

4 Why might people chose to leave their homes and live in another country?

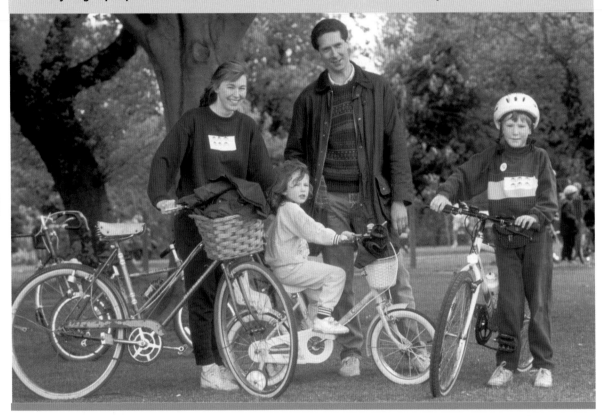

KEY TERMS

Birth rate
The number of live births per thousand of the population in one year.

Death rate
The number of deaths per thousand of the population in one year.

Infant mortality rate
The number of deaths of infants under one year of age, per thousand live births.

Immigration
People coming to live in a country from another country.

Emigration
People leaving a country to live in another country.

Net migration
The difference between the number of immigrants and the number of emigrants coming to and from a specific country.

Life expectancy
A statistical measure which predicts the average number of years a person is likely to live. This could be estimated from any particular age, but is usually expressed as from birth.

Dependent population
The age groups who are dependent on the rest of the population for economic security – young people from 0–16 years, and people over the retirement age.

Population trends and demographic data

Demography is the term used to describe the study of the size and structure of the population. Demographic statistics are used by governments, planners and social scientists to identify changes in population. Some of the things that governments may need to know include:

- the trends in **birth rate** – to inform provision for children and young families

- the trends in **life expectancy** – to inform provision for older people

- levels of unemployment

- regional differences in the size and structure of the populations

- levels of migration, both within countries and between countries.

The census

Every ten years since 1801, with the exception of 1941, there has been a census – a detailed count of the population. The last census was in 2001, and the next is planned for 2011. At the census, every householder is required by law to provide details of everyone staying in their household on the designated night. Included in the census are people in hospitals, hotels, prisons and all other institutions. In addition, there is every attempt to record the number of people who are homeless or in temporary accommodation. This information is used to inform central and local government planning. It is also used by many other independent organisations to help manage their work and target their resources.

The population of the United Kingdom – England, Wales, Scotland and Northern Ireland – on census night 2001 was 58,789,194, of which almost 50 million lived in England. The census website provides detailed information on the census findings. Information includes the following detailed statistical information:

- 11.7 million dependent children (0–16) lived in the UK.

- 22.9% of dependent children lived in lone-parent families.

- 17.6% of children lived in 'workless' households – that is, where there are no adults in work.

- 21% of the population were over 60 years of age.

- 20% of the population were under 16 years of age.

- There had been a big increase in the number of people over 85 years of age – now over 1.1million, or 1.9% of the population.

There is information relating to family size and household structure, levels of education and employment, race and ethnicity, religious adherence, and the quality and sufficiency of housing. The 2011 Census Programme is already in place, preparing for the next census. There are proposed measures to employ staff to follow up areas of low-response rates and, for the first time, to introduce internet response facilities.

The Office of National Statistics

The Office of National Statistics (ONS) is the government department that provides ongoing demographic, economic and other social statistics used by government and other policy-makers to inform planning decisions and to monitor progress. Data published includes the registration of all births, deaths and marriages, and regular publications, including *Social Trends* and *Population Trends*, available in hard copy and electronically.

Voluntary organisations and other independent sources of research

Many charitable organisations will systematically collect data in order to plan and monitor their activities, present information to their funders and to educate and provide statistical evidence to support their causes. Pressure groups and specific-interest groups will present research data to support their cause. Academic researchers will also contribute to the body of knowledge on a wide range of health and care issues. Throughout this textbook you will find evidence drawn from these sources.

When using statistical information it is, of course, essential to record the *source* of data and also to consider the authors' *purpose* when they supplied the data. If the data is supplied by a pressure group, is it presented in such a way that it will be persuasive? If the data is from a newspaper, is it aimed at the particular views and prejudices of its readers? Has there been important data omitted? Do you need to look further for fuller information? Should you consult data from an organisation known to support a different point of view on this issue? Statistics must always be used with caution, and presented with care.

Getting you thinking

1 Describe the stereotypical image of an older man or woman that you have seen presented in a television programme.

2 Do you think that older people are respected members of the community in which you live?

3 Explain how people such as those in the picture can counteract the stereotypical images of retirement and old age that exist in society.

4 What health and welfare needs do you associate with old age?

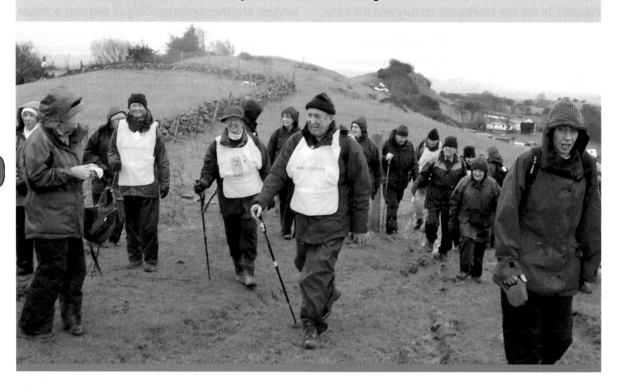

KEY TERMS

Ageism
Attitudes and behaviour which discriminate against people because of their age.

Community care
Provision where people should be cared for in their homes or in small 'family' units rather than in large, less personal institutions.

Age discrimination
Treating people differently (and normally less well) on the basis of their age.

Life expectancy
A statistical measure which predicts the average number of years a person is likely to live. This could be estimated from any particular age, but is usually expressed as from birth.

Extended family
A family group of normally three or more generations who form a close-knit network, and provide support and care for members.

Morbidity
The incidence of chronic ill health and disease.

Nuclear family
The small family unit of two generations – parent(s) and their children.

An ageing population

Earlier in this unit we noted the changing age structure of the population and specifically the increased proportion of older people in our society. In this topic we are going to consider the implications of an ageing population and the sources of support for older people.

'Simply to grow old is not in itself a problem' says Muriel Brown in her book *Introduction to Social Administration in Britain*. Ageing is a natural process that affects us all. It leads to slower physical and cognitive responses, some poorer vision, less acute hearing and some loss of energy and increased frailty. This is *not*, in itself, a problem – but limited support for people in their older life may well be.

Many people in retirement live full and active lives – continuing in paid work, working as volunteers and enjoying their additional leisure time. Those over 85 years of age are more likely to need support. For those with poor health, and especially if they are on low incomes, older age can be lonely and depressing. This is not a comment on old age itself, but rather a comment on the support available and our response to the vulnerable.

In 2003, according to estimates based on the 2001 census, there were over 11 million older people in the population. This is expected to increase to 11.4 million in 2006, and 12.2 million in 2011 – and it will rise to nearly 14 million by 2026 (www.ace.org.uk/Ageconcern). Further, the older population is ageing. Within the population aged 65 and over, the proportion of people aged 85 and over has increased from 7% in 1971 to 12% in 2004 (ONS www.statistics.gov.uk/cci/nugget.asp?id=881).

In many societies, older people (the elders) have high status and have an important role in the family and in the wider community – notably in China, India and many parts of Africa, and within Muslim, Hindu and Sikh communities. In modern Britain, however, it could be argued that older people are less central to our way of life, both in the family and in the wider community.

In 2004, Age Concern, in partnership with the University of Kent, undertook a research programme exploring the extent of prejudice and discrimination about age and ageing. They found that:

- More people (29%) reported suffering **age discrimination** than any other form of discrimination.

- From age 55 onwards, people were twice as likely to have experienced age prejudice than any other form of discrimination.

- Nearly 30% of people believed there is more prejudice against the old than five years ago, and that this will continue to get worse.

- One third of people thought that the demographic shift towards an older society would make life worse in terms of standards of living, security, health, jobs and education.

- One in three respondents said they viewed the over 70s as incompetent and incapable.

How ageist is Britain? Age Concern 2004

There has been no legislation in place to prevent discrimination against people on the basis of their age, but the European Directive on Equal Treatment (2000/78/EC) will require all member states to pass legislation which will outlaw discrimination in employment and training on the grounds of age This is scheduled to be implemented in October 2006, extending further the equality legislation in the UK.

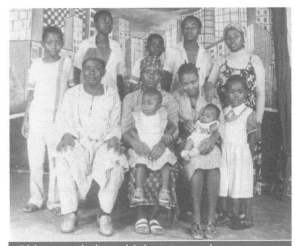

Older people have high status and an important role in African families like this one.

Figure 11 *Life expectancy and healthy life expectancy at birth: by sex*			
United Kingdom			
	1961	**1991**	**2003**
Males			
Life expectancy	67.8	73.2	76.2
Healthy life expectancy	...	66.1	...
Females			
Life expectancy	73.6	78.7	80.5
Healthy life expectancy	...	68.5	...

Source: Government Actuary's Department; Office of National Statistics

The family and the care of older people

In the societies and cultural groups where older people are particularly well respected they often live in an **extended family** – where a wide kinship network is expected to provide support for the family. In modern Britain, however, the likelihood of living alone increases with age. In 2002, 48% of those 75 years of age and over were living alone, compared with 12% aged 25–44 (www.ace.org.uk/AgeConcern). Changes in our society have arguably, however, made it more difficult for families to easily provide support for the dependent elderly, for several reasons:

- Families are smaller than they used to be. The average number of children in families has fallen (*Social Trends*). There are fewer adult children to share in the responsibilities of care and support.

- There have been changes in the position and status of women in society. Far more women are in paid employment and unable to provide daily care for dependent relatives.

- Far fewer families live near their elderly relatives than was the case 50 years ago, and this provides serious difficulties in providing care for the frail and vulnerable.

- The proportion of adult children who live with their parents or other older family members is very small.

- The complications and stress that arise from the increase in family breakdown and divorce make caring for the vulnerable elderly more difficult.

- There was, arguably, some change of attitude towards the care of older people in the years following the Second World War, with the development of a welfare state. It was assumed that older people would be cared for by the state. It was not necessary for adult children to be relied on for their care.

- The cost of caring for older people by adult relatives has not been fully addressed by the state. Benefits for carers have never been sufficient to compensate for the loss of potential earnings.

- Housing policy has not addressed the potential need for caring for older relatives. Three-bedroom houses with a 'through lounge' are not well suited to caring for elderly relatives.

- Employers are not required by law to agree flexible working arrangements for employees who are also caring for vulnerable relatives.

Gordon Lishman, Director General of Age Concern England, is quoted as saying:

' ...carers are caught in a no-win situation. If they give up work they face poverty. If they keep their jobs, they must struggle with unrelenting hours'

(www.ageconcern.org.uk).

Poverty and older age

There have been numbers of studies pointing to the higher incidence of poverty amongst older people compared to the population as a whole. On reaching retirement age, most people give up their full-time employment and are then dependent on income from their pensions and from savings.

Economic well-being in older age is closely linked with prosperity whilst in employment. Those who have enjoyed good wages, little unemployment, and occupational pension plans enjoy greater financial security in older age than those who have had interrupted employment and lower wages. Because of this, women, who make up the larger proportion of the older population and experience longer periods of ill health (**morbidity**) in older age also experience greater financial hardship. They are less likely to be

The lives of the affluent and the poor

Sally, who is 14 years of age has four grandparents all of whom are retired and in their late sixties. Sally's mum's parents seem to be having the time of their life. They were both doctors and had a good income all their life and now have a good occupational pension. They have a beautiful home. They play golf, go on holiday abroad during the winter, take their grandchildren away during the summer holidays and really they just don't seem to age.

Sally's dad's parents, however, are not doing quite so well. Grandad was a steelworker and was made redundant in the 1970s. He managed to get other jobs but they were all poorly paid and there was no occupational pension. Grandma worked part-time as a cleaner but she didn't have a works pension either and she never paid in to the state pension scheme. They still live in the council house that they moved to when they got married. It is damp and difficult to heat. Sally knows that in the winter her dad's parents have to choose between spending their small pensions on eating well or keeping warm. They do manage to go away on holiday for a week in the summer but they have never been on holiday abroad.

entitled to a full state pension or have paid into occupational pensions. Their wages whilst in employment are likely to have been lower and they are likely to have had a more interrupted working pattern. Most women now in older age will have given up paid work when their children were small and are more likely than their husbands to have reduced their work pattern to care for older relatives. The state pension scheme does not compensate people (usually women) who have interrupted their employment to care for adult relatives.

Gordon Lishman (in the same speech as quoted above) said: 'Carers save the economy billions through unpaid work each year, and they need flexible working as much as parents do. At the same time our outmoded pension system needs sweeping reforms.'

Care of the vulnerable old

Most older people do not require any regular practical care support. They live independent lives in the community – often contributing more than they obviously receive. Where they do need help, notwithstanding the comments earlier in this section, the help is most likely to come from family, friends or neighbours. When help is from family, despite changes in attitudes and equality legislation, it is far more likely to be from adult daughters than from sons.

For much of the twentieth century, vulnerable older people whose families were unable to provide the practical help needed were generally cared for in large institutions, very often geriatric hospitals. Many of these hospitals had once been the local 'workhouse' and despite changes, care in the geriatric hospital was often linked with the sadness and stigma of the workhouse. From the 1960s onwards, there were a number of reports criticising the quality of care in these large institutions, but it was not until the 1990 NHS and Community Care Act that there was legislative support and resources allocated for planned care in the community. The system continues to be managed by local social service departments who,

following the assessment of **community care** needs, will purchase care services from a range of statutory, private and voluntary providers. The care for the older people may include home care services, meals on wheels, attendance at a day centre or lunch club, adaptations to their own home, or full-time care in a residential care home. Only very rarely will long-term care be provided in large institutions or hospitals.

Informal carers

Sue is in her late fifties and has just given up work to care for her elderly mother, Grace. Sue herself is not well, she has always suffered from arthritis and gets bad headaches when she is tired. Grace lives a bus ride away from Sue on the other side of town. Sue and her partner Brian live with their son Tom in a two-bedroom terraced house. The bathroom and toilet are upstairs and so it is difficult for Grace to even visit them. Sue has arranged for Grace to receive meals-on-wheels and also a daily home-help during the week. However, Sue and Brian also have to ensure that Grace has proper meals at the weekend and that there is someone there over night because Grace is nervous in the dark when she is on her own. They provide this care for her themselves.

1 **What is meant by the term 'community care'?**

2 **Describe the types of community care services that may be provided for older people who need support with daily living activities.**

3 **Why may there be poverty in older age?**

4 **Explain why, in the twenty-first century, it may be difficult for adult children to provide practical care for older relatives.**

extension activities

1 Using the internet, your library or your local benefits office, list the main welfare benefits available to older people, and describe how they may support care in the community policies.

2 Find out more about the statutory, voluntary and private provision which supports older people in your area.

Discrimination and access to health and care services

Getting you thinking

Paul and Jane are opening a new nursery. They are currently advertising for staff in the local paper.

1 Should Paul and Jane make sure that the staff are from a range of ethnic backgrounds?

2 How do you think parents and carers will react to having a male nursery manager?

3 Should they put up notices at the nursery in a range of community languages, or should they encourage parents and carers to communicate in English?

4 Can you think of an occasion when you felt discriminated against? What did this feel like?

5 Is it too much to ask the nursery staff to meet the individual needs of all the children?

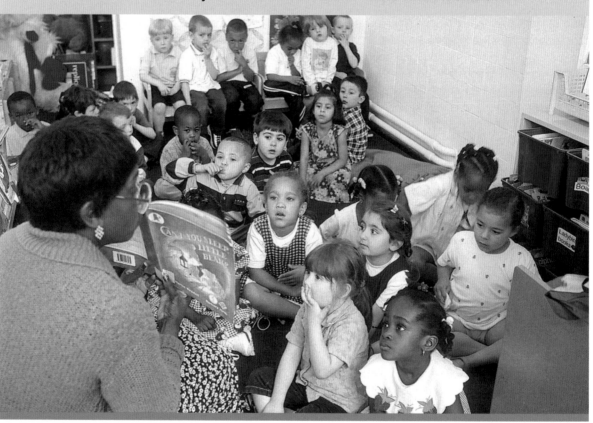

KEY TERMS

Discrimination
Treating people differently, and in this context normally less favourably, on the grounds of inherited or social categories, e.g. race, gender, sexual orientation or age.

Prejudice
Pre-judgements or preconceived opinions and ideas about a particular group, which are not modified in the light of new experiences of that group.

Statutory
Required by law.

Stereotype
An over-simplified image of the characteristics of a particular group, e.g. women are better at childcare than men.

Diversity

Diversity refers to differences, variety and contrast. Diversity focuses on our uniqueness as individuals and the obvious and subtle differences between us. Examples of the differences that are of social significance are differences in age, race and ethnicity, gender and sexuality, physical and sensory ability, religion and marital status. It is in these areas of difference that there has been specific action by governments – but they are by no means the only areas in which harassment and **discrimination** occur. Sometimes particular characteristics are associated with groups of people – that women are natural carers, for example, or that Africans have a great sense of rhythm, or that men are good at mechanics – and then all members of the group are expected to have these characteristics. These descriptions are **stereotypes** – they do not describe real individuals or address the diversity within groups. People who are stereotyped in this way can be discriminated against, because their individuality is not recognised. Each is simply treated as a member of a group with these perceived characteristics, and not as an individual.

In health and care settings, understanding the differences between people is necessary to:

- understand the needs of service users.

- meet the care needs of service users.

- ensure that information is clear and accessible to all service users.

- ensure that staff from diverse backgrounds and with specific individual needs are not isolated or misunderstood at work.

- encourage a wider range of people to work in the health and care services.

Diversity in this context is not about treating everybody the same, but it is about treating everybody with equal respect and care.

Equal opportunities

Views on equality of opportunity may be seen as falling into two main categories – those relating to equality of access to services and valued opportunities in society, and those relating to the possibility of equality of outcomes – that all individuals should be entitled to an equal share of the benefits.

Equality of access

Equal opportunities, in the context of policy making in modern Britain, has been mainly concerned with the first category – equal access for all – to employment and educational opportunities, our political institutions, and to the services that different organisations provide. All social groups should be provided with the chance to make the most of their talents and to use them for the benefit of the wider community. Policies have been aimed at removing the barriers that disadvantaged groups have found in achieving their potential and in accessing services. Across all parties and across the European Union there has been general and legislative support for equality of access. Most significantly there has been equality legislation in the UK:

- The Equal Pay Act 1970

- The Sex Discrimination Act 1975

- The Race Relations Act 1976 and the Race Relations Amendment Act 2000

- The Disability Discrimination Act 1995

- The Special Educational Needs and Disabilities Act (SENDA) 2001

- The Human Rights Act 1998

There have also been directives from the European Union:

- The Equal Treatment Directive 1976 for men and women.

This led, among other things, to the equalisation of retirement ages for men and women.

- The Equal Treatment Directive 2000 for religion or belief, disability, age or sexual orientation.

This led to discrimination on the grounds of religion, belief and sexual orientation in employment to become illegal in 2003 and discrimination on the grounds of age to become illegal in 2006. It is illegal to advertise jobs as open to young people only, and illegal to discriminate on the grounds of age when advertising and recruiting for posts, and in promotion and training.

Equality of outcome

Policies which support the view that everybody should be entitled to an equal share of society's benefits – which might include an equal share of wealth, income, quality of housing and education, and equal power and status – have been rare. There has been little political support for creating an equal society, but policy-makers in most advanced countries and

Getting you thinking

1 'There are plenty of opportunities for everyone. Nobody needs to be poor these days.' Is that how it is?

2 Are we all middle class now?

3 Is it true that we're all far better off than our grandparents' generation were?

4 Are some groups always excluded from the good things on offer?

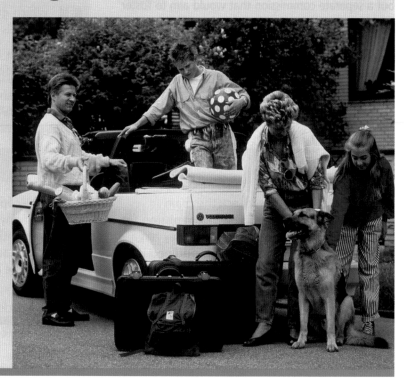

KEY TERMS

Social stratification
The grouping of people together according to their perceived status or rank within society.

Egalitarian society
A society in which everyone is regarded as equal.

Social class
There are many competing definitions of social class. Central to all definitions is the idea that position in society is determined by our economic circumstances, which will then influence our life choices, our opportunities and future prospects

Social exclusion
A term used to describe a situation where people are unable to participate fully in society for a number of related reasons – including poverty, unemployment, poor housing (or homelessness), poor health and poor educational achievement.

Underclass
Coined by Gunnar Myrdal (1969) and closely linked with the idea of social exclusion, this term is normally used now to refer to the people in poverty who are excluded from fully participating in society because of the social and economic changes that are outside their control.

Prejudice
A strongly held attitude towards a particular group which will often persist, even when shown to be unjustified or unfounded.

Discrimination
Treating a person or a group of people differently (usually less favourably) than others.

Stereotype
Defining a group of people – black people or lone parents, for example – as if they all possess the same personal characteristics, ignoring their individual differences.

Labelling
Closely linked with stereotyping. When a person is 'labelled' then usually the stereotypical characteristics of that group are applied to them, and their individual characteristics are ignored.

Inequalities in society

Inequalities in our society are well documented by social scientists, journalists and government statisticians. The observable consequences of inequality, though, are probably all too visible in everyday life. They are seen in the range of housing in modern Britain, the contrasting environments within towns and cities, differences in schools and children's educational achievements, and differences in individual levels of wealth and income. These inequalities are reflected in the fact that:

- Children from manual social backgrounds are 1.5 times more likely to die as infants than children from non-manual backgrounds.

- Babies from manual social backgrounds are 1.3 times more likely to be of low birth weight than those from professional backgrounds.

- Teenage motherhood is six times as common amongst those from manual social backgrounds as for those from professional backgrounds.

- Forty per cent of lone parents are not in paid work.

- Overcrowding is more than three times as prevalent in social rented (local authority and housing association) housing as in owner-occupied housing.

- People of black Caribbean, Bangladeshi and African ethnicity are twice as likely to be out of work (and wanting work) as white people.

(www.poverty.org.uk)

Social stratification

Social stratification is a term that sociologists have adapted from geologists' terminology, where 'stratification' refers to the different layers of rock, one on top of another. Almost all known societies have had a concept of some groups being of higher status than others. In America, before the civil war, groupings in the South were based on race. In feudal Britain, land ownership was a key determinant of status.

Hindus have a strict hierarchy of social 'castes', with the Brahmin (the priestly caste) regarded as the most superior and the Sudras (the labouring caste) considered to have the least status. Beneath the Sudra caste are the casteless – the 'untouchables', a group now theoretically prohibited by the Indian government, but still of considerable actual significance.

Those in the higher social groups are normally more wealthy and have access to a quality of life valued within that society. There have, however, been experiments in establishing unstratified, more

egalitarian **societies**. Probably the best known and most developed example is the kibbutz system in Israel. There are currently about 240 kibbutzim in Israel, with populations of several hundred each. All property and land are communally owned, and all goods are distributed to members according to their need. Children are brought up and educated communally. Money is not normally used. General assemblies are held to discuss and make major decisions. Studies of kibbutzim, however – most notably by Eva Rosenfeld (1957) – have suggested that there is some stratification, particularly between the leaders, elected to run the kibbutzim and the 'ordinary' members who carry out the tasks.

Social class

Most modern societies today are stratified by **social class**, a system based largely on economic factors linked with income and wealth. In modern Britain, most research into the impact of social class on health and well-being has used occupation to locate people's class position. Occupation has long been seen as closely linked with level (and security) of income, and also with people's standing in the community.

Since 1911, the census data has been analysed by class categories, based on occupation. This system, which was usually known as the 'Registrar General's Scale' (the Registrar General being the head of the Office for National Statistics) remained largely unchanged until 1991, and consisted of six 'social classes':

1 Professional occupations, e.g. architect, accountant, doctor, judge, optician

2 Managerial and technical occupations, e.g. farmer, nurse, school teacher,

3 **(non-manual)** e.g. clerical worker, secretary, shop assistant

3 **(manual)** e.g. bricklayer, bus driver, carpenter, cook, police constable

4 Semi-skilled occupations, e.g. bar person, postman, bus conductor, farm worker

5 Unskilled occupations, e.g. chimney sweep, office cleaner, window cleaner.

For the 2001 census a new occupational classification was introduced, which is thought to be more flexible, and which includes those people who are not in paid work:

1.1 Employers and managers in large organisations, e.g. managing director

1.2 Higher professionals, e.g. doctors, solicitors, teachers

2 Lower managerial and professional occupations, e.g. nurses, journalists

3 Intermediate occupations, e.g. clerks and secretaries

4 Small employers and own account workers, e.g. taxi drivers, painters and decorators

5 Lower supervisory, craft and related occupations, e.g. plumbers and electricians

6 Semi-routine occupations, e.g. shop assistants, hairdressers

7 Routine occupations, e.g. cleaners, refuse collectors

8 Those people who are not in paid employment.

These systems of classification – and others which are very similar in structure – have been used to analyse research into levels of poverty and the impact of social class on a wide range of social and economic activities, including the inequalities identified at the beginning of this section.

Social exclusion

Social exclusion is a term closely linked with issues of poverty and deprivation, but it refers to wider issues of participation in society. The Social Exclusion Unit, set up by the Labour Government in 1997, describes 'social exclusion' as a shorthand term for what can happen when people suffer from a combination of linked problems, such as unemployment, poor housing, poor skills, low income, high crime environments, bad health, poverty and family breakdown.

The Social Exclusion Unit was set up to address perceived social problems, which were seen as having interlinked causes, and therefore needed co-ordinated solutions. They were looking for 'joined-up solutions to joined-up problems'. Tony Blair when launching the unit was quoted as saying that social exclusion is 'about more than financial deprivation. It is about the damage done by poor housing, ill-health, poor education, lack of decent transport, but above all lack of work.' (quoted in Tossell, D. and Webb, D. (2000) *Social Issues for Carers*). Unemployment – especially prolonged unemployment – was seen as a crucial factor in individuals and their families becoming excluded from the social, economic and political life of society.

The term 'social exclusion' has come to replace a closely linked concept of the **underclass**, a term you may come across in some sociology and social policy texts. Both these terms are used to describe people who are 'on the edge' of our society, and not able to

take a full part in economic, political and social life.

The overall effect of the interrelated causes and consequences of social exclusion is to 'marginalise' those individuals and groups in our society who are not able to fully participate. Marginalised groups will normally lack the income to take a full part in the economic and social life of our society.

Those groups are likely to be the subject of **prejudice**. This term is not easy to define, but it refers to strongly held beliefs and attitudes about people which often have no basis in factual evidence, but which are held so *strongly* that they are difficult to shift. The beliefs and attitudes are often directed at disadvantaged groups, and usually attribute negative characteristics to them. People who have prejudicial attitudes to specific groups rarely look for robust evidence to support their view – and even when it is presented to them it rarely makes any difference.

This process is closely linked to stereotyping. A **stereotype** is a set of characteristics that members of a particular group are said to possess, e.g. 'that all hoodies are school drop-outs, they often shoplift and they cannot be trusted'. People who have been stereotyped tend not to be seen as individuals but as a typical member of the group. When a stereotype is widely held it is sometimes said that the individual or group has been **labelled**, because the stereotypical characteristics are routinely applied to them.

It will be becoming clear how prejudicial attitudes and stereotyping can lead to **discrimination** or discriminatory behaviour. If we have negative attitudes towards a particular group we are likely to be wary of them and treat them less favourably than other members of society.

Social exclusion will potentially lead to a range of negative consequences for the social, emotional, intellectual and physical development of the people affected. They are likely to become socially isolated because they are marginalised. They also are unlikely to have the income which will support an active social life. This is likely to lead to a poor self-image, low self-esteem and little self-confidence. These social, emotional and economic circumstances will not easily support educational success, and are likely to impact negatively on general health and well-being, and physical health in particular.

Check your understanding

1 Define the terms social stratification, social class, social exclusion.

2 Describe the social issues that the government tried to address through the Social Exclusion Unit.

3 Explain why prejudice may lead to discrimination against disadvantaged groups in our society.

4 Explain why the idea of stereotyping and labelling may be seen as closely linked.

extension activities

1 Working with another member of your group, try to describe how a society could operate if everybody was equal. What would be the advantages and disadvantages of an equal society?

2 The government has identified that people vulnerable to social exclusion include the homeless and people in poor housing, the unemployed, people with poor educational qualifications and people on low incomes.

Find out more statistics on these areas of people's lives. Try to establish whether trends are improving or not. Discuss with other members of your group how you would address the problems.

Getting you thinking

1 Write a list of items that you think are essential – and without which you would be in poverty.
2 Compare this with your friends' lists.
3 In your own words, write a definition of poverty.
4 Which groups in our society do you think are most likely to be in poverty?
5 What are the main consequences of poverty in the United Kingdom?

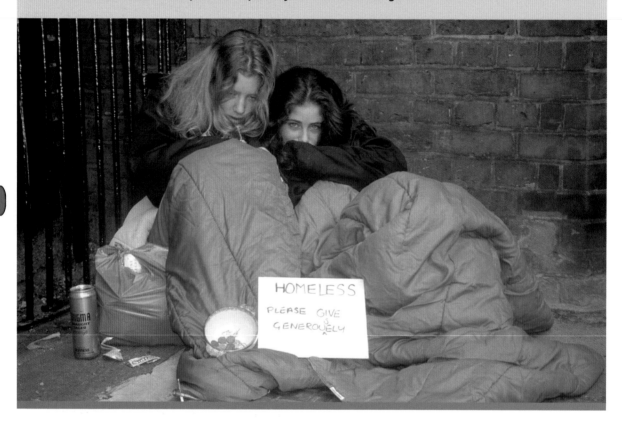

KEY TERMS

Absolute poverty
A level of income below that which will sustain good health.

Culture of poverty
A view that poverty is associated with a particular (and separate) way of life that is passed on from generation to generation.

Means-tested benefits
Welfare benefits that are only available to people if their income and savings are below a certain level, decided by the government.

Poverty line
A term, introduced by Seebohm Rowntree, which set a level of income below which people were said to be in poverty.

Relative poverty
Relative poverty occurs when people live below the standard of living normally accepted in a particular society.

Universal benefits
Welfare benefits to which people are entitled, regardless of their income or savings.

What do we mean by poverty?

In this topic we will discuss what we mean by poverty, and how difficult it is to measure poverty. We will then consider why, in a wealthy nation like ours, poverty still persists and, finally, how governments have responded to the identified needs of the poorest in our society.

It will be no doubt be clear when comparing your lists of 'essentials' that it is difficult to agree on what we mean by 'poverty'. And if we cannot easily define a term, we will have great difficulty in measuring the extent of the problem – or even if the problem exists.

The first systematic studies of poverty in England were conducted by social reformers at the turn of the nineteenth century. Charles Booth (1840–1916) in his study, *Life and Labour of the London Poor*, and the Quaker Seebohm Rowntree (1871–1954) in his study of York, *Poverty: A study of town life*, exposed the existence of widespread poverty in these two cities. These studies were important, not only in their own right, but also in their continuing influence. They provided evidence and an approach to understanding poverty, which has influenced government policies, and also provided an approach to defining and measuring poverty which has influenced the subsequent research in this area.

Booth covered a wide range of issues which have become central themes in studies of poverty, including employment, health, housing, religion and the level of wages. He was probably the first to identify the close links between poor health, disability, poverty, poor housing, unemployment and bad working conditions.

Rowntree (probably better known for his chocolate factory which was a main employer in York at the time) developed a vocabulary for discussing poverty which has informed discussion since. He introduced the idea of a **poverty line** – a concept that is still used by governments, and informs our benefit system today. It identifies a level of income below which people are regarded as living in poverty.

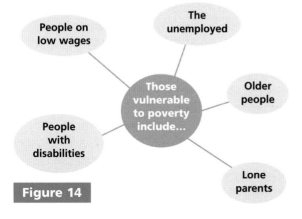

Figure 14

Rowntree defined people as poor if their income was such that the resulting deprivation had a detrimental effect on their health. With the assistance of the British Medical Association, he calculated the income that was necessary for the members of a household to maintain 'physical efficiency'. If their income was below this level they were regarded as in **absolute poverty**. The income allowed a basic diet that would be adequate, but no more. There was no allowance for papers or magazines, or alcohol, or travel. There was no allowance for stamps for writing to children living away from home. Families were regarded as in 'primary poverty' if their income was below the level that would maintain physical efficiency, and in 'secondary poverty' if their income would have been sufficient had they not spent money on items not on his list. This distinction could be seen as pointing to the idea of the 'deserving poor' and the 'undeserving poor'.

Rowntree conducted further studies in1936 and 1950 where the understanding of poverty suggested that there was more to being poor than simply not being able to keep the body intact – social and emotional health were significant too. The 1936 study allowed that, to be above the poverty line, people should have an income sufficient for a radio, newspaper, beer and a holiday.

Later studies of poverty developed further the idea that poverty could be regarded as a level of income below which people were 'not able to participate in the life of the community'. The level, then at which a poverty line may be set would vary from community to community, and at different times in history. In some parts of Africa, for example, to have suitable shelter and regular meals would be regarded as rich indeed. In modern Britain people would normally regard this as not enough to count as playing a full part in the community. Peter Townsend (1979) was key in the development of the idea that the idea of poverty should be related to the society in which people live. He developed the idea of **relative poverty** (relative deprivation), claiming that:

'Individuals, families and groups in the population can be said to be in poverty when they lack the resources to obtain the types of diet, participate in the activities and have the living conditions and amenities which are customary, or at least widely encouraged or approved in the societies to which they belong . . . they are in effect excluded from ordinary living patterns, customs and activities.'

Townsend P. (ed.) (1979) Poverty in the United Kingdom

This approach to poverty was taken further by Mack and Lansley (1985, 1991) in their major studies *Breadline Britain*, defining poverty in relative terms.

They attempted to define poverty by asking their respondents what they considered to be necessities in modern Britain. An item was considered a necessity if more than half the respondents classified it as such. On the basis of this list of 'perceived necessities', Mack and Lansley measured the extent of poverty. In these, they took account of personal choices, asking respondents whether they lacked an item out of 'choice' or 'necessity'. Some people, for example, might choose to not have a television or a telephone in their home. Mack and Lansley found that generally, where people lacked three or more 'necessities' it had little to do with choice. It was unavoidable – they just couldn't afford them. This approach has been used since.

The most recent attempt to update the *Breadline Britain* studies was the 1999 'Poverty and Social Exclusion Survey of Britain' produced by the Office of National Statistics, supported by the Joseph Rowntree Trust. The aim of this study was to:

- Update the *Breadline Britain* surveys.

- Estimate the size of groups of households in different circumstances.

- Explore movements in and out of poverty.

- Look at age and gender differences in experiences and responses to poverty.

Over 90% of the population in this survey regarded a bed and bedding for everyone, warm living areas of the home, a damp-free home, the ability to visit family and friends in hospital, two meals a day, and medicines prescribed by the doctor as necessities.

The researchers found that a quarter (26%) of the British population was living in poverty measured in terms of low income and multiple deprivation of the agreed necessities.

(Adapted from www.bris.ac.uk/poverty/pse.)

A 'working definition' of poverty is still necessary to identify the extent of need, and then to address the issues. Some nations, including the United States, use a 'budget standard', based on the cost of a minimum basket of food (following Rowntree's idea). The UK and other members of the European Union set a poverty line at 50% of the median income. (The median is the mid-point of the full range of incomes in the population.) Those with an income of less than 50% of this amount are deemed to be in poverty.

Despite all these differences in definition, for those people on low incomes – perhaps having to choose between eating well and keeping warm – poverty is all too present.

Culture of poverty

Oscar Lewis, an American writer, is identified as the author most closely associated with the idea of a **culture of poverty**. He thought that poverty was associated with a particular, separate, way of life that was passed on from generation to generation. He thought that in order to cope with their stressful circumstances the poor were unlikely to plan for the future – they rarely saved, they had a less well ordered life, and a more fatalistic attitude to the future. Their culture and way of life was different to the mainstream in the society. A similar idea was developed in the 1970s through the concept of the 'cycle of deprivation' in which it is said that the lifestyle of the poor was passed on from one generation to the next. There is, however, little evidence to suggest that the poor have values and aspirations that are significantly different from the rest of society. They shop largely in the same high street, they are subject to the same advertisements, and similar demands are made by their children. As a result, they have a keen sense of being amongst the least well off in modern Britain.

Welfare benefits concerned with poverty

This section considers the benefit system aimed at supporting those identified as being in financial poverty. The structure of the benefit system can be traced back to the system set up following the Beveridge Report, and specifically to addressing issues of 'want'. Writing at a time of almost full employment, he saw poverty as generally caused by two things – first, the loss of income caused by the old age, unemployment, ill-health, or death of the family's main wage earner (at that time almost always the man) and, secondly, the cost of children.

The benefit system was to be largely financed by a new 'National Insurance' scheme to which people would contribute when they were in work and from which they were able to claim when they were unable to work. This meant that they would claim retirement pension when they were too old to work, sickness benefit when they were too ill to work, and unemployment benefit (now Job Seekers Allowance) when unemployed. They would be entitled to these benefits because they had paid into the National Insurance scheme and they met the life circumstances criteria – they had reached retirement age, for example. These benefits were not related to a person's income, neither were they charity – they were an entitlement. They were **universal benefits**, available to all who had paid into the scheme and met the life circumstances criteria.

In addition to the National Insurance benefits (often called 'contributory' benefits, because they depended on payment of National Insurance contributions) there were **means-tested benefits** for people who had not paid into the scheme, normally because they had not been in consistent employment – and, of course, there would always be people who had *never* worked. Eligibility for means-tested benefits depended on people's level of income and their level of savings. Those unable to work, who had not paid into the scheme, would be entitled to benefit only if their own resources fell below a certain level – the level that the government thought adequate to keep them out of poverty. This approach, therefore drew on Rowntree's concept of a poverty line. The benefits today that are means tested include Income Support, Housing Benefit, Educational Maintenance Allowance, and the non-contributory Jobs Seekers Allowance – paid to the unemployed who have not paid sufficient contributions to the National Insurance scheme.

The take-up of benefits

Of particular interest (and concern) to social workers is why, despite poverty, a significant proportion of the benefits aimed at the poorest in society is not claimed, including benefits aimed specifically at older people. The benefits with the lowest take-up rates are the means-tested benefits. There are many possible reasons why this might be the case:

- The benefit system is very complicated, and people are often not clear of their entitlements.

- The forms that need to be completed are long and often complex.

- The questions asked and the information required can be seen as an invasion into privacy, and too much of an intrusion into personal circumstances.

- Some claimants are too proud to claim their benefit, particularly the means-tested benefits. Some older people in particular still see this as charity rather than an entitlement.

- Some people feel that there is a stigma attached to claiming their benefit.

- Claiming means-tested benefits often requires visiting the Benefits Office, and some feel that there is a stigma attached to this as well.

Poor take-up of benefits

Martha is seventy five years of age. She lives on her state retirement pension and is finding it difficult to manage. An advice worker who visited the day centre she attends explained to Martha that she could also claim Income Support and additional Housing Benefit. Both of these are means-tested benefits. Martha became quite annoyed and impatient at this advice. She said "I don't want the social prying into my private business. I haven't claimed anything in my life before and I'm not going to start now. Anyway it's so complicated. They want to know everything. And what if I get it wrong? I could be all over the newspapers if I claim too much".

In the mean time Martha is depressed and worried. She is frightened to put on the heating in the winter because she cannot afford the bills. Her diet is poor and her general quality of life declining.

Check your understanding

1 Define the terms 'primary poverty' and 'secondary poverty', as introduced by Seebohm Rowntree.

2 Explain the difference between universal benefits and means-tested benefits.

3 Which groups in our society are most vulnerable to poverty?

4 Identify the likely reasons why there is a lower take-up rate for means-tested benefits than for universal benefits.

e x t e n s i o n **a c t i v i t i e s**

1 Using the internet, your local library, Citizen's Advice Bureau, or Benefits Office, list and briefly describe five universal benefits and five means-tested benefits.

2 Universal benefits are available to the most wealthy members of the community – who could quite well manage without them. Is this a good use of taxpayers' money? Discuss this with reference to Child Benefit.

Getting you thinking

Your local health authority is planning to open a hostel in your area for people with mental health problems.

1 Write down your initial feelings about this plan.

2 Compare your thoughts with other people in your class

3 How do you think the people who live nearby will feel?

4 Try to identify two reasons in favour of this plan, and two reasons against it.

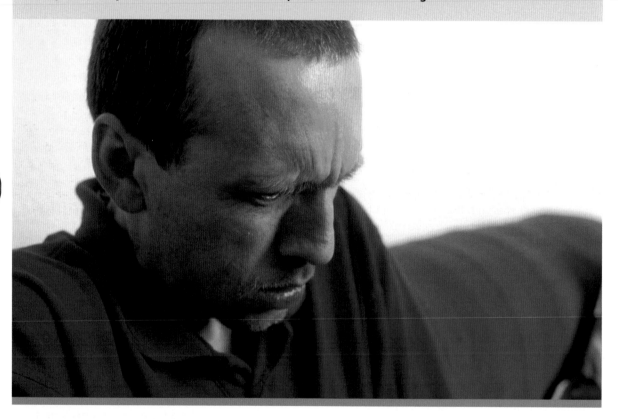

KEY TERMS

Institutionalisation
The process of becoming dependent on the rules and routines of large organisations.

Labelling
The process of attaching stigmatising stereotypes to particular groups of people who are then seen as all sharing negative characteristics.

Multi-disciplinary team
A team of care workers from a range of professional backgrounds. The team may include doctors, nurses, social workers and occupational therapists, for example.

Stigma
A term closely related to labelling which refers to the impact of negative attitudes and behaviour on the health and well-being of marginalised groups, e.g. offenders, the mentally ill or travelling families.

Total institution
A large, highly organised residential establishment where people live their lives completely separately from the wider society, e.g. a prison or an army barracks or a large mental hospital.

How do we measure the health of the nation?

In Unit 9 there is a fuller discussion of what we mean when we describe somebody as 'healthy'. A favoured definition by health and care workers is the World Health Organization's view that health is 'a state of complete physical, mental and social well-being, and not the absence of disease or infirmity'.

Measuring how far this has been achieved across all sections of the population, however, and how that compares with other societies and across other historical periods, is a challenge. In order to measure well-being statistically there has to be a clear definition that is, in itself, measurable – a challenge indeed.

Most research – and hence most statistical information – on the healthiness of nations describes levels of *ill-health*. There is, for example, detailed data available on the numbers of GP and hospital appointments, the take-up of immunisation programmes, the incidence of diagnosed mental illness, levels of morbidity and mortality, including suicide rates. All this data has been analysed by social class, occupation, geographical region, ethnicity, age, sex and occupation – variables that are far easier to define and measure than levels of well-being. To measure our own level of well-being is challenge enough, so comparisons with others are not easily open to objective study or statistical analysis.

What is mental illness?

Mental illness is very common (and we will discuss the statistics that support this claim later) but there is a great deal of controversy, discussion and uncertainty about what we mean by a mental illness, what are the causes and how people can be helped to recover. There are difficulties of definition. What is seen as 'normal' and 'abnormal' behaviour varies between societies, and at different times in history. Further, there can be considerable difficulties in diagnosis and appropriate support when doctors, carers and clients are from different cultural or religious backgrounds.

Psychiatrists have, however, categorised different forms of mental illness. Amongst the most common are depression, anxiety, panic attacks, phobias, obsessive–compulsive disorders and schizophrenia. Identifying a condition helps, of course, with decisions on forms of treatment and the ongoing care needed. Doctors, however, may disagree on the diagnosis. Giving a specific diagnosis *can* lead to some negative consequences – sometimes referred to as **labelling**.

Labelling someone as 'a depressive' can lead to this becoming the defining characteristic of that person. It is seen as their main characteristic, and other aspects of their life – as a parent, teacher, lover and friend – are overlooked. The condition becomes a label that they have great difficulty leaving behind, even when the symptoms have gone.

This lack of clear definition and certain diagnosis could be seen to underpin the ignorance, fear and anxiety about issues of mental health, and the prejudice faced by many people with mental health problems.

The causes of mental illnesses

The causes of mental illness and distress are also not fully understood. They are part of a wider discussion of the link between nature and nurture – that is, whether our personalities are shaped by our genetic make-up or the result of our life experiences. It is likely that mental distress is the result of a combination of factors drawn from our inherited characteristics (our genes), ongoing changes in our biochemistry (e.g. hormonal changes) and life experiences, including our family background and the consequences of stressful life events. It is possible that some people, because of their genetic make-up, are more vulnerable to mental illness than others, and that the illness is triggered by stressful or traumatic life events, such as divorce, redundancy or the death of a partner.

Figure 15

Possible causes of mental illness: Genetic factors, Changes in bio-chemistry, Brain injury, Stressful life events, Family and relationship problems

How common is mental illness?

It is very difficult to accurately calculate the levels and incidence of mental illness. There are readily available statistics on the frequency of mental health problems in the UK, but these statistics need to be treated with caution.

The number of people identified as suffering from a mental illness will often be based on the number of people presenting themselves for treatment. But there are many people with mental health problems who do not seek professional help – for a range of reasons. They may not realise that they are ill. They may

Ability and disability

Getting you thinking

1 How would you define the term 'disability'? Compare your definition with those of other people in your group.

2 How easy is it for a person in a wheelchair to go shopping in the High Street that you normally use?

3 Imagine that you needed to use a wheelchair. How easy would it be for you to attend school or college and follow this course?

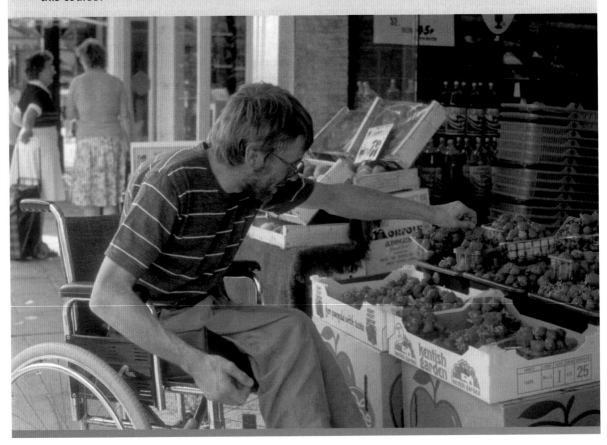

KEY TERMS

Direct payments
Cash payments made to people assessed as needing community care services, so that they can select the specific support they need.

Disabling environment
An environment in which adaptations are not in place to ensure that people with impairments can take a full part in day-to-day life.

Impairment
The limitations that may be made on an individual due to physical, mental or sensory dysfunction.

Institutionalisation
The process of becoming dependent on the rules and routines of large organisations.

The difficulties of definition

As in so many areas of social care and social policy, terms relating to people with physical disabilities and impairments are used in different ways by different writers. It is important when considering these issues to be clear exactly how you are using the terms. In many ways there is no clear dividing line between people with disabilities and the rest of society. Most of us will suffer disabilities at some point in our lives, and the same condition may create serious problems in day-to-day life for some people but not for others. Some may therefore regard the condition as a disability, whilst others may not.

Accurate figures of the number of people with disabilities are not known. This is partly because of the difficulties of definition and partly because the registers of people with disabilities kept by local authorities are incomplete. There is little agreement over who should be identified as 'disabled'. In 2005, the definition used in the Disability Discrimination Act was extended to protect more people with HIV, cancer and multiple sclerosis, and the requirement that a mental illness should be clinically 'well recognised' was removed. The government is currently revising its guidance on the definition of disability.

The Disability Discrimination Act !995 defines a person with a disability as 'someone who has a physical or mental impairment that has a substantial and long-term adverse effect on his or her ability to carry out normal day-to-day activities'. 'Long-term' normally means that the effect of the impairment 'has lasted or is likely to last for at least 12 months'. Normal day-to-day activities includes things like eating, washing, walking and going shopping.

A helpful distinction can be made between the terms '**impairment**' and 'disability'. Impairment is seen as the limitations that may be made on an individual, due to physical, mental or sensory dysfunction – with a focus on the individual. Disability, on the other hand, is seen as the restricted opportunity to take part in the normal life of the community, due to physical, social or attitudinal barriers.

The medical model of disability

Images of people with disability often show restricted mobility – people using wheelchairs, for example, or white canes. But there are many physical conditions, of course, that may be 'disabling' but are not visible – such as back pain, heart conditions or asthma. The medical model views disability as a dysfunction or an impairment located within the person's body. They have multiple sclerosis, for example, and their

Medical model of disability

Aziz became blind as an adult as a result of diabetes. He cannot read Braille. He has had very little support to develop skills for daily living. He is very nervous of using kitchen equipment and, in fact, cannot even make a cup of tea with confidence. Aziz is never sure that the house is clean and this bothers him quite a lot. Although he has a white stick to use outside Aziz is very nervous of going out of the house. The roads are very busy where he lives and the pavements are uneven. Aziz also feels personally vulnerable. He knows that anyone could take advantage of him. He's usually quite frightened when he goes out. Aziz has explained this situation to his GP. Unfortunately his GP says that Aziz just has to adapt to his new situations. He tries to impress on Aziz that he has a serious disability and that he needs to adapt his life to this.

difficulties in day-to-day living would be seen as a consequence of their condition. It would thus be seen as the individual's responsibility to adjust to the limitations that may follow.

The physical consequences of a medical condition or impairment, however, will vary. The age and personal circumstances of the person will impact on its effect, for example, and people's attitudes to the condition will affect its impact on day-to-day life.

The psychological approach to disability

The psychological approach to disability also has its main focus on the individual, with a particular concern that individuals should adjust to their condition. This approach will address the individual's mental response to their impairment and the therapy given may be concerned with developing coping strategies.

The social model of disability

In contrast to the medical and psychological models, the social model locates disability within society. If someone is in a wheelchair – but there is 100% access to all amenities – then proponents of the social model would feel that they no longer had a disability. They would have an 'impairment' but this would not impact negatively on their day-to-day life. The social model therefore locates the problems not with the individual, but in the physical environment, and in people's attitudes and practices. Here the onus is put on society to adapt to the needs of people with disabilities. The

Carl, aged 25 is a solicitor's clerk who has multiple sclerosis. He can now only walk short distances. He always uses walking sticks and often a wheelchair to get around his home and workplace. His house has been adapted so that he can carry out all normal day-to-day activities. The doors have been widened for his wheelchair, the electricity points are now at waist height and he has had a stair lift, adapted bath and shower fitted. Carl's employer has also tried to help by providing him with a laptop so that he can often work from home. Carl now has an adapted car and is able to visit his family and friends quite easily as well as go on holiday and plan an active social life of his choice. He has impairments but the adaptations to his home and work environment mean that he rarely feels 'disabled'.

focus of this model is on the **disabling environment**.

It is probably more helpful to consider the valuable insights of all three models rather than to just see them as three competing ideas. It is necessary to understand the likely physical impact of a condition in order to make appropriate environmental changes and organise appropriate support. It's helpful to use the insights of psychology to support people in their adaptation to change. However, it could be argued that social care workers need to particularly embrace the social model if they are to ensure that people with impairments are going to fully participate in their communities.

Government responses to disability

The growth of separate institutions to care for people with disabilities started in the Industrial Revolution when more and more people started working away from their homes – in factories and mills. Most people with disabilities who could not be cared for at home by their family or friends lived in hospitals and other institutions – some of them one-time workhouses. This system of care had its roots in the medical model of disability. The people diagnosed as disabled were cared for by medical , nursing and care staff. They were separated from the wider society and vulnerable to the **institutionalisation** discussed in Topic 7. There was no thought that society could or should adapt so that they could be included in the social and economic life of the time. This approach persisted through much of the twentieth century.

The 1944 Disabled Persons (Employment) Act required local authorities to establish the number of people with disabilities in their area, and Part 3 of the 1948 National Assistance Act placed a duty on local authorities to arrange services for disabled people. This measure largely resulted in people going into residential care rather than living independently in the community. The 1970 Chronically Sick and Disabled Persons Act required local authorities to establish the number of people with disabilities in their area, compile a register of people with disabilities and provide for their needs. The response to this requirement, however, varied across the country. The register did not clearly guide provision, which was less than adequate – and in some areas it was ignored. Further, the services available were not well organised from the point of view of the user. There was insufficient coordination of provision, and navigating the systems was complex, and often disheartening. This legislation had attempted to address individual care needs but it did not, in itself, address the *wider issues* – access to employment, education, public services and many public buildings. The existence of the 'disabling environment' was still largely ignored. Not until the passing of the Disability Discrimination Act 1995 was there legislation that required employers, public authorities and care workers to organise and adapt their provision to meet the diverse needs of the population .

The NHS Community Care Act 1990, as its name suggests, was a key point in the development and delivery of care services outside institutions and within communities. It required local authorities to assess the

Mohammed is sixty-one years of age and has Parkinson's Disease. Tamsila, his wife is his main carer. Because she has arthritis, Tamsila is not very strong, finds walking painful and so she doesn't get out much. Tamsila feels pessimistic about the future and is quite depressed. Neither Mohammed nor Tamsila speaks very much English and they feel quite socially isolated.

Mohammed needs considerable help with daily living activities. He and his wife have recently been assessed by the local social services department for a range of community care services. They are going to receive a direct payment for these services so that they can choose their own care providers and pay them directly. Tamsila would like to use people from the Mosque whom she knows and with whom she fees comfortable.

needs of people requesting community care services – and money was made available to the local authorities to finance the provision. At the same time, the larger institutions were closing. Community care provision could include social work support, home care workers providing practical support with daily living activities, day centres providing social, educational, recreational and other therapeutic activities, and physical adaptations to living accommodation. In complex cases, the 1990 Act requires the appointment of a 'care manager' to plan, monitor and review the provision for users and their carers. In 1995, the Carers (Recognition of Services) Act gave informal carers – usually unpaid family and friends – the right to a separate assessment of their needs too.

The 1996 Community Care (Direct Payments) Act allowed local authorities to make cash payments to people who have been assessed as needing community care services. This has been in part a response to the view that people with disabilities should make their own decisions about how their care needs are met, who provides them and how the services are delivered. They use their cash payment to pay for their chosen services.

It was not until the passing of the Disability Discrimination Act (1995) that there was a shift in policy towards 'rights' for disabled people. The Act gives disabled people rights in the areas of:

- Employment

- Access to goods, facilities and services

- Buying or renting land or property.

The proposed Commission for Equality and Human Rights, discussed in more detail in Topic 4, is expected to replace the Disability Rights Commission in 2007. It is expected that the work carried out by the Disability Rights Commission will continue through the new combined commission.

Check your understanding

1. **How does the Disability Discrimination Act define 'disability'?**

2. **Define the term 'impairment'.**

3. **Describe the three main models of disability – the medical model, the psychological model, and the social model.**

4. **During the twentieth century, why might people with disabilities have become institutionalised?**

5. **Briefly describe the measures introduced by the NHS and Community Care Act 1990.**

6. **In what areas of economic and social life did the Disability Discrimination Act 1995 give people rights?**

extension activities

1. Using your local library, advice bureau or social services department, research the range of community care services in your area for people with disabilities.

2. Using the internet, find four groups that support people with disabilities and summarise their aims and activities.

Topic 8 Ability and disability

THIS UNIT LOOKS AT SOME OF THE FACTORS THAT INFLUENCE PEOPLE'S BEHAVIOUR. Care practitioners often need to understand the behaviour that people show in social and health care contexts in order to help them. Why, for example, do people sometimes not take their medication? Care practitioners also need to understand how their own behaviour can be helpful or unhelpful to their service users.

We begin by looking at some of the ways that psychology can help in care practice. It can help practitioners understand, for example, why some people decide they are ill and need to see their doctor, and why others do not. It also helps practitioners understand problem behaviour and how they might help someone with their feelings or their behaviour.

We then look at some of the factors that affect the way people behave. Early experiences are especially important, providing the foundations for later development, but we also look at how people can be affected by events that happen later in their lives.

The idea of a theory is introduced in Topic 3. What can a theory do that 'common sense' can't? The next four topics then go on to look in detail at the four major approaches in psychology: behavioural, cognitive, psychodynamic and humanistic. Learning about the key ideas of each of these approaches should allow you, confidently, to go on to further study in psychology, if you choose to do so. While the unit gives you the chance to learn about psychology, it also gives you the chance to see how psychology is used in real-life situations. The aim is that you too should be able to think about issues in the way that a psychologist might do.

To help you do this, we introduce in Topic 3 the sort of framework that a psychologist (or other care practitioner) might use when faced with a problem. This is a simple framework which works through the various stages – assessment, making sense of the information that assessment provides, deciding on an intervention, and then reviewing how well it has worked.

You will see this framework being used in practice in each of the approaches. This is often done through scenarios where we 'sit in' on a discussion between a therapist or counsellor and a client or service user. These case studies are based on real situations, but the identities of the people involved have been disguised. They illustrate many of the key ideas of the theory and they show how it can be applied by someone with the proper skills and training.

Care practitioners make choices about which approach they'll use when faced with an issue or a problem. It is important, therefore, to look at the strengths of each approach, the weaknesses it has, and when a care practitioner might use it. You should begin to think about this as you study the four approaches, but the evaluations have been collected together in Topic 8 to allow comparisons to be made. (You might like to refer forwards to Topic 8 as you come to the end of each of the approach topics.)

As you work through the different theories, you will see how each of them makes different assumptions about what drives behaviour. They come to different conclusions about how much control people have over what they do, and also say something about how care practitioners might themselves behave in a social or health care context. This takes us into a discussion about the values that underpin care practitioners' work – the 'care value base'.

The unit ends with four longer case studies which show how the key terms that were introduced in earlier topics would apply and be used in a real-life context. The case studies also illustrate how care practitioners go about their work – the main approaches they use, how they use them, and some of the ethical dilemmas they face in their work.

Understanding Human Behaviour

Key questions

By the end of the unit you should be able to use the knowledge and understanding that you develop to answer the following questions:

1 How can a knowledge of psychology help care practitioners in their work?
2 What are the four major theories in psychology that help care practitioners to understand – and perhaps change – behaviour?
3 How do care practitioners decide which approach to use in any particular situation?
4 How do they put theory into practice?

Topic 1 | Using psychology in care work

Getting you thinking

Sam is 3 years old and hasn't started to speak. His parents are worried.

Ruksana is deaf. She is 16 and wants to go to college but isn't sure she'll manage.

Mark is 20. He suffered head injuries in a road accident and now wants to get his life back.

Jean is 88. She has dementia and doesn't want to move into residential care.

1 How would a knowledge of psychology help the care practitioners who will meet Sam, Ruksana, Mark and Jean?

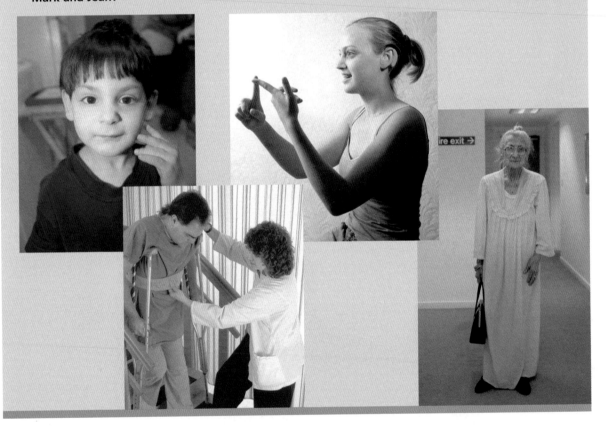

KEY TERMS

Psychology
The systematic study of how people think, feel and behave.

Diagnosis
The way care practitioners identify and classify a disorder or a disease.

ICD
International Classification of Diseases.

DSM-IV
The fourth revision of the Diagnostic and Statistical Manual of the American Psychiatric Association. It has nearly 300 categories of mental disorders.

Counselling
The process of helping someone (a client) to look at issues around their feelings or their behaviour.

Therapy
Treatment.

Care value base
The values and ethical principles that care practitioners apply to their work. These are based on beliefs about the proper way to treat service users.

How does psychology help care practitioners in care work?

Psychology sets out to explain how people think and feel. Psychologists are also interested in how people learn and develop, and how they behave. So psychology can help care practitioners understand behaviour, and it can also give them ideas about how behaviour can be changed.

Psychology has a lot to offer to care work. You may have found this for yourself when you tried the 'Getting you thinking' exercise. The links are sometimes direct and obvious. Perhaps a care worker wants to help someone to change their behaviour. This might be:

- Helping a child with autism to improve their social skills.

- Teaching a young adult with learning disabilities to use public transport.

- Working with an older person who is unhappy or depressed.

In these examples, a care worker could look to psychology – and to psychological theories – for ideas about what to do. Here are a few statements about thinking and feeling which illustrate where psychology can help in care work. Just take few moments to think about these, and try adding some more of your own.

- I think I need to see a doctor.

- I think people discriminate against me because I have a disability.

- I feel depressed.

- I feel a lot better now than I did last week.

- Kelly has learned how to dress herself.

- Adam has learned to throw tantrums to get his own way.

- Adam's social worker is learning how to communicate more effectively.

Which care practitioners might use ideas from psychology in their work?

Many care practitioners will use ideas from psychology directly in the work they do with service users. These include:

Health

Health visitors
Mental health workers
Speech and language therapists
Occupational therapists
Physiotherapists
Clinical psychologists
Some doctors and some nurses

Social Work

Foster carers
Residential care workers
Social workers

Education

Early years workers
Learning assistants
Class teachers and specialist teachers
Educational psychologists

How psychology can help care practitioners understand health and illness

Ideas from psychology can help care practitioners to understand how people deal with physical illnesses. If you think about your friends or members of your family, you will probably know some people who never seem to complain about feeling ill. If they have a cold or the flu, they just seem to keep going. Then there are others who always seem to be going to the doctor, and if they do catch a cold they will be off school or away from work for days on end.

Am I really ill?

Research in the area of health psychology suggests that there may be five questions we ask ourselves when think we are becoming ill. Here are Kate and Emma who both seem to be coming down with a cold. Look at the questions they could be asking themselves and at the answers they might give.

Kate and Emma have exactly the same symptoms, but Kate seems to have decided that she's ill and she will be going to see her doctor. Emma on the other hand is just getting on with it. So psychology can help to explain why some people define themselves as 'ill' when someone else may not.

	Kate	Emma
• What might be wrong with me?	It's probably flu.	It's just a runny nose.
• What has caused me to feel like this?	It must be a virus.	I'm just a bit run down.
• How long will this last?	It might last for days.	I'll feel better tomorrow.
• How will it affect me?	I won't be able to go to work.	I can probably shake this off.
• Can it be cured?	I need to see a doctor. I need medicine.	I just need a bit of rest.

I am ill, but I'm dealing OK with this!

Psychology can also help care practitioners to understand how people react when they are ill.

Pat and Brenda have just met at the Breast Clinic. They have identical breast lumps but they have different thoughts and feelings. Pat is anxious, but Brenda is quite beside herself with worry. Why do you think they might feel differently?

There could be many reasons for this, which might include some of the following factors:

- What they actually know about breast cancer.
- Whether other women in their families have had breast cancer.
- Whether they are normally optimistic or pessimistic in their outlook on life.
- What else is happening in their lives, and what they have to look forward to.
- The support they are getting from their friends and family.

In any event, the doctors and nursing staff who will help Pat and Brenda will need to take their feelings into account when they draw up care plans for them.

I've been to the doctor, but I'm not taking my medicine

Psychology can also help care practitioners understand why many people go to the doctor but don't then follow the doctor's advice or take the medication they've been prescribed. (Some studies have shown that about half of the patients with illnesses such as diabetes or high blood pressure don't take their medication as they should.) There may be three factors that contribute to this:

- Were they *satisfied* with the consultation, in particular with the emotional support and understanding they got from their doctor?
- How much did they *understand* of what the doctor told them?
- How much did they actually *remember* when they left the health centre?

The whole area of doctor–patient communication has attracted a lot of attention in recent years. Can you think why?

Problem behaviour

Psychology, as we have seen, can give care practitioners insights into the behaviour that people show in health contexts. It also gives them ways of understanding 'problem behaviour'.

Problem behaviour is an interesting concept. It raises questions such as, 'Who is this a problem for? Is it the person themselves? Is it their carers or family who experience the problem? Or is it people like teachers or residential care staff who have a problem managing the person's behaviour?' You can see how this can raise some dilemmas for care practitioners.

Maggie is 93 and lives in a residential care home. She is incontinent but this is not a problem for her. She accepts it and gets on with her life. It is, however, a problem for Jenny, the care worker who has to look after her. Jenny wants something done about Maggie's incontinence but Maggie refuses to even discuss it.

Jenny will probably want to discuss her feelings with the manager of the care home and they will check any course of action against the home's care value base.

Recognising 'abnormal behaviour'

There are four main approaches to defining what is normal and what is abnormal behaviour.

The first is a statistical one. This asks how frequently the behaviour occurs within the population as a whole. Behaviours which are less common are more likely to be seen as abnormal. On this definition, some quite common problems (such as depression) would not be seen as abnormal.

The second approach is based on deviation from social norms. With this definition, behaviour is abnormal if it breaks the rules (implicit or explicit) about how people ought to behave. But there are problems with this definition. It would seem to define criminal behaviour as abnormal and, of course, social norms change from culture to culture and over time.

The third approach assumes that there is an ideal state of mental health and that behaviour is abnormal or problematic if we deviate from this. This ideal state was defined by the American psychologist Marie Jahoda in terms of:

- having a positive attitude about yourself

- being able to rely on your own inner resources

- being resistant to stress

- having an accurate and realistic view of the world

- being able to adapt flexibly to the situations we find ourselves in, and the ability to fulfil our potential.

These criteria are difficult to meet (especially the last one) and they seem to express Western values rather than universal values.

A final approach simply asks if people are able to

function adequately. Their behaviour might be unusual – it might seem to be abnormal to other people, but if they are able to carry on with their lives then their behaviour is not dysfunctional, and not a problem. This leaves it up to the person concerned (or to their family) to decide whether or not to seek help. Many care practitioners are happy to work with this definition, provided that the person is not a danger to themselves or to others.

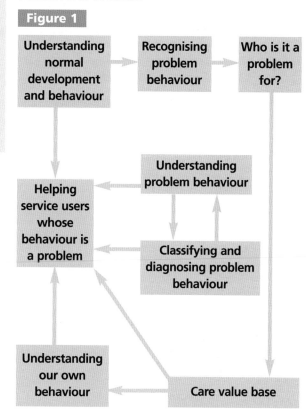

Figure 1

Classifying and diagnosing psychological problems

People who work within a medical model usually want to go further than just *recognising* abnormal behaviour. They want a way of classifying and diagnosing it. This, they argue, gives them a common set of terms when they are discussing their clients' problems with colleagues. It allows them to collect data on the incidence of the problem, and it is also useful when carrying out research. Having a **diagnosis** may also help the clinician decide what treatment to offer.

There are two major systems in use:

- The International Classification of Diseases (**ICD**)

- The Diagnostic and Statistical Manual of Mental Disorders (DSM).

The ICD is a classification system (which you met in Unit 9). The second system, DSM, not only classifies conditions but suggests how a doctor might diagnose them.

The DSM is now in its fourth edition and is more properly referred to as **DSM-IV**. It classifies mental disorders into three main categories:

* Clinical disorders

* Personality disorders

* Mental retardation.

Each has a number of subcategories. The subcategories of clinical disorders, for example, include:

– Schizophrenic and other psychotic disorders

– Mood disorders

– Anxiety disorders

– Sexual and gender-identity disorders

– Eating disorders

– Impulse control disorders

– Delirium, dementia and other cognitive disorders.

The subcategories of personality disorders include:

– Antisocial personality disorder

– Paranoid personality disorder

– Borderline personality disorder

– Avoidant personality disorder

– Dependent personality disorder

– Obsessive–compulsive personality disorder.

There are other subcategories besides these, but this should give you an idea of how DSM-IV looks. Individual conditions like autism, Tourette's Syndrome and Attention Deficit Hyperactivity Disorder (ADHD) fall into one or other of these subcategories.

Counselling

Psychologists are not medically trained in the way that psychiatrists are. They cannot prescribe medication but might, with appropriate training, offer **counselling** to their clients. You don't have to be a psychologist to become a counsellor. Nurses, social workers, teachers, and workers in the voluntary sector all train to be counsellors.

Counselling is a general term which is often used to mean the same as therapy. It refers to a process where the counsellor forms a supportive relationship with the client, and collaborates with them in addressing the problems they are experiencing. Counselling is not the same as giving advice or telling people what to do. The Year 9 student who is sent to the Head of Year for 'counselling' is more likely to be going for a serious telling off than for anything resembling real counselling!

Counselling can be thought of according to the sort of people and issues it tries to deal with. So we would find, for example:

* Adolescent counselling

* Relationship and marital counselling

* Post-traumatic stress counselling

* Addiction counselling for drug and alcohol misuse.

There are many different approaches to counselling. The main approaches we will look at in this unit are:

* Person-centred counselling

* Cognitive-behaviour therapy

* Psychoanalysis

* Transactional analysis.

Each of these is based on a different underlying approach to understanding human behaviour, and you will see some of these in action in the case studies. In practice, many counsellors will swap between approaches, depending on what the issues are for their client.

Looking at care practitioners' behaviour

So far we have looked at some of the ways in which psychology can help to explain the behaviour of service users. However, psychology also provides a way of looking at care practitioners' behaviour. What do they think and feel about the work they do, and about the people they work with? How do they behave towards their service users, and how do the service users perceive the care practitioners?

This is an important idea to finish with. Care practitioners work through a relationship with service users – and they bring their own thoughts, feelings and values to these relationships. Do they demonstrate an understanding and care for them? Do they listen actively and communicate well? Does their behaviour suggest that they will treat service users with respect?

Can you think of any examples where a care practitioner's own thinking, feelings or behaviour might not be helpful to their service users? One example might be thinking in stereotypes – that deaf and hard of hearing people are stupid, for example. Believing that older people deserve less of a service would be another – 'What do you expect? Your mother is 85'. And behaving in a discriminatory way would be yet another. Care practitioners with a strong **care value base** will be aware of these factors, and will work hard to eliminate them from their own behaviour.

Check your understanding

1 Give three examples to show how knowledge of psychology can be helpful to a care practitioner.

2 Why do some people cope better with illness than other people do?

3 Describe the four main approaches to defining abnormal behaviour.

4 Explain what the ICD and DSM-IV are.

5 What are some of the common reasons why people might seek help from a counsellor?

6 Why is it important for care practitioners to examine their own behaviour when they are working with service users?

extension activities

1 List some of the ways that psychology might help a care practitioner who is working with service users in each of the following settings: health, early years (care and education), care of older people, individuals with specific needs.

2 Suggest how each of these care practitioners might use psychology in their day-to-day work: health visitors, mental health workers, speech and language therapists, clinical psychologists, nursery nurses, teachers (including specialist teachers), educational psychologists, foster carers, social workers.

3 How could you test, through an experiment or other kind of study, the accuracy of the diagnoses that psychiatrists make?

Factors affecting our behaviour

Getting you thinking

Tom has just received his school report. He hasn't done well, and his parents don't look pleased. Turning to his father, Tom says, 'So what do you reckon the problem is, Dad? Heredity or environment?'

1 What does the term 'heredity' mean?

2 Describe two personality features that you think you share with one or other of your parents.

3 Explain why children born to the same parents can have different types of personality.

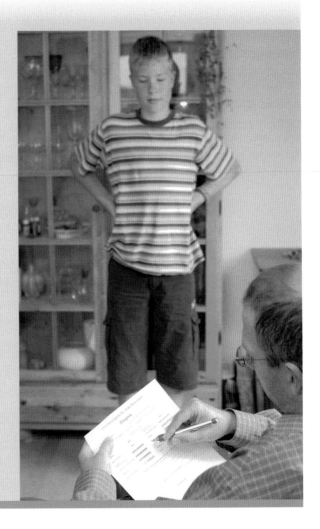

KEY TERMS

Sociology
The study of how society functions.

Socialisation
The process of learning how our society works, its expectations and rules.

Social class
A system of classifying people according to occupation and income.

Secure attachment
A strong and reliable bond, where a child feels safe and secure with their preferred carer.

Insecure attachment
Loose and unstable bonding, which may be a result of parental separation or the death of a parent.

Instinct
Ways of behaving that we are born with, and which everyone shares.

Cognitive development
Development in how we are able to think and understand.

Bereavement
Suffering loss as a result of someone dying.

Bullying
Deliberate and repeated attempts to hurt or upset another person.

Unfair discrimination
The unjustified and less favourable treatment of a person or a group, perhaps as a result of prejudice.

What makes us who we are?

Tom (who received the poor school report) knows about the nature–nurture debate, and you've met this already in this course. The basic idea is that whatever we are – and whatever we become in our lives – is a consequence of two things:

- the genes we inherit from our parents (nature)

- the experiences from our family and social environment that shape our lives (nurture).

We can argue about which set of influences is more important, but we won't have that debate here. Tom, however, is on firm ground. His parents have been responsible for his genetic inheritance *and* for many of the important environmental influences on him. So, could it be them and not Tom who is to blame for his poor school report!

Genes or environment?

Janice and Brian have just had their first child, Thomas, who has been born with Down Syndrome. This is a genetic condition – children with Down Syndrome inherit an extra chromosome, and it is more common among children born to older mothers.

Dr Singh, their paediatrician, arranges for them to have genetic counselling. They learn that there is a high chance that their next child will also have Down Syndrome. They know that Thomas will almost certainly have a degree of learning difficulty, and they learn that around 40 per cent of children with Down Syndrome have a significant heart defect.

Genetics is an important area of work. It helps care practitioners understand how some diseases come about, and why they are more common in some families and communities than in others. Gene studies can also help care practitioners find treatments for some diseases, and they may even prevent the disease occurring in the first place.

Most care practitioners, however, focus on the influences that come from their client users' environment. They have to. Someone's genetic make-up may be the whole reason why they need help, but there is nothing care practitioners can do to change it. They can, however, do something about the environmental influences – the experiences their service users will have which might create a feeling of

wellbeing and enhance their lives. Let's follow this idea through in the next part of the case study.

Janice and Brian see Dr Singh again. She says that she would like to monitor Thomas's health and development closely, and she asks Janice and Brian if they would like to be referred to other services. In time, they will be introduced to a physiotherapist and an occupational therapist who will help them encourage Thomas's gross and fine motor skills. Later they will see a speech and language therapist and a specialist pre-school teacher who will visit them at home. They will also meet their local educational psychologist. In due course they will begin to think about Thomas starting school.

These care practitioners can do nothing about Thomas's genetic make-up. However, they can all suggest ways of giving him new experiences – of changing his environment in some way – to help him develop new and useful skills.

Figure 2 *Why do people have problems?*

Types of problems	Examples
Problems that may result from genetic or biological factors	Syndromes such as Down Syndrome Schizophrenia Autism and dyslexia
Problems that result from an accident or single event	Brain damage following a road traffic accident Cerebral palsy Post traumatic stress
Problems that result from environmental factors	Many mental health problems: low self esteem; depression Slow cognitive development, delayed language

Environmental influences

The rest of this topic focuses on how our behaviour might be shaped by the influences that come from our environment. These influences can be divided into two groups.

The first group are those influences that would be of interest to a psychologist. For example, what is the influence of our early experiences and early **socialisation**, and other things that happen to us within our lives? The focus for psychologists is on the person as an individual.

The second set of influences is of interest to sociologists. These influences arise from our membership of certain groups within society. These are

Insights from sociology

So far we've taken a psychological approach to understanding behaviour, but **sociology** also has insights to offer the care practitioner. Sociology is the study of how society itself functions. It does not try to describe and explain people's behaviour at an individual or personal level but takes a different and wider view. It looks at the major social groupings that exist within our society – social class and ethnicity, for example – and uses these as the bases of its analyses and explanations. It asks big questions – like how our ethnic background might affect our attitudes to health and illness, or how health outcomes are related to social class.

You have, of course, met these ideas before (at AS level and here, in units 7 and 11). You will know how gender, ethnicity, and social class are related to the use of health services and life expectancies. There is no need to go over this again – the relationships and the inequalities are clear and well established by sociological research. Citizens or taxpayers may have views about these inequalities, and service managers or elected politicians may want to take action to address them.

Most care practitioners are not in this position, however. They are more likely to be working with individual service users, and so they need to be aware of the influences of class, gender and ethnicity that might impact upon them. Although we are all unique individuals, we are likely to share many life experiences with people who are in the same social class, gender and ethnic group as we are. These factors may shape, for example, the way we bring up our children, the expectations and ambitions we have for ourselves, and the social roles we play within our communities.

Just pause for a moment to think about some of the other ways that a sociologist might group people – other ways of dividing the population up into groups who might have similar life experiences. We have already mentioned social class, gender and ethnicity. You might add age, sexual orientation and the presence or absence of a disability. The question the sociologist asks is whether there are life experiences and influences, attitudes or ways of behaving which are common within the group and different to some extent from other groups.

The care practitioner needs to be aware of how wider social factors might be influencing their service users' lives – and influencing how they view their lives. For example, white, older and middle-class males are likely to have a number of attitudes and experiences in common, and these are likely to be different from the

attitudes and experiences of young, black and working-class women. The sociologist describes these things in general terms. What may be true for many in the group will not be true for all of them. Care practitioners need awareness, sensitivity and the ability to communicate well, and this should be part of their care value base. They also need to be aware of how social forces have shaped their own attitudes and behaviour.

Dealing with distress

Patsy is a Year 12 student and has been called to see Ms Parkin, Head of the Sixth Form, because of her lateness and absence from school. Patsy usually puts on a hard front but this morning she is really distressed. She tells Ms Parkin that she's finding it hard to cope because she has to look after her mother who has multiple sclerosis. She has to help her wash and dress, she does all the shopping and housework, and also has to care for her two younger brothers. She wants to do well at school but she is so tired. She's worried that her mum will have to go to a care home, and that her brothers will be taken into care. She hasn't told anyone else about this but she's in tears now and hopes Ms Parkin will be able to help her.

Ms Parkin thinks quickly. She hadn't expected any of this and her mind is racing. What can I do as a teacher? What can we do as a school? What would Patsy want us to do? And is there anything we really must do? Who else can help here … the GP perhaps? What about a Young Carers organisation or social services? She tries to form a plan. What might that look like?

Bringing about positive change

In this topic we've looked at how behaviour may be shaped by early experiences – and by later experiences. It is important in care practice to know about service users' early experiences. This can help care practitioners to understand how issues and problems have developed. The care practitioner must not, however, ignore later experiences as these may have the greatest impact in the here and now.

In a real sense the most important experiences are the future experiences that care practitioners can offer to their service users. This is how they bring about change, and that has to be the focus and the reason for their work. How can new experiences, offered as part of a care package, bring about positive changes in clients' lives?

Other factors operate to shape our behaviour. Culture and ethnicity, gender and sexual orientation, our economic status and the social class we belong to. The care practitioner may not know what these influences are and how they operate for any one service user, but their care value base should give a sound basis to their relationship and their work with that person.

Check your understanding

1 Explain why most care practitioners focus on the influences that come from people's environment, rather than those that come from their genetic make-up.

2 Which environmental influences would be of interest to a psychologist and which would be of interest to a sociologist?

3 Write down three key points you have learned about 'bonding'.

4 Explain how early experiences may be important in language and cognitive development.

5 Describe, in your own words, the stages a person goes through following a bereavement.

extension activities

1 Imagine you are a care practitioner and you work with a group of people, half of whom are white, older, working-class women. The other half of the group are black, younger, mainly middle-class men. Explain whether you would use the same or a different approach to working with the different types of people in the group.

2 Find out more about 'early bonding' and the effect it has on a person later in life. Explain why research evidence on bonding is contradictory.

Getting you thinking

Mrs Campbell has brought up a large family, and her granddaughter, Jane, often asks her for advice about her baby.

1 What kind of advice do you think Mrs Campbell would be able to offer Jane?

2 How might the advice and guidance provided by a health visitor, social worker or psychologist be different to that offered by Mrs Campbell?

3 Why do you think that the advice of professional care workers is often seen as having more authority than that of lay people in health and social care situations like this?

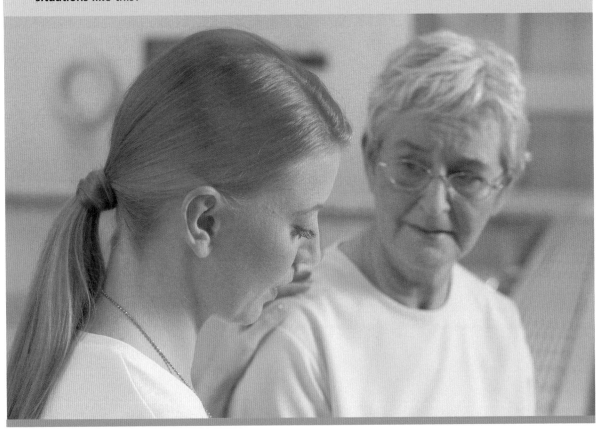

KEY TERMS

Theory
The set of linked and abstract ideas used to understand and explain things. Some theories allow practitioners to predict and control events.

Assessment
Used in this unit to mean the process of collecting information.

Working hypothesis
An attempt to understand what is causing or contributing to a problem.

Intervention
The strategies used to try to resolve a problem.

Review
Checking to see how well the intervention has worked.

What can theories do for practitioners?

Theories help people understand what is going on around them. This might be a physical event like the behaviour of atoms and molecules, or it might be something closer and more personal like the behaviour of a friend or a service user. In each case, a **theory** might help someone

- understand and explain what is happening now
- predict what might happen at some point in the future.

Some theories can also help in solving problems. If a theory helps care practitioners understand why something has happened, and what has gone wrong, perhaps it can help them when they try to put things right.

What's wrong with common sense?

Care practitioners are sometimes criticised for using theories when all they need is a bit of 'common sense'. This is an interesting sort of argument, and worth looking at in a bit more detail.

What we call 'common sense' is built up from observations of what we see happening around us, and how events seem to be linked. These observations are not made in any systematic way, and the conclusions are not always very logical.

Let's look at an example. Let's imagine that Asha's baby is crying. Her mother says the baby must be hungry. 'That's just common sense. Babies cry when they are hungry,' she says. So Asha feeds her baby and he stops crying. It looks like Asha's mother has been proved right.

But hold on. The baby stopped crying when Asha fed him – but does this mean that he was hungry? No, not necessarily. Perhaps he was uncomfortable in his cot. Maybe he just wanted to be picked up. Perhaps he needed some reassurance from his mum. We've made an observation, but we've been careless in the conclusions we've drawn for it.

Theories are also built up from observations, but these are likely to be careful and systematic. They might also be based on experimental studies. The conclusions will also fit together in a logical way.

If we wanted to develop a more complete theory about why babies cry and how we should respond to them, we would need a much wider range of observations. We might look at a range of situations

where mothers (and fathers and strangers) respond to babies by lifting them, giving them attention, feeding them, and so on. We would probably come to the conclusion that there are lots of reasons why babies cry, and being hungry is only one of them.

Theories give us ways of examining common sense, and there are times when common sense is not so very different from what a theory might tell us. However, theories also allow us to think about, understand and deal with problems that common sense has no answers for.

Who can I ask?

This is Asha's first baby and she is worried that he seems to cry a lot. There are lots of babies in her extended family but her sisters and cousins seem so confident and their babies seem so contented. Asha wonders if she is failing as a mother but feels she can't ask her mother or her sisters for advice.

Instead Asha plucks up courage to discuss this with her health visitor and says she wants to find out more about children's development and how to meet their development needs. Her health visitor has a number of ideas. Perhaps Asha and her baby might join a mother and toddler group where mothers share their experiences and support one another. Maybe she could join some of the sessions for new parents at the local Sure Start Centre. Outside speakers come and talk about feeding, teething, toilet training and tantrums. Or perhaps Asha might like to do a course in child development at her local college. She leaves these ideas with Asha. She wants Asha to make the choice for herself.

Theories about behaviour

Theories in psychology are different from theories in physics or chemistry, in a number of ways. One of the most striking differences is in the sheer number of theories that psychology seems to have. There seems to be lots of theories which set out to explain much the same sort of thing. There are many theories, for example, which try to explain how children develop language, how they learn to read, how their personalities develop, and so on. Physics and chemistry, on the other hand, seem to get by with far fewer theories.

There are several reasons why psychology is like this, and we will look at them when we start to consider the four main approaches to understanding behaviour that are covered later in this unit:

- behavioural approaches

- cognitive approaches

- humanistic approaches

- psychodynamic approaches.

Each of these approaches has areas where their theories work well, and areas where they don't. For example, psychodynamic theories are useful and work well with people who have good language and communication skills. But psychodynamic theories don't work so well with young children or with people who have learning disabilities, for whom a behavioural approach might work better.

This means that care practitioners often have a choice of which theory they might use to help them resolve a problem for a service user. They are likely to choose the theory that seems to fit the problem best – especially if it has been helpful in a similar case in the past. They are also likely to reject theories that do not fit with their own care value base.

A problem-solving framework

This unit is intended to be practical. While it is important to know about these theories, you should go further and try to put the theories into practice. You should start thinking in the same way that a psychologist or mental health worker would do when faced with a real-life problem. Below is a framework – a model – to help you understand how a mental health worker goes about their work.

This simple model has four stages and it is cyclical. In other words, it can loop back on itself – you can go back to the start and round the loop again as often as necessary. You will have seen something like this before in the Care Planning Cycle.

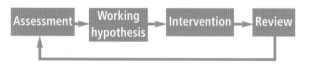

The first stage is **assessment**. Here the psychologist collects information about the problem. This might be done through:

- interviews with the service user, their family, or with other people who have worked with them

- observing the service user's behaviour in different contexts

- checklists, questionnaires, or through some specially designed tasks or tests.

How this is done depends on what kind of problem is being dealt with, and how much is already known about the person and the problem. The sort of assessment that's done also depends on the sort of theoretical approaches that the psychologist finds helpful. If she prefers to use a behavioural approach, her assessment will involve careful observation. And if she uses a psychodynamic approach, her assessment will be based on interviews. (These might be difficult ideas to grasp for now, but we'll come back to them later.)

In the next stage, the psychologist draws up some kind of **working hypothesis**. This is an attempt to understand what might be causing or contributing to the problem, and it might just be a first stab. In doing this the practitioner draws on

- their assessment of the problem

- their experience of similar problems in the past

- a range of theories that might explain this behaviour.

The psychologist then decides on an **intervention**. If she has an idea about what is causing the problem, what can she do or what can she change to make things better? This would usually involve discussions with the service user, and maybe their family and other workers. The intervention might involve:

- something that the service user can do for themselves

- some counselling or other therapeutic (treatment) work by the psychologist

- action by the people who care for the service user in some way.

If the intervention looks like it might be helpful, and if the people who will be involved agree to it, it can then be put into effect.

Just pause for a moment. If you've met these psychological theories before, can you see how the sort of theory the psychologist is using might influence the working hypotheses and the interventions that they suggest? Psychologists who like to use a behavioural approach will have one sort of idea about how to help a service user. Those who use a psychoanalytic approach will have very different ideas. We'll see how this happens when we look at examples later on in this unit.

Putting an intervention into place is not the end of the matter. The next stage is a **review**, ideally set some time in advance. At the review, the psychologist and the service user will get together with the carers and other workers to decide whether or not the intervention has been successful.

If the intervention has been well designed, it will have included:

- some kind of recording and some ongoing monitoring

- some targets, stating what would be expected to have happened by the review date.

This allows the people at the review to decide whether the intervention has worked. It may have been completely successful and no further intervention will be needed. Life is seldom as simple as this, however! For example, the review might show that the intervention had been partly successful – or it might not have worked at all.

Suppose the intervention hasn't worked, what happens next? The psychologist simply goes around the cycle again. She may decide to carry out a different or more detailed assessment – and the intervention, the monitoring and review will already have given her more information about the problem. New information and insights might then suggest a different working hypothesis, and this might give her better ideas for her intervention. So she runs the intervention, and then reviews it. She might then have resolved the problem, or she may need to go round the cycle one more time.

The model is a simple one, and we will use it again in this unit. It allows you to study some important ideas, and in particular the way that theories can be linked to practice. You will see this, for example, in:

- the assessment stage – where different theories have different ideas about what information should be collected.

- working hypotheses – where different theories can lead to quite different ideas about why a problem exists, and what causes it.

- interventions – where different theories provide very different ideas about what might be done to help someone.

Where does diagnosis fit in the framework?

Is there something missing from this framework? When you go to the doctor, you get an examination and a diagnosis, and then you get treatment. These 'working hypotheses' are all very well, but wouldn't it be better to have a proper diagnosis? And a proper diagnosis would lead to some proper treatment!

Some psychologists and mental health workers would agree with this. Others, however, would disagree strongly and would argue that diagnoses are unnecessary and even unhelpful. Let's look at some of their arguments.

They might say, first, that the diagnostic procedures and categories here are often quite vague. For example, there is no definitive test which identifies whether a child is autistic, and experts still disagree about what autism actually is. In other areas of health care, however, there are simple tests which lead to clear diagnoses. A blood test, for example, will tell a doctor whether their patient has diabetes.

They might go on to say that a diagnosis doesn't actually explain what should be done to help the service user. If a child does have autism, that doesn't

Understanding Peter

Peter has autism and learning difficulties. He attends a day centre where the staff describe him as 'aggressive and violent'. They've recently called in Alison, a clinical psychologist, to help them.

As part of her **assessment**, Alison discusses Peter's behaviour with his family. They say that they experience no problems of this sort. She then speaks with staff at the day centre. They describe frequent and unpredictable outbursts. She asks the staff to keep a record of these and spends some time observing Peter for herself.

Alison forms a **working hypothesis**. It seems that Peter's outbursts occur when he is asked to stop one activity and go on to another. This is not a problem at home where he follows routines that he knows. However, the centre offers a very varied

programme and her hypothesis is that Peter has problems coping with change.

Alison's **intervention** will involve a visual timetable. The activities available for each day will be shown to Peter using photos. He will choose what he wants to do, and the photos will be put in order on to a board. As one activity is completed, Peter will remove the photo and move on to the next activity. This way he always knows what is coming next, when dinner is, and when it's time to go home.

After two weeks they review the program. It's been a success. Peter's outbursts have reduced from an average of ten a day to an average of two a day.

Figure 4

Social interaction

- Problems relating to others
- Few friends, often alone
- Problems with sharing and taking turns
- Doesn't understand social rules
- May seem obstinate and rude.

Communication

- May have no speech and little communication
- Perhaps late in starting to talk
- Simply repeats what you say
- Literal understanding and use of language
- Speech sounds stilted or pedantic
- Can't engage in the to and fro of a conversation.

Imagination and flexibility

- Needs routines and structure
- Upset by changes
- Repetitive play
- Obsessional interests
- Little creative ability
- Unable to see the other person's point of view.

Autism and Autistic Spectrum Disorders (ASD)

Thinking about labels and labelling

Look back at the *Understanding Peter* case study. Was Peter's behaviour 'aggressive and violent' or was he 'frustrated and upset'? Let's look at how these labels might lead to different end points.

Here is one script:

- Peter's behaviour is aggressive and violent.
- Peter is an aggressive and violent person.
- That's not our responsibility.
- And we shouldn't have to put up with this.

And another:

- Peter seems to be frustrated and upset.
- So what might be upsetting or frustrating him?
- It's probably something we're doing here in the day centre.
- So what could we do to make this better?

problems for which no useful diagnosis can be given. Either there isn't a diagnosis, or the diagnosis simply a way of describing the person's behaviour without adding anything to an understanding of it. Saying that someone has a 'conduct disorder' might be an example of this. They might even say that all these categories (like the ones you saw in DSM-IV) don't exist in a real sense. They are simply an attempt to make sense of the complicated world that psychologists work in.

A final argument concerns the harmful effects of labelling people. It is sometimes argued that a label, like 'autistic', causes other people to respond in stereotyped and unhelpful ways, rather than responding to the person as an individual in their own right.

These are interesting arguments and there is probably a degree of truth in all of them! However it can be argued in return that a term like autism can be used as a working hypothesis. It's not a label, it's a signpost – showing psychologists where they might look to find interventions that have a better chance of working.

In addition, diagnoses – even tentative diagnoses – can be helpful to service users and their families. It gives them a way to understand their problems and explain them to other people. It also suggests where they might look to find out more for themselves, and can link them up with local support groups and other voluntary organisations.

actually tell the practitioners what to do next. Children on the autistic spectrum are unique people, and they need to be responded to as individuals. This is different from the diabetes example: the patient with diabetes needs a course of insulin, and the doctor can work out from the test results what dose to give them.

The next argument is that people often have

Moving on

Over the next four topics we will look at some of the major approaches in psychology, and as we do so, keep the problem-solving framework in mind. We'll use lots of case studies to illustrate these approaches, and this should help to bring them to life.

Knowing about these approaches is useful to anyone working in the health and social care field. Importantly, however, you should be able to apply them in a range of health and social care contexts. It is the practical applications that are important to service users, and they will be important when you come to take your exam!

Check your understanding

1 How do theories help care practitioners' work?

2 Name the four stages of the problem-solving framework. Describe what happens in each stage. Explain why this can be described as a cycle.

3 Explain why some people believe that having a diagnosis is important in helping people who have mental health problems.

4 Why do other people think that a diagnosis is sometimes not helpful?

extension activities

1 Chi, who is three years old, goes to nursery. He stays for lunch – but he never seems to eat anything. Sally, who runs the nursery, is concerned about him not eating. She wants to find out more, to make an assessment, and work out how she might be able to help Chi.

Work with a partner and make a list of the things she might do as part of her assessment. There are no right and wrong answers here – but what observations and interviews might help her?

2 Having a diagnosis may not be important to some care practitioners, but it is often important to parents. Think about children who might have autism or Attention Deficit Hyperactivity Disorder (ADHD). Why might having a diagnosis be important to the parents of these children?

Getting you thinking

Jamie is three years old and has just started going to playgroup. Sara, his mother, has been having some problems with him at home. She's worried because Jamie is always on the go. He never seems to be still, and she wonders if he might have Attention Deficit Hyperactivity Disorder (ADHD). Sara hopes that the staff at the playgroup will be able to help her with ideas and with practical support.

Lorna manages the playgroup. She arranges a meeting with Sara two weeks into Jamie's placement there and she asks Sara to share her concerns with her. Lorna is very experienced in working with young children and likes to take a behavioural approach, at least as a first step, when she is dealing with problems.

1 What does the acronym ADHD stand for?

2 How would you expect a child with ADHD to behave?

3 What can be done to help children with ADHD?

4 How would you deal with behaviour like that shown in the picture?

This topic will work through this case study, to help to show you what a behavioural approach might involve.

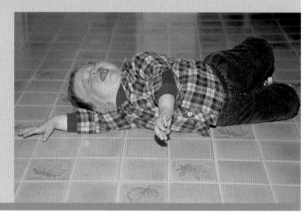

KEY TERMS

Behavioural approach
An approach that says that most of our behaviour is learned. It can be unlearned and re-learned, using reinforcement (rewards).

Behaviour modification programme
Using behavioural approaches to change someone's behaviour.

Reinforcement
Something (like a reward) that follows someone doing something, which makes that behaviour more likely to happen again.

Positive reinforcement
Reinforcement by something pleasant happening.

Negative reinforcement
Reinforcement by something unpleasant stopping.

Punishment
Something unpleasant starting.

Social reinforcement
Praise, attention, or recognition from others.

Shaping behaviour
Building up complex patterns of behaviour gradually, in small steps.

Extinguishing behaviour
Eliminating unwanted behaviour.

Time out
Removing someone from all sources of social reinforcement.

Schedule of reinforcement
How often the behaviour is reinforced.

Token economy
Using tokens (stars, smiley faces) as reinforcement. These have no value in themselves, but can be exchanged for something the person wants.

Vicarious reinforcement
Indirect reinforcement.

ABC approach (Behavioural)
Looking at the Antecedents, Behaviour and Consequences of behaviour.

An outline of the behavioural approach

Behavioural approaches can be traced back to an American psychologist called B. F. Skinner. Skinner began to publish his work in the 1930s, and his thinking is still important today. The theory is very simple. It proposes that

- most behaviour is learned

- learning takes place as a result of rewards (Skinner called this **reinforcement**)

- people repeat behaviour if it will lead to a reward of some kind.

The approach is described as 'behavioural' because Skinner was only concerned with people's external, observable behaviour. He was not interested in what might be going on inside a person's head. It was not necessary to ask what the person might be thinking or feeling. What really mattered was what they were actually doing. This is very different from the other approaches we will be looking at.

Practitioners who like to use a behavioural approach are sometimes described as 'behaviourists' and the techniques they use to influence and change behaviour are often referred to as '**behaviour modification programme**s'.

Describing behaviour

Behaviourists don't like people to use fuzzy words such as 'aggressive', 'disruptive' or 'co-operative'. They want to know exactly what a term means – what behaviour it refers to. So if a child is described as 'aggressive', a behaviourist might ask 'When she is being aggressive, what would I actually see her doing?' The answer might be 'Well, she would be taking toys away from other children, and pushing and hitting them.' This approach has now identified the specific behaviour that might need to be changed.

The behaviourist's next question might be 'And what should she be doing instead?' to which the answer might be 'Playing alongside other children and sharing her toys with them.' This has taken the process a step further – identifying the behaviour to be changed, and the behaviour to be put in its place.

So let's go back to our playgroup case study and see what Lorna is planning to do.

Think back to the framework, introduced in the last topic. The first step involves doing an assessment of some sort. From what you have already learned about the behavioural approach, what sort of assessment might Lorna be planning?

She's thinking about carrying out an observation of Jamie. She will need to identify some behaviour that can be clearly defined and easily observed, and she'll watch to see where, when and how often this behaviour occurs.

Jamie's mother, Sara, spoke about him never being still. Lorna's first idea is to count 'the number of times he runs around the classroom' but she decides that this isn't going to work. What exactly would she be counting – what exactly does 'run' mean? When does a fast walk turn into a run? And should a short run count the same as a long run? She decides instead to record the amount of time Jamie spends sitting down, either on his own or with another child. Because it would be difficult to do this over the whole morning, she decides to observe Jamie for 15 minutes every morning, just after the children have finished their orange juice.

Lorna does her observation – her assessment – over five days. She records how much time Jamie spends sitting down, working or playing at the table. This averages two minutes in a typical 15-minute period. This gives Lorna a baseline against which she can measure Jamie's progress, once the intervention starts.

She also makes some notes about what he is doing when he is not sitting down, and she notes how other people are responding to him.

Positive and negative reinforcement

Reward (reinforcement) is a key idea in all behavioural approaches – if a piece of someone's behaviour is reinforced, they are likely to repeat it.

Figure 6

Antecedents — What's happening before the behaviour occurs?

↓

Behaviour — What does the person actually do?

↓

Consequences — What happens next? Could it be rewarding and reinforcing the behaviour?

changing the consequence – thus taking the reinforcement away. The behaviour might then extinguish over a period of time. That reinforcing event could also be used to reward a different and incompatible piece of behaviour. So one piece of behaviour is extinguished, and replaced with another!

The main features of the behavioural approach should now be becoming clear:

- The relevant behaviour has to be defined clearly and objectively, without 'fuzzy' language.

- Assessment will involve careful observation of the behaviour … and remember the ABC model.

- The working hypothesis is likely to focus on what is reinforcing the behaviour; and on how to reinforce the new behaviour wanted instead.

- The intervention will say quite specifically what is to be done. In fact it is often written out, and everyone might be given a copy.

- The intervention is likely to involve people like parents, carers, and staff in doing things – more so than the service user themselves.

- It is likely to include quite specific targets, and these will be used to measure change.

- Change can be gradual, and new behaviour can be shaped up over a period of time.

Lorna's observations

Let's see how Lorna does this. Lorna's observations don't reveal any obvious antecedents for Jamie's behaviour, except that he seems to run off most often when there are no adults close to him – and he never runs away when an adult is actually working with him.

As for the consequences, Lorna notices that the playgroup staff respond very quickly when he runs off. Sometimes they even run after him – in case he should fall or knock someone over. This makes him run even faster. It looks as though he might be enjoying this.

What do you think Lorna's working hypothesis might be? Lorna thinks that Jamie's running about is simply a way of getting adult attention. It's this – the attention that adults give him – that could be reinforcing his behaviour.

Lorna decides to check this idea out with Sara, Jamie's mum. Sara is not sure about this, but she's very happy to plan an intervention with Lorna, on the assumption that it might be right.

So, what might Lorna and Sara decide to do? There are a number of possible answers to this question, but Lorna and her staff decide:

- Not to run after Jamie if he runs off. Instead they will take him quietly back to where he ought to be. So he gets no attention for his 'running behaviour'.

- In addition, they will look for every occasion when Jamie is sitting down doing something he ought to be doing, and they will give him lots of praise and attention for this.

- Finally, they will target Jamie for an extra small-group session with two children and an adult every morning. This will give him attention for sitting and working, in the company of other children.

The intervention will run for two weeks. Jamie's behaviour will be observed in the 15 minutes after juice, and the target is to increase the amount of time he spends sitting and doing something appropriate.

Lorna and Sara meet to review Jamie's progress. The intervention has been successful up to a point. Jamie is now spending five minutes in every 15 sitting and behaving appropriately, and this is similar to one or two other children in the group. Lorna decides that she would like to run the intervention, unchanged, for a further four weeks and they will meet again to review progress. Sara is happy with this and now has some ideas to try at home.

Check your understanding

1 Explain the ideas of positive reinforcement and negative reinforcement.

2 What's the difference between negative reinforcement and punishment?

3 Explain how a piece of behaviour can be 'shaped' using reinforcement.

4 What is vicarious reinforcement?

5 What happens in a token economy?

6 In the ABC approach to observation, what does each of the letters stand for?

extension activities

1 Try to turn these 'fuzzies' into objective and observable descriptions of each person's behaviour (hint – what would you actually see them doing?):
'Jane is really naughty.'
'Norah has excellent table manners.'
'Peter is very difficult in the mornings.'
'Ann is really fun to be with!'

2 Now take your description of Jane's behaviour or Peter's behaviour. How could you observe and record that behaviour?

3 Finally, think of someone you know whose behaviour can be inappropriate at times. Can you think of some of the things that might be reinforcing that behaviour? (Hint – think of the consequences. What happens after the behaviour occurs?)

Getting you thinking

1 Wayne has said, 'Hi' to Ali, but Ali didn't answer him. Wayne now believes that Ali doesn't like him. Is this conclusion correct?

2 Can you think of other situations where people jump to the wrong conclusions?

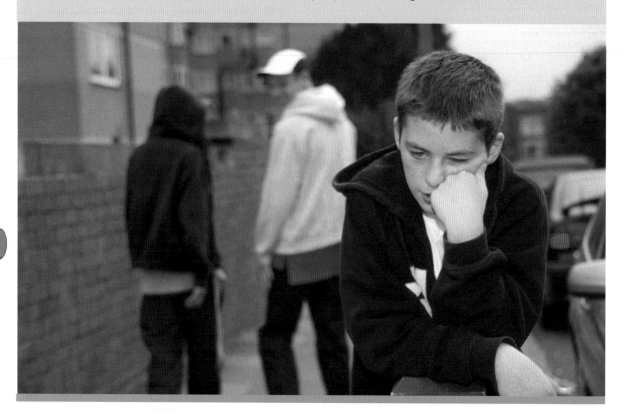

KEY TERMS

Cognitive
To do with thoughts and thinking.

Cognitive primacy
The view that what we think determines what we feel and do.

Information processing approaches
Ways of understanding our behaviour which look at how we deal with information – what things we attend to, what we ignore, and what we can remember.

ABC approach (Cognitive)
Analysing behaviour in terms of the Activating event, Beliefs (which may be irrational or dysfunctional) and the emotional or behavioural Consequences.

Functional beliefs
Ways of thinking that are helpful to us.

Dysfunctional beliefs
Beliefs that are faulty and unhelpful.

Schemas
How we bring together and organise information about ourselves and things around us.

Schematic thinking
Thinking using schemas.

Cognitive-behavioural therapy (CBT)
Using a cognitive approach to help people change the way they feel and act.

Homework
Tasks the client is asked to do – things to practise until they see the counsellor again.

What's happened to thinking?

When you were working on the last topic on behavioural approaches, did you begin to worry that people's ability to *think* didn't seem to figure anywhere in the behaviourist's model? The behaviourists said that they didn't need to ask about what might be going on inside a person's head. But things do go on inside people's heads: they think, they understand and they make choices. So if care practitioners want to help people change their behaviour, perhaps they should ask about what they think, as well as looking at what they do.

If you were thinking along these lines, you're in good company. Two Americans – the psychologist Albert Ellis and the psychiatrist Aaron Beck – came to much the same conclusion, and went on to develop the '**cognitive**' approach to understanding problem behaviour (cognitive – because it focuses on thinking).

Remember the behaviourists' ABC model, where:

A is the antecedent – the stimulus that might set the behaviour off

B is the behaviour itself – the response to the stimulus

C is the consequence – what happens next by way of reinforcement.

The cognitive approach says that thinking and feeling come in between the stimulus and the response. And in order to help people who have a problem with their behaviour, practitioners need to help them examine what they think and feel.

Rational thinking and distorted thinking

The cognitive approach assumes that much of the time, what people think and what they believe are quite rational. Sometimes, however, their thinking is distorted and this can lead to social, emotional and behavioural difficulties.

Rational thinking	Distorted thinking
Thinking is based on good evidence.	Thinking is based on limited evidence, or on no evidence at all
Conclusions are logical, and based on the evidence.	Conclusions are irrational and are not supported by the evidence
This leads to functional beliefs. These are useful and helpful.	This leads to **dysfunctional beliefs** which are unhelpful.
Result: happy, competent and effective people.	Result: problematic behaviour: fears, anxieties and depression.

Cognitive primacy

Cognitive primacy is a psychologist's way of saying that thoughts and beliefs are important – that what people think and believe determines what they feel and do. So, if a service user has a problem with their emotions (their feelings) or with their behaviour, the therapist will try to uncover their distorted thinking and help them to examine their **dysfunctional beliefs**.

Information processing

We make some mistakes in our thinking because of the way we process information. For example, our attention is selective. There is usually lots going on around us but we are not aware of all of it. We notice and attend to things that are important to us, things that we expect to see, and things that we want to see. We often think by sorting things into categories (**schemas**) and our thinking is not always logical. We remember some things and forget others.

Distorted thinking

Beck identified a number of ways in which our thinking can be distorted. Here are some examples. Do these ever apply to you or your friends?

We make inferences and draw conclusions where we have no evidence. For example, 'James hasn't phoned me. That means he doesn't like me.' Sometimes these inferences get chained together, for example, 'I expect he's gone out with Emma or Caroline instead, and no one will ever want to go out with me. And that just proves how ugly and unattractive I am.'

We sometimes over-generalise and draw sweeping conclusions from very limited evidence. For example, 'I've just failed my driving test and there's no point in taking it again. I'll never pass. I'm useless.'

We sometimes think in categories that can be absolute, inflexible and opposite. Beck called this 'dichotomous' thinking. For example we might divide people into 'those who like me' and 'those who hate me'. There are no shades of grey here. If somebody doesn't seem to like me, then they must hate me.

Another kind of distorted thinking is when people personalise things and assume that if something goes wrong, it must be their fault. For example, 'Amir is in a bad mood. I must have upset him.'

Beck described this kind of thinking as 'automatic thoughts'. Automatic because we don't ever examine them, and they've become to reflect the way we see the world. Notice how they tend to be self-critical.

Schemas and schematic processing

Automatic thoughts could also be described as schemas [the plural is sometimes written as *schemata*]. Schemas are the ways in which we bring together and organise information about ourselves, other people, and things around us. It's like we've got the world sorted into ready-made categories, on the shelf and available when we need them. Like any sorting system, schemas tend to simplify things that might be quite complex. They cause us to focus on some details at the expense of others – but they speed up our ability to process new information, and allow us to interpret, remember and evaluate new information. Thinking in schemas is described as schematic processing.

More distorted thinking

Ellis also suggested that words like 'should', 'ought to', 'need to' and 'must' often reveal irrational and distorted thinking. Examples might be:

'He should enjoy spending time with me.'

'She ought to phone me.'

'I need to lose weight.'

'I must live up to my parents' expectations.'

These are all very strong statements, but how many of them are supported by good evidence? Let's check one out, the one about living up to parents' expectations. If you heard someone saying this, you could try asking questions like:

'Why must you live up to your parent's expectations?'

'What would happen if you did?'

'What's the worst that would happen to you if you didn't?'

'What evidence do you have that leads you to believe any of this?'

Cognitive-behavioural therapy

The approach we've described as the 'cognitive approach' is also known as the 'cognitive-behavioural approach'. People who use these approaches to help others change their behaviour practise cognitive-behavioural counselling, or **cognitive-behavioural therapy** (CBT).

Let's look again at the three main ideas in cognitive-behavioural therapy before seeing how it might work in practice:

- What people think and what they believe determine how they feel and how they behave.

- Emotional problems are the result of negative and distorted thinking – they arise out of dysfunctional beliefs.

- If care practitioners can change this negative and distorted thinking, they will help people to overcome their emotional and behavioural problems.

Another ABC model

The first stage in cognitive-behavioural counselling is to make some assessment of how the client sees their situation. The counsellor has a framework for doing this and, rather confusingly, it's also an ABC model.

- **A** is the activating event. Something happens. Let's say that one of your classmates had just passed you in the corridor without acknowledging you.

- **B** refers to the beliefs you have about this. You might think, 'She's just ignored me, probably she doesn't like me, and it's so awful because I need people to like me.'

- **C** stands for consequences, and these might be emotional or behavioural consequences. An emotional consequence might be that you get upset and depressed. A behavioural consequence might be that you will ignore this student in future, because you believe that she ignored you.

John is 23, he is single and lives at home with his parents. He finds it difficult to go out socially and although he has a girlfriend at the moment, he thinks she will dump him. John experiences panic attacks when he is in crowded places, and buses and trains are especially difficult for him.

Jenny, the counsellor, greets John warmly, and asks him to talk about himself and his difficulties. She encourages John through 'active listening'. This could involve prompting questions – 'Tell me a bit more about that' – and reflecting ideas back and checking them out with him – 'Would I be right in thinking then that …?' Throughout the interview, she is making a note of:

- A: the activating event

- B: the beliefs and thoughts about A

- C: the emotional and behavioural consequences of B.

JENNY: So, let's talk about that time on the bus. Can you tell me how you felt?

JOHN: Well, everyone was looking at me, and I felt tense – sort of sick – and I just wanted to get off.

JENNY: The consequence was that you felt sick and you wanted to get off. Is that right?

JOHN: Yes.

JENNY: OK, so people were looking at you. I'll put that down as an activating event. And what thoughts did you have at the time?

JOHN: I just thought, they must think I'm weird.

JENNY: Hmm. That sounds to me like a dysfunctional belief.

Jenny has identified the activating event and the consequences – the (A) and the (C) – but the (A) doesn't cause the (C). She needs to identify John's beliefs – the (B) – because it's the (B) that causes the (C).

In a real counselling session, the therapist would explore a number of other emotional episodes but Jenny's assessment is already leading to a working hypothesis: John believes other people think he's weird and look down on him, and this has led to a poor self-concept and low self-esteem. So he finds it difficult to go out and mix socially.

At their next meeting, Jenny will start working on an intervention with John and this will involve a number of steps. Like other cognitive-behavioural therapists, she will explain her approach carefully to John. She will teach John to monitor:

- things that happen to him – the activating events (A)

- how these things make him feel – the consequences (C).

She will also help him to:

- understand that he has beliefs (B) about (A) that make him feel (C)

- examine the evidence for these beliefs. Is his thinking distorted and are his beliefs dysfunctional?

Finally, she will:

- invite John to try interpreting the activating events (A) in other and more rational ways

- ask him to try out some things for 'homework'.

This should lead to different beliefs (B) and to different feelings and behavioural consequences (C). Let's listen in to one of their sessions:

JENNY: You said, John, that everyone on the bus was looking at you? Was that everyone?

JOHN: Well, that's how it seemed at the time.

JENNY: How it seemed?

JOHN: Hmm. Some people were looking at me, but I guess some didn't really notice me.

Jenny is beginning to get John to look at the evidence, at the activating event (A). She continues:

JENNY: OK. Some people were looking at you. Now tell me again, why was that?

Jenny wants John to find the belief (B) that leads to his feelings of low self-esteem (C).

JOHN: It's obvious! They think I'm weird. That's why they look at me.

JENNY: OK, but there are other reasons why we look at people. Yes?

JOHN: Yes. Well, sometimes.

JENNY: Reasons like …what?

JOHN: Well, some people look interesting. Attractive maybe.

JENNY: Well maybe that's why some of the people on the bus looked at you. Maybe some of them thought you were interesting. Is that possible?

JOHN: It's possible. But it's not very likely.

Jenny is offering John another belief (B) about the event (A). If he believes that he might be interesting (and not weird) then he will feel better about himself, and may start to mix more. But John's not convinced, so Jenny goes back to look at the connections between (A) and (B).

JENNY: Let's see if I've got this right. Some people weren't looking at you?

JOHN: That's right.

JENNY: And for those who were, what's the evidence, John, that any of them thought you were weird?

JOHN: Well, that's what I assumed. I can't prove it. But I certainly felt weird!

JENNY: OK. But could you agree that maybe some of them thought you were … interesting?

JOHN: It's possible, I suppose.

JENNY: And if some people thought you were interesting, would that make you feel interesting?

JOHN: That's a bit much to hope for, don't you think!

Can you see how Jenny is starting to challenge John's distorted thinking and inviting him to accept a different set of beliefs? John isn't convinced, but Jenny isn't surprised by this. John has had these beliefs about himself for many years.

Cognitive-behaviour therapy isn't just about talking. Clients are asked to do something, some kind of homework between their sessions. This could be a way of exploring or testing out some new belief (B) to see what the consequences (C) might be. Jenny decides to give John a choice here.

JENNY: OK, John, There's a couple of things I'd like you to try out before next week. I'd like you to go back on the bus, and I'd like you to look around and notice the number of people who are not looking at you. Could you do that?

JOHN: I get it! You want me to examine the belief that everyone is looking at me?

JENNY: Well done, John. That's it exactly.

JOHN: Anything else?

JENNY: If you can manage it, I'd like you to choose someone, perhaps an older person, and say to yourself, 'Maybe they think I'm interesting.' Then hold eye contact for a count of three, and just make a mental note of how that feels to you. Could you do that?

John decides he could do the noticing task, but doesn't think he could hold eye contact with anyone. So they agree that he will just do the first bit of homework, and he'll tell Jenny how it feels next time they meet.

Thinking back to our problem-solving framework, Jenny has done her assessment, she has a working hypothesis, and she has started on an intervention. She will review this next time she meets John.

Depression

Beck was especially interested in using cognitive-behaviour therapy with people who have depression. There are some special challenges here for the therapist. For example,

- The client's thinking will be very negative, particularly their beliefs about themselves. 'I'm just no good any more.' It may be difficult to get them to consider any alternative, positive beliefs.

- They may also have negative views about the future, and think that things will never change. As a result, they may find it difficult to commit to making the changes that they need to make. 'What's the point?'

- They may also lack the energy to change. 'I couldn't manage this week's **homework**. I was just worn out.'

- Finally, they may get depressed by their inability to cope, and this just makes them more depressed. This has been described as 'depression about depression'.

The counselling process will be similar to what Jenny did with John, but the counsellor might place a bit more emphasis now on 'homework'. If she can get the client to change their behaviour, even in a small way, then she might break this cycle of being depressed about being depressed.

Two symptoms of depression are apathy and inactivity, and so the counsellor might decide to work

	Monday	Tuesday
8.00–8.30	Take a shower	
8.30–9.00	Have breakfast	
9.00–10.00	Read the newspaper	
10.00–11.00	Do the ironing	
11.00–12.00	Go shopping	
12.00–1.00	Have lunch	
1.00–2.00	Do the dishes, clean the kitchen	
Etc.	Etc.	
8.00–8.30	Plan tomorrow's activities	
8.30–11.00	TV then bed	

with the client to make up a timetable, a list of things they will do in a day. This will be carefully graded – nothing too difficult to start with – and it will include things that they might enjoy (or used to enjoy before they became depressed). This will be written out, the client will tick each activity off as they finish it, and perhaps write down on a scale of 1–10 how much they enjoyed it.

Doing homework keeps clients involved in their therapy between sessions, and a 'to do' list such as this one helps the depressed person see that they can manage their lives. This challenges some of their dysfunctional beliefs about not being able to cope, and not being able to change. The counsellor will review this with them at their next meeting.

We will look at the strength and weaknesses of the cognitive approach when we come to Topic 8.

Check your understanding

1 Why is this called a 'cognitive' approach?

2 Why does this approach place such stress on what we think and believe?

3 Give some examples of distorted thinking and suggest why these might happen.

4 What are dysfunctional beliefs?

5 Cognitive-behaviour therapists use an ABC approach. What do the letters stand for?

6 Why are clients asked to do 'homework'?

7 What other things will the therapist need to be aware of when working with people who are depressed?

extension activities

1 Dave has passed Natasha in the corridor and didn't speak to her, and Natasha is really upset. She often gets upset over things like this.

Imagine you are a cognitive-behavioural counsellor working with Natasha. How might Natasha's thinking be distorted and what dysfunctional beliefs might she have? How could you help her to examine these? What homework might you set for her?

2 Choose another problem – an invented one – and role-play this with a partner.

269

Topic 5 Cognitive approaches

Getting you thinking

1 What kind of emotions do you think this girl is feeling?

2 How might knowing something about her past help you to understand what she is feeling now?

3 Why can't we always explain why we think, feel and act the way we do?

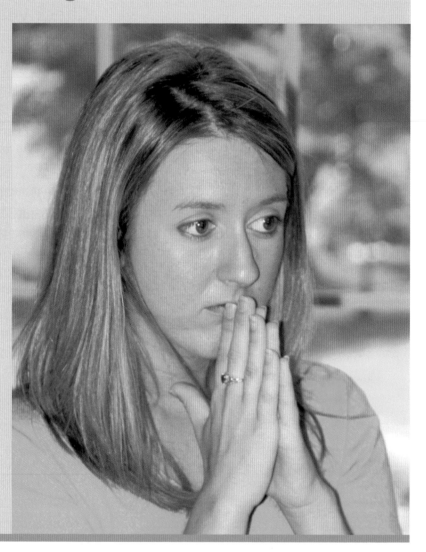

KEY TERMS

Psychodynamic approaches
Approaches based on the idea that our thoughts and feelings are the result of unconscious processes.

Conscious
What we are aware of.

Unconscious
Thoughts and feelings that we are not aware of.

Id
The part of our mind that contains our basic instincts, and aggressive and sexual drives.

Ego
The part of our mind that is rational and based in reality.

Superego
The part of our mind that represents ideals and values – our conscience.

Ego defence mechanisms
The ways the ego can protect itself from the urges of the id (repression, for example).

Transactional analysis (TA)
An approach to understanding behaviour through interpreting the interactions people have.

Psychodynamics, psychoanalysis and Freud

Psychodynamic approaches to understanding human behaviour date from the end of the nineteenth century, and begin with the work of Sigmund Freud (picture opposite). Freud was a doctor who set up a clinic to treat nervous diseases in Vienna in 1886. He had come across a kind of treatment where people were cured of their symptoms by talking about them, and this became the basis of his own approach. As his patients talked about their lives and their fears and anxieties, Freud came to form his own theory of how our personalities develop. He also developed a distinctive way of helping his patients which is known as psychoanalysis. The terms psychoanalytic and psychodynamic are sometimes used interchangeably, but it would be more correct to say that psychoanalytic theories are examples of a larger group of psychodynamic theories.

Conscious and unconscious

Is our behaviour influenced by things we are not aware of? People who take a psychodynamic view believe it is. Freud, for example, distinguished three states of mind:

- The 'conscious' is what we are aware of, in the here and now.

- The 'preconscious' consists of things we can bring back easily, into consciousness, from our memories.

- The 'unconscious' is the store of all the thoughts, feelings and ideas we have had during our lifetime. Although these cannot be brought easily into awareness, they can have a major influence on our feelings and our behaviour in the here and now.

Freud was particularly interested in the unconscious part of the mind. His techniques of psychoanalysis tried to reach repressed thoughts and memories and bring them safely into consciousness. That way his patients would be able to gain insight into their difficulties and, with the psychoanalyst's support, deal with any painful memories and unresolved conflicts. This should bring them to a better state of mental health.

The id, the ego and the superego

Through his clinical work, Freud came to believe that the mind consists of three interrelated systems. These don't exist in a physical sense but they were, for Freud, a useful way of thinking about how our personalities develop.

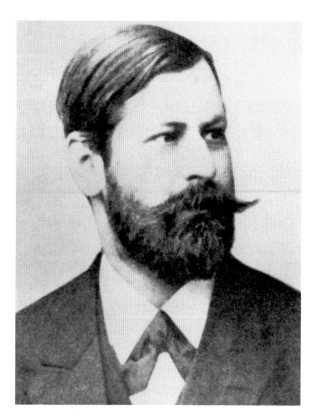

The energy for the whole system comes, he said, from the **id**. This is a mass of powerful pleasure-seeking instincts, which demands immediate satisfaction. The id operates according to the 'pleasure principle'.

Clearly we cannot have all our wants and desires met. We have to fit in with the world around us, and so the id has to be kept in check. This is a job for the **ego**. The id requires immediate satisfaction, but the ego advises self-control! The ego operates according to the 'reality principle' and has to find safe and acceptable ways to satisfy the id's basic demands and desires.

The final piece in the jigsaw is the **superego**. The superego is rather like our conscience. It is concerned with right and wrong, and it incorporates the moral values which we learn initially from our parents, and then through the society we live in. The supergo operates according to a 'perfection principle' and it will try to persuade the ego to adopt its moral and idealist goals rather than the realistic goals the ego normally pursues.

These three systems – the id, the ego and the superego – are constantly in tension with each other. You can see, for example, how the id and the superego will be in direct conflict with each other, and how the ego has to act like a kind of referee. A strong ego allows both the id and the superego to express themselves in socially appropriate ways, and at appropriate times. This makes, in Freud's terms, for a balanced and healthy individual.

Sometimes, however, the ego is not strong enough to control the id or the superego. If the ego is weak, the

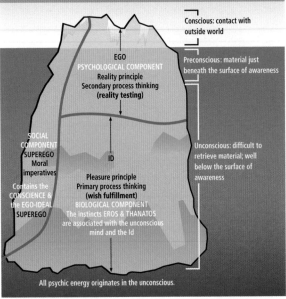

Figure 7 The mind was seen by Freud as being like a partly submerged iceberg.

Conscious: contact with outside world

EGO
PSYCHOLOGICAL COMPONENT
Reality principle
Secondary process thinking
(reality testing)

Preconscious: material just beneath the surface of awareness

SOCIAL COMPONENT
SUPEREGO
Moral imperatives
Contains the CONSCIENCE & the EGO-IDEAL
SUPEREGO

ID

Unconscious: difficult to retrieve material; well below the surface of awareness

Pleasure principle
Primary process thinking
(wish fulfillment)
BIOLOGICAL COMPONENT
The instincts EROS & THANATOS are associated with the unconscious mind and the Id

All psychic energy originates in the unconscious.

impulses from the id might dominate a personality and this could lead to dangerous, destructive or immoral behaviour. If the superego comes to dominate, a person may become overly moral and deny themselves very ordinary and acceptable pleasures. This could lead to anxieties, phobias and neurotic behaviour in later life.

Ego defence mechanisms

According to Freud, our unconscious mind contains all sorts of thoughts and feelings – some of them so awful that we cannot safely admit them to ourselves. As a result, we need ways of defending our conscious mind (our ego) from these thoughts and we have a number of **ego defence mechanisms** which do this for us. These defence mechanisms have a number of things in common:

- They deny or distort reality in one way or another.

- They operate unconsciously, so that we are not aware of them.

- They allow us to cope with the demands of life.

Here are some of the more common ego defence mechanisms in Freud's theory.

Repression is the fundamental defence mechanism in Freud's theory. It occurs when unacceptable thoughts, desires and emotions are blocked so that they do not become conscious.

Projection occurs when we attribute our own feelings of guilt or inadequacy on to another person, and then we blame them for the very faults we have ourselves. For example, we might describe someone we know as mean and stingy when it is really us who is mean and stingy.

Sublimation happens when we shift our thoughts and desires into an activity which is socially acceptable. It is claimed, for example, that our aggressive drives are sublimated and expressed in playing sports. Competitive games, especially contact sports, offer a socially acceptable outlet for our aggression. It has also been claimed that artistic pursuits – singing, painting, and so on – are a way of expressing our inhibited sexual desires!

Regression occurs when we display childish behaviour, behaviour that might have been effective for us when we were much younger. This can happen when we're anxious. Mostly it passes unnoticed as, for example, when we suck a pencil, or suck our thumb. Sometimes, though, it can be a problem. For example, a child might start wetting the bed if she is going through a difficult time at school.

Getting to the unconscious

Freud was particularly interested in what was happening in our unconscious, but you might have noticed a problem with this. How can the psychotherapist explore a person's unconscious mind when the person themselves doesn't know what's there? And it gets even more difficult if the person has strong defence mechanisms to keep the most difficult and painful thoughts at an unconscious level and out of awareness. Some special techniques will be needed here. The case study about Sasha (opposite) will show it can be done.

Did you notice a common thread here? Whatever Sasha says or does has to be interpreted by the psychotherapist for some underlying meaning. It may not be accepted at face value.

Attachment

John Bowlby, a British psychoanalyst, was particularly interested in the bonding, or attachments, we make with significant people in our lives. Our first attachments are usually with our parents. Bowlby argued that if children are separated from their parents, or if they do not make a secure bond with them, they will have problems making close and stable relationships with other people. The child might either cling on to relationships in later life – or they might avoid making close relationships altogether. If the family provides the child with a secure base, however, the child will be able to make deep and lasting relationships, and go out into the world confidently.

Bowlby's work has been very influential in care practice. For example:

- Hospitals now make it easier for parents to visit and stay with their children.

Reaching Sasha's unconscious

Sasha is 5 years old and is in her first year at primary school. She doesn't like going to school. She cries every morning, and she complains of feeling sick. If she ever gets as far as the school gate, she throws a huge tantrum and refuses to go in.

Sasha's parents have met the school's educational psychologist, who tried a behavioural approach to the problem. This involved rewarding (reinforcing) Sasha for getting dressed without crying on school days, and for walking closer to the school gate each day. This intervention was partly successful but Sasha still refused to let go of her mum's hand.

The educational psychologist refers Sasha to a psychotherapist who, as part of her assessment, will explore some of Sasha's unconscious thoughts.

She begins by asking Sasha to talk about herself and about school. She will listen carefully to what Sasha says, and try to identify any patterns in what Sasha tells her. Is Sasha, for example, defending herself by distorting or avoiding some areas? Sasha, however, is very defensive and will not talk about school at all.

At their next meeting she lets Sasha say whatever comes into her mind. The psychotherapist calls this 'free association'. She hopes that some of Sasha's unconscious thoughts or fears may slip out if she relaxes and starts to drop her defence mechanisms. This doesn't work. Sasha is only 5, her language skills are not well developed, and the psychotherapist finds it hard to interpret what Sasha is telling her. With an older child, she might have tried hypnosis but she rules this out for the same reasons.

She then asks Sasha if she can remember any dreams she's had. Freud said that dreams were 'the royal road to the unconscious'. He thought that the things we dream about represent people and situations in our waking life. We are not aware of the connections, but the psychotherapist may be able to interpret this for us. Sasha tells the psychotherapist about a dream where she is in a busy shop, lost and crying because she cannot find her mummy.

At their next meeting, the psychotherapist tries something different. She asks Sasha to draw some pictures of herself and the people in her family. She also brings out some dolls and Sasha plays with them, acting out some of the things that are happening, or might be happening in her life. Sasha enjoys this. The psychotherapist watches her closely and tries to interpret what Sasha's behaviour might be telling her.

Until now, everyone has assumed that Sasha is afraid of something at school. This assessment – especially the drawings and the doll play – leads the psychotherapist to a different working hypothesis. She thinks that Sasha isn't afraid of anything at school. She's simply afraid to leave her parents, especially her mummy, in case she's not there when she comes back from school. Sasha's parents now remember a time when Sasha's mum had to go into hospital for a few days. This upset Sasha and she has repressed it. Her drawings and her doll play have brought this out, and this will lead to a very different intervention from what has been tried before.

Why is Amy so anxious?

Sasha's classmate Amy is also experiencing problems at school. The teaching assistant has noticed that, most days, she has wet herself by late afternoon. She discusses this with the class teacher and they decide to observe Amy closely. They notice that she never seems to go to the toilet and she is wet nearly every afternoon.

They call to see Amy's mother, Mrs Kerr, at home. They notice how very clean and tidy the house is – almost excessively so. Mrs Kerr is very proud of her home and says the toilets at school are 'very dirty and smelly'. They begin to notice how very rigid Mrs Kerr is in her opinions about children

and they suspect that Amy's toilet training was a harsh and punitive experience. They learn that Amy is punished and sent to her bedroom for coming home wet from school.

The School staff suspect that Mrs Kerr has a very strong superego and that she operates on the 'perfection principle'. They decide that they need to help her move towards a position of reality. They will explain to her that many five-years-olds wet themselves at school, and they will show Amy that the school toilets can be used quite safely.

- Social workers try hard to keep children with their birth parents.

These changes in care practice recognise the importance of early attachments.

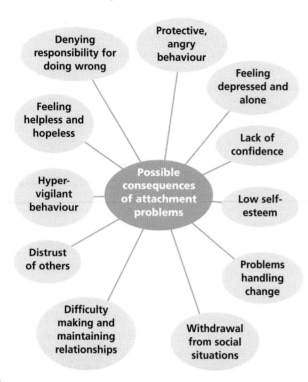

Figure 8 Possible consequences of attachment problems

Presenting problems from the past

Tom is 43 and lives with his partner Pat. Their relationship is running into difficulties and Pat wants them to go to counselling together. During discussion with the counsellor it emerges that Tom has always had problems sustaining close relationships, and the counsellor wonders if this could be the result of his experiences as a child. He learns that Tom's mother had problems looking after him, he was taken into care, and passed through a large number of foster placements. Along the way, Tom formed no real attachments with anyone, either at home or at school. It wasn't worth the effort, he said, as nothing ever seemed to last. He just got moved on to a new home and a new school. With every failed relationship, Tom became less willing to commit to the next one and this became a vicious circle which he really wants to change.

Bowlby suggested that people develop their own 'internal working model' of the world. This is represents the way we think about ourselves and the significant people we are attached to. Because this is organised and not haphazard, a psychotherapist could explore this with a service user. How do they see the world? Why do they see it that way? And are there any other ways in which they can see and understand it?

Transactional analysis

A number of other 'therapies' have been developed out of psychoanalysis, including transactional analysis (TA). This approach was developed by Eric Berne, an American psychiatrist. (Berne originally trained as a psychoanalyst but his application to practice was turned down on the grounds that he was not 'ready'. It was felt that he needed to spend several more years under analysis himself.)

In TA, the word **transactions** means, roughly, the interactions we have with other people. These transactions (interactions) need to be analysed (interpreted) before we can understand what they really mean.

One important idea in TA is that we give each other recognition or 'strokes'. Young children get a lot of physical strokes (hugs and cuddles). Adults exchange verbal strokes (like praise for example) – and strokes can be negative as well as positive (criticism and put downs.) Berne said that people need to have strokes, and if they cannot get positive strokes, they might work deliberately to get negative strokes. This might explain someone's negative and even self-destructive behaviour.

Another interesting idea is that we exchange strokes through 'games' in which transactions are not always what they seem. Berne explained this in his bestselling book, *Games People Play*. He gave his games interesting names – 'Why don't you … Yes but…', for example. In a conversation like this, one person, Tom, will ask for advice. Jen offers advice, 'Why don't you …' and Tom rejects every suggestion with a 'Yes but …' Tom is playing a game here. He does not really want advice from Jen, what he wants are strokes and this is a roundabout way of getting them.

These are the sorts of transactions that the practitioner will try to analyse but, as you might expect, there is a lot more to TA than this.

Check your understanding

1 **Complete this table.**

	Id	Ego	Superego
Conscious?	No		Yes
Concerned with?			Conscience and moral values
Operates according to?		Reality principle	
If it is not controlled, will lead to what?	Instinctive and immoral behaviour	The ego operates as the controlling system	

2 **List some of the ways in which a psychoanalyst might explore a person's unconscious.**

3 **In TA, what are strokes and games?**

extension **activities**

1 Try an internet search for some of the key terms in this topic. Some of the sites will be quite complicated, but they may help your understanding of the main ideas.

Topic 6 Psychodynamic approaches

Topic 7 Humanistic approaches

Getting you thinking

1 What do you think happens in a counselling situation like the one pictured?

2 Can you tell from the picture which one is the counsellor, and which one is the client?

3 Describe the role that the counsellor is expected to play in a counselling relationship.

4 What qualities and skills do you think a person needs to be an effective counsellor?

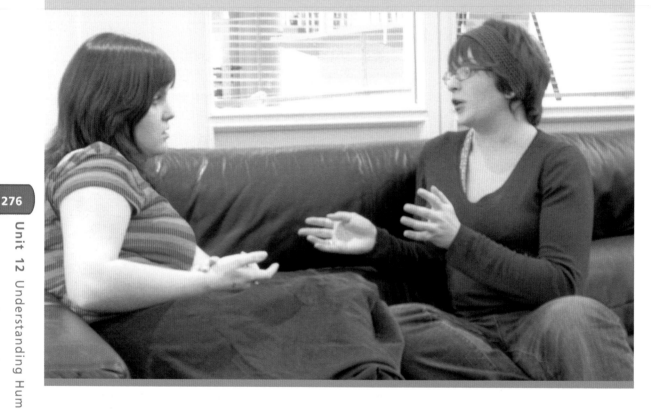

KEY TERMS

Self-actualisation
The process of becoming a whole, complete person.

Organismic self
A version of the self that contains everything we experience, including things we are not aware of.

Congruence
When the experiences that we have fit comfortably with our self-concept.

Locus
The Latin word for place.

Internal locus of control
The belief that we are able to influence events.

External locus of control
The belief that we have little control over events – control is external to us.

Core conditions for person-centred therapy
The relationship the counsellor tries to create, based on unconditional positive regard, empathy and genuineness.

Unconditional positive regard
Acceptance and respect, non-judgemental.

Empathy
The ability to see and feel things from another person's point of view.

Genuineness
Giving something of yourself in a therapeutic relationship.

Unit 12 Understanding Human Behaviour

Person-centred psychology

Humanistic psychology – person-centred psychology – is based on the idea that we have a natural tendency to grow and develop as people. This is not growing in a physical sense, but in a psychological sense. We will look at the work of two key figures in humanistic psychology – Abraham Maslow and Carl Rogers.

Maslow is probably best known for his 'hierarchy of needs'. This draws attention to the needs which have to be met, in order of priority (in a hierarchy) for us to become fully complete as a person. There are six levels of needs:

- **Physiological needs** are our most basic needs – the need for air, water, food, and for some degree of physical comfort. These needs have to be met first, before we can expect to meet any of our other needs.

- **Safety needs**. We need, next, to avoid pain and harm. We need to be safe.

- **Belongingness**. This is the first of the higher-order needs, and it refers to our need to belong and feel secure. This need is likely to be met first within our families.

- **Love needs**. Once we feel secure and we belong, we need to love and be loved in return.

- **Self-esteem needs**. We need, next, to feel that we are worthwhile people, and this is what Maslow meant by our need for self-esteem. Self-esteem develops as we become more competent and independent – and from the recognition we get from other people.

- **Self-actualisation needs**. These needs come at the very top of Maslow's hierarchy, and refer to our need to become a whole, and integrated person. This is a difficult idea, but as it underpins much of the humanistic (person-centred approach) we'll take a bit of time to explore what it means.

Self-actualisation

As we said earlier, the big idea in humanistic psychology is that people have a tendency to grow, develop and to become more complete – through the process of self-actualisation. This is not, however, a passive process – it's not like the way a flower grows or develops. Instead it's something we bring about through our own actions.

Maybe you can get a feel for what self-actualisation means by looking at people who seem to have achieved this. This brings us to a really interesting piece of work and a very original piece of thinking. If psychology only studies people with problems, said Maslow, then what results is a stunted form of psychology. It is only concerned with problems and fails to recognise all that it means to be human. (If you think of psychoanalytic theory – a theory built up from people with problems – you might agree with Maslow about this.) So, he said, why don't we study people who *don't* have problems and, in particular, people who have achieved a state of self-actualisation?

Maslow then identified a group of self-actualising people: people who had realised their potential to the fullest extent. Some of these were historical figures (like Abraham Lincoln and Beethoven) and others were living at the time of his study (like Albert Einstein). Maslow then tried to discover what features they shared, which made them a bit different from people in general.

He came up with a list of features – about fifteen in all, but this shorter list gives a sense of what Maslow found:

- Self-actualising people are spontaneous and unconventional.

- They identify with others and genuinely want to help them.

- They tend to have very close relationships with a few people only.

- Their appreciation of people is fresh, not stereotyped.
- Their sense of humour is based on seeing jokes in everyday things.
- They have strong views on what is right and wrong.
- They are creative, rather than conforming.

Although many of the people in Maslow's sample were gifted and talented, he did not believe that we have to be highly intelligent to become self-actualised people. Very few of us have the intellectual and creative gifts of Einstein or Beethoven, but we self-actualise when we make the very best of the possibilities we do have. This might be in an artistic or creative field, or it might be more intellectual, in terms of what we know and understand about ourselves and the world around us. It might also be in developing our interpersonal and social skills.

The idea of the 'self' in humanistic psychology

The word 'self' has been used several times now, so perhaps we should explore in a bit of detail what this actually means. In fact, there are at least four ways that the word self is used within the humanistic (person-centred) approach:

- The first is the **ideal self**. This is not how we are, but how we would like to be.
- The next is the perceived self (our **self-concept**). This is the person, the self, that we are actually aware of. It's the answer we would give to the questions, 'Who am I? What do I think and feel? What do I believe and value?'
- The third is the **organismic self**, which is made up from everything we experience, and this includes experiences that we are not aware of. If these experiences fit comfortably with our self-concept, if we can make sense of them, we call this **congruence**. If the experiences don't fit, we will deny or distort experiences and push them out of our awareness. This unpleasant situation is called **incongruence**.
- Finally there is the **integrating self** (perceiving self). The job of the integrating self is to try to create congruence between our experiences (our organismic self) and our self-concept.

You might ask yourself, 'What actually causes this incongruence?' Or put more simply, 'How is it that we can end up with a view of ourselves (our self-concept) that is so at odds with our experiences?'

One answer is that we might have grown up in an environment where people (such as our parents) show approval only when we meet their conditions or expectations. So far as *we* can see, we're doing well. We feel we're being successful – but we're not worthwhile in their eyes because we haven't met their expectations. Humanistic approaches describe this as 'conditions of worth'. The opposite of this, which is discussed below, is unconditional positive regard.

Person-centred counselling

What happens to our personal growth if we experience emotional problems?

A fundamental idea within the person-centred approach is that we all have the resources within us to solve these problems for ourselves. We may need a therapist or counsellor to help us, but their role is 'non-directive.' In other words, they will not advise us, or tell us what to do. Instead they will help us discover the resources we have within us, so that we can help ourselves, and take charge of our own lives.

Locus of control

The idea that we all have the resources and power to make changes in our lives is similar to the concept of 'locus of control':

- Some people have an internal locus of control. (The word 'locus' is just the Latin word for 'place'.) People with an internal locus of control think that

Who can control and change their behaviour?

Janis and Susan have just been told by their doctor that they are pregnant. They are both heavy smokers and the doctor suggests that it's really time to stop smoking.

Janis has an internal locus of control. She knows stopping will be hard but she knows she can stop if she really wants to. 'There are no excuses,' she says. 'No one's forcing me to smoke. Stopping is down to me, and will-power!'

Susan has an external locus of control. Stopping, she says, would be really stressful and this would cause problems between her and her partner. If he was more supportive, well maybe she could stop … but now's not a good time. 'Anyway,' she continues, 'what's going to happen is going to happen whatever you do. And smoking never did my mum any harm, or me for that matter.'

they have the ability to influence events, because control is internal to them. As a result, they are likely to make the effort to change things.

- Other people have an external locus of control. They are more likely to think that events occur through chance, or because of things external to them that they have no control over – 'It's just fate' or 'I blame the system!' They are less likely to take control in their lives.

One of the tasks of the counsellor is to help their clients shift towards more of an internal locus of control.

Core conditions for person-centred therapy

The other three approaches we've looked at all use special 'techniques' of one sort or another. For example, cognitive behaviour therapy has techniques for examining and challenging our beliefs, psychodynamic approaches have techniques for interpreting our experience to find deeper meanings, and behavioural approaches work through carefully analysing and changing the environment through the use of reinforcement.

Person-centred therapy is different. It does not rely on techniques. What is important is the relationship between the therapist and the client. Carl Rogers identified three features (or core conditions) of this relationship: unconditional positive regard, empathy and genuineness.

Unconditional positive regard

Rogers believed that the counsellor must express unconditional positive regard for the client. This is something like warmth and acceptance. The counsellor accepts and respects the person as they are at that moment in time, and this is done without reservations. The counsellor does not make judgements and does not express approval or disapproval.

You can probably see how showing unconditional positive regard would be helpful in care practitioners' work with many service users outside of a counselling relationship. It sets a kind of emotional tone in which the service user feels themselves to be valued and a person of worth.

Empathy

Empathy involves trying to step into the client's shoes, to see and experience the world as they do. This requires intense concentration and careful, active listening. Can the counsellor see the world in the same way, and begin to feel what their client is feeling?

Skilled counsellors are able do this, but this is only half the story. It's not enough for them to *feel* empathy – they need to share this, to *express* their feeing of empathy back to the client.

A counsellor might express their empathy through non-verbal signals. For example you might see the counsellor leaning slightly forward to show that they are attentive and listening. They might also 'mirror' the posture of their client – doing the same things with their hands, crossing and uncrossing their feet and so on. We all do this, and for most of the time we are not aware of doing it.

The counsellor will also express their empathy through the way they respond to what the client says. This might be non-verbal – through nods or facial expressions – or the counsellor might say something that shows they are on the way to understanding the client's feelings. Sometimes the counsellor might summarise what the client has said and check that they understand it:

COUNSELLOR: It sounds as though Alisha left you feeling a bit stupid. Would that be right Sarah?

CLIENT: Hmm. Yeah.

This shows the counsellor has been listening and trying to feel what the client has been feeling. Sometimes the counsellor might do nothing more than repeat a word or a phrase that the client has just said:

CLIENT: So when she did that, I was left feeling really angry.

COUNSELLOR: Feeling really angry?

The counsellor has said just enough for the client to feel listened to, and to know that they've been 'heard'. The client can elaborate and say more if they want to, but as this is a non-directive approach, they are not asked or obliged to do so.

Sometimes the counsellor might express empathy through not breaking a period of silence – just waiting till the client feels they want to go on. One silence, in one of Rogers's counselling sessions, was timed at 17 minutes.

Empathy, therefore, builds up in a cyclical process:

- The counsellor tries to get in touch with what the client feels.

- The counsellor expresses their awareness of this to the client.

- The client senses the counsellor's understanding.

- The client then continues in a way that gives feedback to the counsellor on how accurate their awareness is.

Getting you thinking

1 Why might each of these people be crying?

2 What approaches might be used to help them?

3 Explain why the same approaches wouldn't work for all of them.

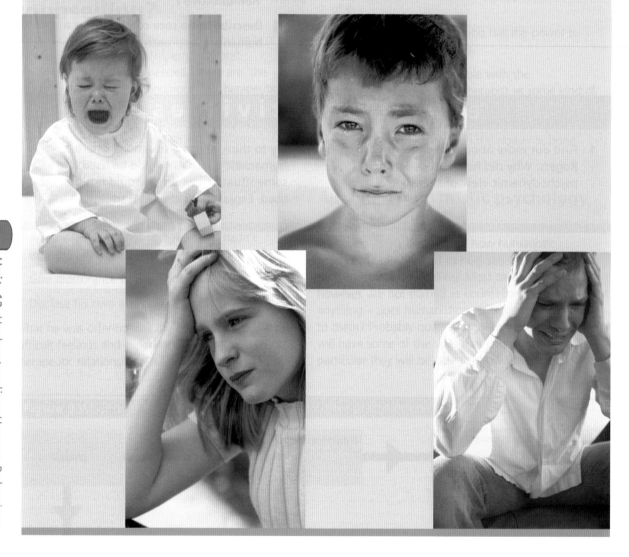

KEY TERMS

Deterministic theories
Theories that see our behaviour as being caused (determined) by things we have no control over. These kind of theories would say that we have no free will. We think we make choices – but we don't.

Symptom substitution
This happens when one behaviour (e.g. nail-biting) is extinguished, only to be replaced by another (e.g. bed-wetting).

Rogerian counselling
Person-centred counselling, in the style of Carl Rogers.

Four approaches to choose from

You've now had the chance to look at four of the major approaches that psychologists have used to understand human behaviour. These are:

• Behavioural approaches

• Cognitive approaches

• Psychodynamic approaches

• Humanistic approaches.

We are now going to evaluate these approaches – looking at their strengths and weaknesses – and we'll ask why a care practitioner might choose to use one approach rather than another. Let's listen in to Sasha discussing this with Jane. Sasha is studying Health and Social Care, and Jane is a clinical psychologist.

SASHA: When you're working with your clients, do you always use the same approach?

JANE: No. Sometimes I use one approach and sometimes I use another.

SASHA: What does it depend on?

JANE: Well, it depends on a number of things. In the first place, it depends on who I am working with. If the client is very young, I'll probably use a behavioural approach. If they're older and have good understanding, I might use one of the 'talking therapies'.

SASHA: Does the approach you choose depend on what sort of problem you're dealing with?

JANE: Yes, up to a point. The behavioural approach is useful when the client needs to learn new behaviours, but the others … they all deal with the same sorts of problems, really.

SASHA: So what other things affect your choice?

JANE: I think there are a number of other factors. I'll usually start with an approach which has worked for me with similar cases in the past, and I'll change approaches if what I'm doing isn't effective. Maybe I need a new working hypothesis, and a new approach will give me that. I also try to choose approaches that give quick results. We have long waiting lists here, and long-term therapy may not be cost-effective.

SASHA: Does your care value base affect your choice?

JANE: What do you mean exactly?

SASHA: It's about treating people respectfully, supporting their individual rights, and behaving ethically.

JANE: Ah. I see what you mean. We prefer to talk about professional ethics, and there is a Code of Conduct for Chartered Psychologists. It is important to me. In practice it means avoiding anything that infringes the client's rights, and especially anything that might cause them harm. I also try to choose approaches which the client and their families can understand.

SASHA: Why?

JANE: Well, our Code of Conduct says that the client should give their 'informed consent' to any interventions and I don't think you can give informed consent if you don't understand what is going to happen to you.

SASHA: Are there any approaches that you don't use?

JANE: I don't use the psychodynamic approach. I'm not trained to use that.

Evaluating behavioural approaches

Behavioural approaches have been very influential in the past, and people who favour behavioural approaches often say things like these:

The basic idea is very simple to understand. 'If behaviour is reinforced, we tend to repeat it.' The key terms are clear (although people sometimes confuse negative reinforcement and punishment) and many people find that the theory makes sense for them.

Behaviourists can show that this basic idea is true, at least some of the time. A lot of early experimental work was done with animals using food as reinforcement, and many experiments have been done with people using social rewards (like praise) and token economies (star charts for young children for example.) Behaviourists can show how behaviour changes, using reinforcement, to bring about learning.

The behavioural approach is objective in the sense that everyone can see the relevant behaviour and can agree when it is happening. There are two reasons for this. First, behaviourists are only interested in people's observable behaviour, and secondly, 'fuzzy' words (like over-active or aggressive) get defined in terms of what the person is actually seen doing.

The approach is easy to put into practice. The behaviourist would say that all of us use reinforcement quite naturally and spontaneously in our day-to-day lives. For example we give out social reinforcement as we interact with other people, and this influences the behaviour of other people towards us. Sometimes we use reinforcement more knowingly, like the parents who praise and cuddle their child the first time she uses a potty. All that is happening in a behaviour-modification programme is the application of the principles of reinforcement in a more deliberate and consistent manner.

The approach works – it does change the way people behave – and the results may be quick, thus avoiding long and expensive courses of counselling or therapy. Because it does not rely on any direct communication between the worker and the client, it can be used with young children and with people who have learning disabilities, where 'talking' approaches might not work. Behavioural approaches are also used to help people who are anxious and who have addictions.

Because the behavioural approach assumes that nearly all of our behaviour is learned, it can be used to 'shape' behaviour very gradually and help people develop new behaviours and new skills. This is different from all the other approaches: there are things that only the behavioural approach can do.

The behaviourists might say, finally, that this approach does not describe people as 'abnormal'. They don't say, 'Sue is neurotic', they ask instead about the specific behaviours that Sue needs to change. So they avoid the effects of labelling.

Critics of the behavioural approach would say, first, that behaviourists are making a big mistake by ignoring what goes on inside people's heads. The approach is therefore very narrow and limited. If care practitioners know what people think, and why they think the way they do, then they can help them to achieve change for themselves.

The critics go on to say that the model only deals with the symptoms and not the causes of people's problems. For example, practitioners might use a technique like systematic desensitisation to help an anxious child overcome their fears about starting school. They might be successful in the short term, but the problem might well start up again after the next school holiday. Alternatively, the child might display their anxiety in other ways – perhaps nail-biting or bed-wetting. This is sometimes referred to as '**symptom substitution**'.

Critics have also objected to some of the methods used in behaviour-modification programmes. The use of 'time-out' can be upsetting for children and critics might object to the way that time out rooms are used in some specialist facilities. People are removed from the company of others for short periods and get no attention (reinforcement) for their inappropriate

behaviour. How is this different from punishment and solitary confinement?

Critics also argue that the approach is manipulative and dehumanising. It provides a very bleak view of people as organisms, which simply respond to, and repeat things which give them pleasure.

We'll come back to this when we think about the care value base. One of the questions we need to ask ourselves is whether the ends (what care practitioners can achieve for people) justify the means (what the care practitioners do with people).

Evaluating psychodynamic approaches

People who favour a psychodynamic approach say that this approach, unlike the behavioural approach, really does get to the root cause of people's problems. This might involve a long period of therapy (analysis) that could take the person back to things they had forgotten or repressed from their childhood.

They might go on to say that the approach is effective because it gives the client insight into why they think or feel the way they do. This allows the person to think about and to change many aspects of their lives – not just single pieces of surface behaviour as the behavioural approach might do. They might also say that giving people insight into their problems is a very respectful way for care practitioners to behave, and that this should be part of everyone's care value base.

Supporters would also say that this approach has been around much longer than any of the others. It has stood the test of time because it works across a wide range of problems, including depression, eating problems, and sexual disorders.

Critics (and especially those from the behavioural camp) would argue that these theories are much more complicated than they need to be, and difficult to make sense of. Psychotherapists need years of training and have to go through analysis themselves as part of their training.

They might go on to say that it is hard to find any independent evidence that supports psychodynamic theories. These theories are not 'scientific'. The theories and the techniques of psychoanalysis are not based on any direct evidence. They are not based on what the client says, but on what the psychotherapist thinks they meant. The emphasis on the unconscious and the need to analyse and interpret what people do or say causes problems for many people. If motives are unconscious, can we ever know for sure what they are?

Some people claim that psychoanalysis can be harmful if the insights it is supposed to give are more than the person is able to handle. The insight may be more distressing than the problem it is connected with. One recent controversy surrounds the so-called 'false memory syndrome' where people undergoing analysis claim to have recovered memories of traumatic and abusive episodes from their childhood – episodes that didn't happen.

It is also said that psychodynamic theories – just like behavioural ones – take a very deterministic view of people. This is another way of saying that these theories assume that we have little control over how we are and what we do. The behaviourist says that we are shaped by how we have been reinforced over our lifetime. The psychodynamic approach sees us as being the product of early (often childhood) influences that are unconscious and that we are not aware of.

Some critics argue that the psychoanalysis is often a very lengthy process and it is therefore not cost-effective. Others have gone further, and claimed that psychotherapy doesn't actually work. Many studies have been done to assess the effectiveness of psychoanalysis. However, because the methods of psychoanalysis are complex and because it is hard to measure how much better people become, it has proved very difficult to design a properly controlled study.

Critics also ask whether these theories have any relevance to modern times and to different cultures. Freud, for example, worked with middle-class patients in Vienna at the end of the nineteenth century. Are any of his insights – which were only his interpretations – relevant now?

Evaluating cognitive approaches

The cognitive approach – the cognitive-behavioural approach – is being used increasingly in health and care contexts. It shares a number of features with the behavioural approach, and Jane – the clinical psychologist talking to Sasha – would probably move between these two approaches quite comfortably. Like the behavioural approach, this is a very structured way of understanding and changing behaviour. The key ideas of the theory are clear, and the process of therapy is easily understood. Like the behavioural approach, many people find that it makes sense to them.

The cognitive approach (in common with the psychodynamic approach) pays careful attention to what the client says. This reveals, in a very direct way, what they think and believe. The therapist can then look for any faulty or dysfunctional beliefs which affect how the client feels and how they behave. The cognitive approach differs from the psychodynamic approach in saying that the therapist can accept what the client tells them, without needing to interpret it to find other and hidden meanings.

Some people see this directness as a strength of the cognitive-behaviour approach. It makes the approach easy to learn and apply without lengthy training, and it also means that clients can learn the techniques for themselves. This is a deliberate part of the therapy. Once clients know what the techniques are and how to use them, they should be able to apply them to other areas of their lives. It is sometimes said that people who are seen by a psychotherapist become dependent on their therapist. Cognitive approaches aim for independence, and it might be argued that 'empowering' the service users in this way should be part of everyone's care value base.

Cognitive behaviour therapy is widely used in health and care settings. It is used in a range of situations where people have difficulty coping with life, with issues such as stress, depression, anxieties and anger management. It is claimed to be relatively quick and therefore cost-effective.

Critics would say that the approach is not suitable for everyone. Because this is a 'talking therapy', it would be difficult to use with clients who have very limited language skills. The client needs to be able to understand what the counsellor is saying, and have the skills to put their own thoughts and beliefs into words that the counsellor can understand. The approach would also be difficult to use with people who find it hard to follow a rational line of thought.

Critics might argue from a psychodynamic viewpoint, and claim that cognitive approaches do not deal with the underlying causes of people's problems. It's a bit like the criticism they make of behavioural methods. The cognitive-behavioural therapist may have to sort out one dysfunctional belief and then another, and another. The psychodynamic approach, by contrast, tries to work out why these irrational beliefs arise in the first place.

The key question is whether the approach works. Some studies have shown it to be very effective, very quickly, when compared with no therapy at all. Other studies have been less clear-cut. For example, in treating people with depression, some studies show it to be more effective than drug treatments while other studies have found no difference. Drugs, however, can have undesirable side effects, and people often relapse if they stop taking their medication. This, it is claimed, would not happen with cognitive-behavioural therapy.

Evaluating humanistic approaches

Humanistic (person-centred) approaches have had a huge influence, especially in the area of counselling. The growth of Rogerian, person-centred counselling may be taken as one measure of its effectiveness. In common with the other 'talking therapies', however, it has been difficult to show how effective the approach actually is.

Person-centred approaches are often described as 'non-directive'. Counsellors are not intrusive. They meet their clients as equals and do not set themselves up as 'experts'. Training as a counsellor does not depend on any other professional qualifications, but there is as yet no uniformity in the length and quality of training that counsellors receive.

Person-centred counselling, in common with cognitive-behaviour therapy, does not require any kind of diagnosis, and it avoids labelling people.

Critics have pointed out that some of the key terms are difficult to understand. What exactly is the 'organismic self'? How does 'congruence' occur? And how would anyone know how close they were to 'self-actualisation'?

Humanistic psychology, and care value bases

Perhaps the most important feature of humanistic psychology, and its greatest contribution to practitioners' work in health and social care is the values and the principles which underlie it and which it expresses.

Most people who work as care practitioners are not counsellors or therapists. They may be early years workers, learning assistants, or speech and language therapists. They may be nurses, doctors, or carers. What does humanistic psychology have to offer to people working in these sorts of roles?

This question can be answered in a number of ways. First, we can look at the way care practitioners behave. Remember the three 'core conditions' of person-centred counselling. These were:

- Unconditional positive regard – the counsellor accepting and respecting the client as they are.

- Empathy – the counsellor trying to experience the world in the same way as the client does.

- Genuineness: the counsellor bringing something of themselves, appropriately, into the relationship.

These are qualities that many care practitioners bring to their relationships with all their service users. Think, for example, about the worker in the care home who treats all the residents with respect, and who seems to understand their view of the world. They may not be aware of it, but they are using some key ideas from humanistic psychology. If they were asked why they show this sort of respect to their service users, they might say that it:

- Acknowledges individuals' beliefs and identities

- Promotes and supports their rights

- Promotes anti-discriminatory practice

- Promotes effective communication.

You will have met these ideas before when you studied the values in care, and you might recognise these as part of the care value base. People who put the ideas of humanistic psychology into practice are likely to be expressing many of the ideas found within the care value base. And vice versa – someone who uses these care values in their work is likely to be using ideas that we also find in humanistic psychology.

Perhaps the most fundamental questions are about what it means to be a person. Some people believe that we are entirely shaped by events outside of ourselves, and some theories in psychology seem to support this view. Behaviourism, in its most extreme form, says that we are simply the consequence of how our past behaviour has been reinforced. This makes our future behaviour entirely predictable – what we do in any new situation is simply a reflection of what we did in similar situations in the past, and how that behaviour was reinforced. In fact, the behaviourist could say, we don't actually have a choice about how we behave. Our reinforcement history determines how we will behave. We think we have a choice – but we don't really. Behavioural approaches could be described as 'deterministic', as could many of the psychodynamic approaches. In these theories, our behaviour is shaped – determined

Figure 10

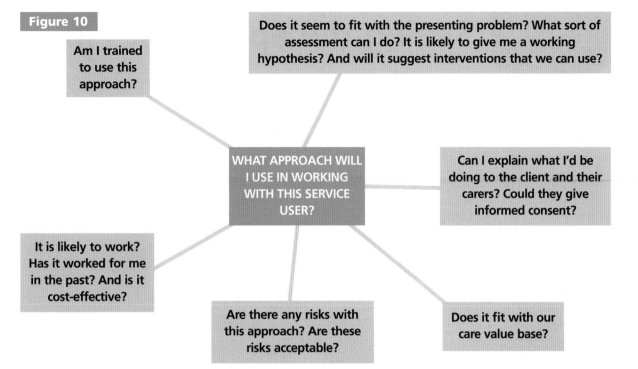

Figure 10

Am I trained to use this approach?

Does it seem to fit with the presenting problem? What sort of assessment can I do? It is likely to give me a working hypothesis? And will it suggest interventions that we can use?

WHAT APPROACH WILL I USE IN WORKING WITH THIS SERVICE USER?

Can I explain what I'd be doing to the client and their carers? Could they give informed consent?

It is likely to work? Has it worked for me in the past? And is it cost-effective?

Are there any risks with this approach? Are these risks acceptable?

Does it fit with our care value base?

– by our early experiences and our unresolved conflicts and traumas – and it needs an expert to sort this out for us.

Humanistic psychology takes a very different view. Humanistic psychology says that people have the power to make choices and changes in their lives. We can overcome the effects of early bad experiences, and we can become something much more than we are now. Remember the highest levels of Maslow's hierarchy of needs – the need for self-esteem and for self-actualisation? The humanistic approach also says that care practitioners can help people find direction and make choices and changes – but they do it from a position of equality and not as 'experts'.

These humanistic principles are also found among care values. Are these the sorts of principles that would be important to you, if you were a care practitioner?

Check your understanding

1 Explain why clinical psychologists have a code of conduct. What similarity does this have to the care value base?

2 Give two advantages of a behavioural approach to therapy and two disadvantages.

3 Explain what is meant by a 'false memory syndrome' in psychodynamic therapy.

4 Describe when a cognitive-behaviour approach might be used in a health and care setting.

extension **activities**

1 Describe one similarity and one difference between behaviour modification and cognitive-behavioural therapy. Discuss the statement, 'Behaviour modification is only for the young and cognitive therapy is only for the old.'

2 Make up a table to show the key features of all four theories. Imagine that you are explaining it to someone who knows nothing about psychological approaches. For each approach, describe a situation where you think the approach would work well, explaining why.

Topic 9 | Seeing the approaches in practice

Getting you thinking

Dr McNeil has set up this meeting to discuss Mrs O'Brien's care plan. (See page 292.) There are workers here from health, social services and a charity (or a voluntary agency).

1 What are the advantages of a group of care workers getting together in this way?

2 How might their different professional backgrounds and training affect this group's ability to work together?

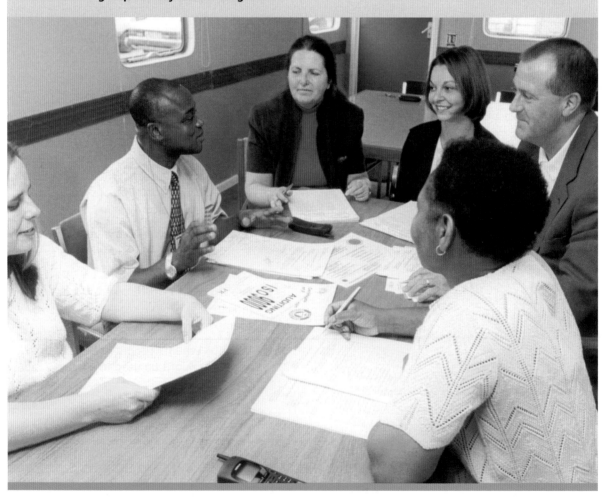

This final topic is based around a number of case studies. These will allow you to revisit the main ideas covered in this unit, and to see how these can be applied in real-life contexts.

This could be an important part of your learning on this unit and it should also help you when you come to take your exam. The exam questions are likely to be based around real-life situations. So how would a care practitioner deal with these?

The behavioural approach in action

Robbie is three years old and lives with his mother, Sharon. He goes to a local playgroup three mornings a week. He finds it difficult to separate from his mother and he can be quite aggressive towards the other children. Sharon asks Salena, the playgroup supervisor, if she can help. What might Salena decide to do?

Here is a mind map showing Salena's thinking.

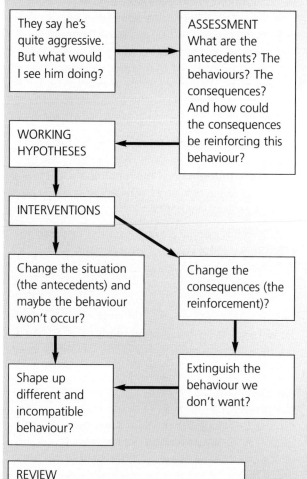

They say he's quite aggressive. But what would I see him doing?

ASSESSMENT
What are the antecedents? The behaviours? The consequences? And how could the consequences be reinforcing this behaviour?

WORKING HYPOTHESES

INTERVENTIONS

Change the situation (the antecedents) and maybe the behaviour won't occur?

Change the consequences (the reinforcement)?

Shape up different and incompatible behaviour?

Extinguish the behaviour we don't want?

REVIEW
Decide on some targets and set a date.

Salena's mind map

Salena will start by doing an **assessment** of the problem. She will then decide what **approach** (behavioural, cognitive, psychodynamic or humanistic) she will use. Salena decides on a **behavioural approach**. This is a good choice with young children where they may have to learn some new behaviour, or where nothing else would work. Salena also likes this approach because it avoids labelling and stereotyping.

She then does some further assessment, based on Robbie's **observable behaviour**. She needs to define what 'quite aggressive' means. It's a 'fuzzy' term so she defines it as hitting or pushing other children, and she will count how often this happens. She uses the **ABC** approach: **antecedents**, **behaviour** and **consequences**. She is looking for consequences that might be reinforcing Robbie's behaviours.

Salena needs a **working hypothesis**. She notices that Robbie gets a lot of attention from the other workers when he hits children, and this may be **positive reinforcement**. He could also be getting **negative reinforcement** for his behaviour because he gets to leave a situation with other children which seems to cause him some anxiety.

Salena then designs her **intervention**. This is a **behaviour-modification programme**. She will try to **extinguish** Robbie's hitting and pushing by **shaping** new behaviour which is **incompatible** with this. So the playgroup staff will be gently firm with him if he pushes another child, they will not remove him from the situation; and they will give him lots of attention whenever he shows signs of joining other children. Salena checks that what she proposes is consistent with her **care value base**. She decides on the targets she hopes to achieve (to reduce hitting and pushing to no more that two occasions each morning) and sets a date for a **review**.

Cognitive approaches and cognitive-behaviour therapy

This case study is from a health context – a referral from a GP to a community psychiatric nurse:

> 'My patient, Ann Winter, is 16. She has an eating disorder. She eats very little, and her weight is dropping. I believe she is anorexic and I would be grateful if you could work out a suitable treatment programme for her.'

Ken, the community psychiatric nurse, receives the referral. Let's look at what he does.

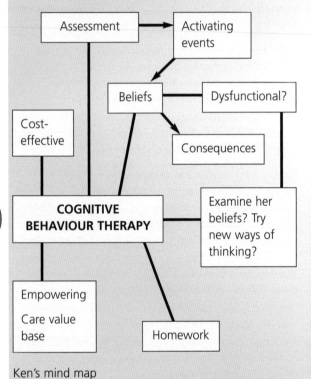

Ken's mind map

Ken decides to use a **cognitive (cognitive-behavioural)** approach. He has recently done some **training** in **cognitive-behaviour therapy (CBT)** and he has good **experience** of using this approach. CBT sometimes produces results quickly and as Ken's team has a long waiting list, this is a **cost-effective** approach.

He wonders if the **diagnosis** of anorexia will help him understand Ann's problems. Is it just a **label**, a fancy way of saying that Ann doesn't eat very much? Ken thinks the diagnosis will help. He has found in the past that this diagnosis has pointed him towards interventions that seem to work.

His **assessment** involves an **ABC** approach, but this time the letters stand for the **activating event**, the **beliefs** the person has (usually about themselves), and the emotional **consequences**. CBT says that it's not the activating event that causes the emotional consequences, it's the beliefs the person has about the event (and about themselves) that are important. So Ken needs to find out what Ann's beliefs are.

Ken's **working hypothesis** will be that Ann's thinking is **distorted** in some way. She will have **automatic thoughts** and **dysfunctional beliefs** and these lead to the emotional and behavioural consequences of not eating.

Once Ken has identified Ann's distorted thinking, he needs to work out what his **intervention** will be. He will help Ann to examine her beliefs. He might challenge her – is there another way of looking at this? Ken will point out other ways of thinking, and he will invite her to try out a different set of beliefs. He will also set her some **homework** – some tasks to do. He will **review** how well Ann has managed these tasks when they next meet.

Ken likes to use CBT because of the way it **involves the service user**. It gives them techniques that they can use to change their own lives and many service users find this **empowering**. Ken believes this is an ethical way to treat people. It fits with his own **care value base**.

Comparisons

You should be able to see a pattern emerging in what Salena and Ken are doing. Although their approaches are different, they've both gone through the same cycle of assessment, working hypothesis, intervention and review. Care practitioners really do think this way, so have this framework in mind when you are thinking about a case study of your own.

Each of the four approaches makes different assumptions about why we behave in the ways we do. This is evident in how they deal with assessment where:

- the behavioural approach looks at observed behaviour.

- the cognitive and humanistic approaches listen to what the person says.

- the psychodynamic approach interprets what the person says or does.

Each approach leads to different working hypotheses, and the interventions in the four approaches are very different.

All four approaches build in a process of review. This allows the care practitioners to check how successful the intervention has been, and to decide on what needs to happen next. The service user would be involved in the review, and perhaps their families, and any other workers who are involved.

A final thing to note is how important the care value base is to Salena and to Ken. It leads them to have preferences for some approaches and some interventions over others.

They might also rule out some interventions as unethical – because they are not appropriate for this issue, with this client, in these circumstances.

The next case study will revisit and reinforce some other ideas. Don't forget what has just been covered, however, because it will be relevant to the other case studies.

Psychodynamic approaches and family therapy

Joan is 57 and is seriously depressed. Her GP, Dr McNeil, has prescribed antidepressant medication, but this hasn't really worked. She has now referred Joan to Keith Wood, a **psychotherapist** at the local hospital. Keith uses a **psychodynamic** approach in his work.

By the end of their first session, Keith is beginning to get a picture of what is happening in Joan's life. Joan's father died when she was young and Joan wasn't able to go through the normal **grieving** process. Her mother had a strict, no-nonsense view of this. 'Folks like us just have to get on with our lives,' she told Joan. This was the **culture** of their times, and these views were common among people of their **social class**.

Because of this early **loss**, Joan has found it hard to form **secure attachments** with other people. Keith thinks that she has an **unconscious motivation** which prevents her getting really close to people in case she loses them. He thinks this is why Joan has problems in her relationship with her husband, Peter.

There are also problems in Joan's relationship with her mother. Their relationship has always been distant and cold but her mother, Mrs O'Brien, is now quite elderly and she needs a lot of care. Keith thinks that Joan's **superego** and **id** are in conflict over this. Her superego works on the **perfection principle** and says that 'good daughters have to look after their mothers'. Her id, working on the **pleasure principle**, says that Joan should 'look after number one'. Joan's ego cannot resolve this conflict – her **ego defence**

mechanisms are not strong enough and she cannot **repress** any of these feelings.

Keith decides that working with Joan on her own will be of only limited benefit. He wants to work with Joan, Peter and Mrs O'Brien together. This is **family therapy**. It's an approach that Keith has used successfully when people are stuck in unhelpful relationships – where everyone needs to look at their feelings and at how other people are affected by their behaviour. When Keith thinks about this further, he decides that it would not be proper to include Mrs O'Brien in this work. She is elderly and confused, and this could be painful and difficult – and it would be of no real benefit to her. Keith talks this over with his line manager. She has the same **care values** as Keith, and she agrees with him.

This case study illustrates some of the key ideas in the psychodynamic approach. It also brings out some real dilemmas. Shouldn't Keith have at least tried to include Mrs O'Brien in family therapy? Why did he assume that this would be too painful for her? Did anyone ask her? In any case, his first responsibility is to Joan not to her mother, and this could have been really helpful for Joan. It could also have been helpful to Mrs O'Brien. Perhaps she would have welcomed the chance to talk about her feelings, and to repair her relationship with her daughter in the last years of her life.

The learning point here is that values are really quite personal things. While a professional group may share a care value base, and may even have a formal Code of Conduct, this will not resolve all the difficult ethical issues that they are likely to face. Different people will interpret the Code in different ways, and there may be areas of practice which the Code or the care value base does not address at all.

Bringing a humanistic perspective to care work

The final case study is about a care-coordination meeting at Mayfield Health Centre.

Dr McNeil is chairing the meeting, and they happen to be discussing the care of Mrs O'Brien, Joan's mother. This is a **multi-agency meeting** – involving a number of different professionals from health, social services and the voluntary sector. Dr McNeil finds that this is an effective way to assess needs, to make plans and to deliver services. By working together they make the best use of everyone's skills and time. Gaps in services can be identified, and overlaps can be avoided.

As we join the meeting, Rita Valvona is speaking. Rita works for Crossroads, a voluntary agency that provides care for Mrs O'Brien at home. Rita has got to know Mrs O'Brien well. She knows that Mrs O'Brien lost her husband many years ago, and that she has one daughter, Joan, who rarely comes to visit. Rita brings a **humanistic** approach to her work and shows **unconditional positive regard** and **empathy** to Mrs O'Brien. She accepts and understands Mrs O'Brien without making judgements about her. Rita does, however, find Joan's behaviour difficult to understand and accept. Rita comes from a large and close Italian family where this would never happen. In fact there are many differences between her life experiences and Mrs O'Brien's – there are differences in **age**, **culture**, and **social class**. Rita has to be aware of these

differences and then tries to put them to one side. She does, however, share some of her own experiences with Mrs O'Brien. This is **genuineness**, the third **core condition** in **person-centred counselling**.

Mrs O'Brien has told Rita that Joan has **bullied** her for many years. Rita feels that this explains why Mrs O'Brien has such a **negative self-concept** and **low self-esteem**. She is not well off, and because of her **economic status**, she has found it difficult to go out and join with older people in her community. This has left her feeling **marginalised** and **socially excluded**.

Kate Buchanan, the social worker, wants to talk about Joan's behaviour, but Dr McNeil feels uncomfortable with this. She is the only person present who actually knows Joan. She knows from Keith what Joan's own problems are and, following her own **care value base**, she believes that she should keep these **confidential**.

Kate goes on to say that Rita's person-centred approach seems to be working with Mrs O'Brien. She has seen a number of positive changes over the past few weeks. She explains these changes using **Maslow's hierarchy of needs**, and thinks that Rita is helping Mrs O'Brien to meet her **self-esteem needs**. She may not meet her needs for **self-actualisation**, but she is a lot happier than she was.

The meeting decides that other workers should adopt the same approach, and they agree to meet again in six weeks to **review** Mrs O'Brien's **care plan**.

These four case studies illustrate many of the key terms you came across earlier in this unit. The case studies are based on real-life events and should give you insights into the way that care practitioners go about their work – the framework they use to plan their interventions, the main approaches they might use, and the ethical dilemmas they face on a daily basis.

Check your understanding

1 You are working in an early years setting and Mr Thomson, a parent, asks you to explain how 'rewards' or 'reinforcement' can be used to change behaviour. Mr Thomson wants his son Jim to play more co-operatively with Jane, his younger sister. Explain the basic ideas of the behavioural approach simply, and in your own words to Mr Thomson.

2 You were introduced to an ABC approach when you learned about behavioural approaches. You came across another ABC approach when we looked at cognitive approaches. What do the letters stand for in each approach?

3 Read back through the case studies, look at the key terms, which are in **bold type**, and try to explain what each of them means. Use your own words if you can.

extension activities

1 Look back at the case study where Keith works with Joan. Could you draw a mind-map which illustrates how Keith is thinking about Joan's problems and how he plans to tackle them? There is no right answer – but what do you think this would look like?

2 Now imagine that you are Dr McNeil. She has mind-mapped the discussion that they had during their meeting to discuss Mrs O'Brien. What might that look like?

3 Dr McNeil decided to say nothing to the meeting about Joan's depressive illness and about the part her early experiences with her mother may have played in this. Was she right to do so?

4 At the meeting, Dr McNeil learned, through Rita, that Joan may have been bullying her mother for many years. Should she pass this information on to Keith? Or is it confidential to Mrs O'Brien? What do you think?

ABC Approach (Behavioural) – This is a strategy for analysing behaviour. It involves looking at the Antecedents, Behaviour and Consequences of specific behaviours.

ABC Approach (Cognitive) – This is a strategy for analysing the links between thinking and behaviour. It involves analysing behaviour in terms of the Activating event, Beliefs (which may be irrational or dysfunctional) and the emotional or behavioural Consequences.

Absolute poverty – A level of income below that which will sustain good health.

Accountability – Being responsible to someone or for something. Registered health and social care practitioners are accountable, for example, to their professional body, as well as their employers, for the quality of their care practice.

Aetiology – The study of what causes a disease.

Age discrimination – Treating people differently (and normally less well) on the basis of their age.

Ageism – Attitudes and behaviour which discriminate against older people.

Aim – A person or an organisation's focus or intention. It refers to what they intend to achieve.

Alzheimer's disease – A form of dementia that leads to progressive degeneration of the brain and is the commonest cause of dementia in people of all ages.

Assessment – In health and social care, the assessment process typically involves identifying and judging a person's care needs or personal skills and abilities. In a broader sense the term can refer to the process of judging the importance or effectiveness of something (such as assessing a drug treatment or a health promotion activity).

Atheroma – Fatty plaques that form inside the lining of arteries.

Audit – The monitoring of current activity, practice or policy against predefined standards.

Bacterium – A single-celled micro-organism, capable of reproducing on its own.

Behavioural approach – This approach says that most of our behaviour is learned; it can be unlearned and re-learned using reinforcement (rewards).

Behaviour change – A change in the way someone acts or functions.

Behaviour modification programme – This involves using behavioural approaches to change someone's behaviour.

Beneficence – Acts of charity or generosity that go beyond what people are normally expected to do.

Benign tumour – A discrete lump of cells that is harmless.

Bereavement – Suffering loss as a result of someone dying.

Birth rate – The number of live births per thousand of the population in one year.

Bullying – Deliberate and repeated attempts to hurt or upset another person.

Care planning cycle/process – A multi-stage cycle used by care practitioners to produce and implement individualised care plans.

Care value base – The values and ethical principles that care practitioners apply to their work. These are based on beliefs about the proper way to treat service users. Confidentiality, respecting a person's beliefs and behaving in a non-discriminatory way are all examples of care values.

CAT scan – This refers to Computed Axial Tomography which is a diagnostic technique that involves taking X-rays linked up to a computer.

Census – A national headcount of people and households carried out within a given population.

Central government – The national, as opposed to the local, level of government.

Charters – Documents that set out the targets and standards of service that a care organisation seeks to achieve in its work with service users.

Client centred – This involves focusing on the individual needs, wishes and preferences of clients to maximise their involvement in and control over their care.

Clinical features – The signs and symptoms of a disease.

Clinical governance – The process of improving the quality of care services by controlling and improving work systems in a care organisation.

Clinical trial – An experiment that tries out a potentially helpful procedure on human volunteers in order to find out how well the procedure may or may not work. A clinical trial also attempts to discover and assess risks that may occur during and/or after the procedure.

Cognitive – This term refers to thoughts and thinking.

Cognitive-behavioural therapy (CBT) – A form of treatment that uses a cognitive approach to help people change the way they feel and act.

Cognitive development – The development of thinking and understanding skills.

Cognitive primacy – The view that what we think determines what we feel and do.

Commission for Social Care Inspection (CSCI) – This body monitors, inspects and regulates standards of care in the social care sector in England.

Commissioning – The acquisition or purchasing of care services on behalf of a local population of people.

Communicable disease – A disease caused by a micro-organism which can be transmitted from one person to another.

Community Care – Provision where people should be cared for in their homes or in small 'family' units rather than in large, less personal institutions.

Comparative need – A person's needs in comparison with others in the same situation.

Complementary and alternative medicine – This term is used to describe a diverse range of health-focused practices and treatments, including acupuncture, reflexology and herbal medicine, that are not currently part of orthodox or conventional medicine.

Compliance – The extent to which a patient follows the medical or health advice that they have been given.

Concordance – This term is used to refer to agreement between patient and doctor.

Congruence – This refers to a matching or 'fit' between our experiences and our expectations or self-concept.

Conscious – What we are aware of.

Consultant – A highly skilled, expert care worker who specialises in a particular condition, disease or area of practice.

Control group – A group that is not exposed to a new drug or intervention during a clinical trial but which is compared to a group that is.

Convenience sample – A sample of individuals that is selected for reasons of convenience. That is, the individuals are chosen because they fit the researcher's selection criteria but are not chosen randomly.

Core conditions for person-centred therapy – This refers to the relationship that the counsellor tries to create, based on unconditional positive regard, empathy and genuineness.

Coronary arteries – Blood vessels supplying the heart muscle with food and oxygen.

Counselling – This refers to the supportive process of helping someone (a client) to analyse personal experiences, relationships or issues that are affecting their feelings or their behaviour.

Culture of poverty – A view that poverty is associated with a particular, and separate way of life that is passed on from generation to generation.

Data – Facts that might consist of observations, measurements or other factual information.

Data analysis – The procedures that scientists use to make sense of the data that they collect.

Death rate – The number of deaths per thousand of the population in one year.

Dementia – A group of diseases where there is a progressive loss of brain function.

Demography – The systematic study of the growth, size, distribution, movement and composition of human populations.

Dependent population – The age groups who are dependent on the rest of the population for economic security, namely young people from 0–16 years and those over the retirement age.

Dependency culture – The view that a welfare state will create a society where people rely on state benefits and services rather than working, planning for the future and taking responsibility for their own lives.

Descriptive statistics – Statistics that enable researchers to describe *what* the data are, without drawing conclusions about why this is so.

Deterministic theories – These are theories that see our behaviour as being caused (determined) by things we have no control over. These kind of theories would say that we have no free-will – that is, we think we make choices, but we don't.

Devolved system – Devolution occurs where central government grants power to government at regional or local level. A devolved system is one based on the devolution of power.

DHSSPS – This is an acronym for the Department of Health, Social Services and Public Safety, which has overall responsibility for health and care policy in Northern Ireland.

Diagnosis – The way that practitioners identify and classify a disorder or a disease.

Direct payments – The arrangement whereby a cash payment is made to people who have been assessed as needing community care services. They are then able to select, and pay for, the specific support they need, using the direct payment.

Disabling environment – A physical environment or social situation that presents barriers to access or which prevents participation by certain people.

Discrimination – Treating a person or a group of people differently and usually less favourably than others.

Distributive justice – This refers to the fair distribution of goods and services according to need.

Double-blind assignment – Assignment of people to experimental and control groups such that neither the researcher nor the participants know who is in which group while the research study is being carried out.

DSM-IV – The fourth revision of the Diagnostic and Statistical Manual of the American Psychiatric Association. It has nearly 300 categories of mental disorders.

Dysfunctional beliefs – Beliefs which are thought to be faulty and unhelpful to the person who holds them.

Egalitarian society – A society in which everyone is regarded as equal.

Ego – A term used in psychodynamic approaches that refers to the part of our mind that is rational and based in reality.

Ego defence mechanisms – The ways the ego can protect itself from the urges of the id (the part of our mind that contains our basic instincts, aggressive and sexual drives) – repression, for example.

Eligibility criteria – The requirements or standards that must be met before a person is provided with a care service.

Emigration – This refers to people leaving this country to live in another country.

Empathy – The ability to see and feel things from another person's point of view.

Empirical evidence – Evidence based on direct observation and experience.

Empowerment – A process of supporting and giving choice and decision-making powers to individuals or groups.

Endoscope – A fibre-optic tube for seeing inside the body. This is often used, for example, to examine the state of a person's digestive tract.

Epidemiology – The study of the spread of disease and causes of death and disability in a population.

Ethics – A code of behaviour based on moral principles.

Evaluation – This is the process of finding or judging the value or significance of something. For example, care practitioners evaluate the effectiveness of the interventions and treatments that they use.

Evidence-based practice – Practice that applies the best available evidence, some of it available from research studies, some of it gained from practical experience.

Expectation of life – A statistical measure which predicts the average number of years a person is likely to live. This is often calculated from birth but could be estimated from a particular age.

Experiment – A research procedure that exposes one of two samples to an intervention (e.g. a new medical treatment) in order to see if the intervention has an effect.

Experimental group – A group that is exposed to an intervention.

Exploratory question – A question that encourages an open investigation of a subject or issue.

Expressed need – The needs that people themselves identify and ask for assistance with.

Extended family – This term refers to a family or group, of normally three or more generations, who form a close-knit network and provide support and care for members.

External locus of control – The belief that we have little control over events; where control is believed to be external to, outside of, us. People who believe their future will be decided by 'fate', chance or an 'act of God' rather than by their own actions are likely to have an external locus of control.

Extinguishing behaviour – This refers to eliminating unwanted behaviour through specific steps.

Felt need – What people feel they need.

Functional beliefs – These are ways of thinking that are helpful to us.

Fungus – Usually a multi-cellular micro-organism with a thread-like structure, e.g. mould, but sometimes exists as a single cell, e.g. yeast.

Genuineness – Giving something of yourself in a therapeutic relationship so that there is congruence between what you say, how you present yourself and what you do, think and feel.

Governance of research – The process of applying and monitoring approved research 'rules' and procedures.

GP fund-holding – A funding system where general practitioners are given a budget to spend on purchasing care for patients on their practice list.

Hawthorne effect – This refers to the tendency of participants to behave differently when they know they are being studied.

Health and Social Services Boards – These are the main purchasing or commissioning bodies in Northern Ireland.

Health and Social Services Trusts – These are the main providers of statutory care services in Northern Ireland.

Healthcare Commission – This body monitors, inspects and regulates standards of care in the health care sector.

Holistic assessment – An assessment that focuses on the 'whole person' rather than a specific or partial aspect of their functioning.

Homework – The tasks the client is asked to do – things to practise until they see the counsellor again.

Hypertensive – Having persistent high blood pressure.

Hypotheses – Intelligent but untested propositions.

ICD – International Classification of Diseases.

Id – The part of our mind that contains our basic instincts, and our aggressive and sexual drives (according to psychodynamic approaches).

Immigration – This refers to people coming to live in this country from another country.

Impairment – The limitations that may be made on an individual due to physical, mental or sensory dysfunction.

Incidence – The number of new cases of a specified disease occurring in a given period of time.

Inclusive design (or **Universal design**) – The design of products and environments for use by all people, to the greatest possible extent, without the need for adaptation or specialised design.

Independent living – A philosophy which holds that people with disabilities have the right to live with dignity and with appropriate support in their own homes, to participate fully in their communities, and to have control over their lives.

Independent sector – This term refers to private and not-for-profit voluntary care organisations that are independent of government. A collective term for the private and the voluntary care sectors.

Individualised care – Care that is planned and delivered to meet the specific needs of an individual.

Industrialisation – The development of an economy based on the production of goods in factories, mills and mines rather than agriculture and other cottage industries.

Infant mortality rate – The number of deaths of infants under 1 year of age per thousand live births.

Inferential statistics – Statistics that enable researchers to make inferences from their data to more general conditions.

Informal care – This is care that is provided by relatives and friends of the person who has care needs, on an unpaid basis, outside of the professional care system.

Informal carer – Someone who provides informal care.

Insecure attachment – A situation where someone fails to establish an effective emotional bond or close relationship, usually as a result of parental separation or the death of a parent or loved one.

Instinct – This term refers to those 'inbuilt' or innate ways of behaving and responding that we are born with.

Institutionalisation – This refers to the process of becoming dependent on the rules and routines of large organisations.

Internal locus of control – The belief that we are able to influence and even control events and outcomes in our lives.

Internal market – This is a 'market' in care services that was introduced to promote competition between statutory and other care providers in the early 1990s.

Inter-professional working – This term describes team-working arrangements where care practitioners with different disciplinary backgrounds work collaboratively to meet and manage the care needs of a service user or client.

Interventions – These are the strategies we use to try to resolve a problem or to provide care.

Interview guide – A basic checklist of themes that guides an interviewer on the particular issues that they should explore.

Labelling – The process of attaching stigmatising stereotypes to particular groups of people who are then seen as all sharing negative characteristics.

Laissez-faire – This is a view that the government should not interfere in the workings of the economy nor in the provision of welfare services. The government should 'leave well alone'.

Legislation – A collective term for laws that are passed by Parliament or the EU.

Life expectancy – The average number of years a person is likely to live from a particular point in time. Life expectancy is normally calculated from birth.

Local government – The local, as opposed to national, level of government.

Local Health Care Co-operatives – The bodies that have responsibility for primary care in Scotland.

Locus – The Latin word for 'place'.

Malignant tumour – Lumps of cells that can travel around the body and grow in various organs, also referred to as cancer.

Mass media – This refers to forms of communication, such as television, radio and national newspapers, that are designed to reach a large or mass audience.

Matching – A procedure that helps to ensure that any 'extreme' characteristic in an experimental group (someone with an eating disorder, for example) has a match (counterpart) in the control group.

Means tested benefits – Welfare benefits which are only available to people if their income and savings are below a level decided by government.

Medication – Tablets or other forms of prescribed drugs given to aid recovery.

Meta-analysis – A quantitative systematic review.

Mission statement – A formal statement of a care organisation's aims or objectives. It sets out the organisation's sense of purpose or 'mission'.

Mixed economy of care – A care system that combines public (government), private, voluntary and informal sector services. Each of these types of care is funded in a different way, hence the term 'mixed economy'.

Monoclonal antibodies – 'Magic bullets' designed to 'fight' disease-causing organisms within the body.

Morality – This refers to moral ideas about 'goodness' and 'badness'.

Morbidity – This refers to experiences of ill-health.

Morbidity rate – The number of people who have a particular illness or disease in a given population and at a particular time.

Mortality rate – The number of people who have died from a particular disease in a given population and time.

MRI scan – Magnetic Resonance Imaging, a diagnostic technique using magnetism that produces clear scans.

Multi-agency working – A situation where care practitioners employed by different care organisations (or 'agencies') collaborate to provide care for a particular individual or group of people.

Multi-disciplinary team – A team of care workers from a range of professional backgrounds. This may include doctors, nurses, social workers and occupational therapists, for example.

Multiple Sclerosis – A condition where the immune system attacks and destroys the nerves resulting in the gradual, and eventually terminal, loss of physical functioning.

Myelin sheath – The insulating material that surrounds the nerves.

National Service Frameworks – These are service standards for specific areas of care practice that are defined by government. Care organisations are expected to provide and achieve levels of service delivery that meet these standards.

Need – Something a person requires or could benefit from. People have physical, intellectual, emotional and social needs.

Negative reinforcement – The removal of an aversive or unpleasant stimulus.

Net migration – The difference between the number of immigrants and the number of emigrants.

New Right, The – A view that the government should play a minimal role in the provision of welfare. Taxes should be low and people should decide how they spend their money, making their own provision for health and welfare needs.

Non-communicable disease – A disease not caused by a micro-organism and not usually passed from one person to another.

Non-invasive technique – A diagnostic or treatment procedure that does not involve piercing, cutting or entering the body.

Normative need – Established or expected levels or definitions of 'need', typically defined by academic 'experts' or professional practitioners.

Northern Ireland Assembly – The body (currently suspended) that is due to take on central government responsibilities in Northern Ireland.

Nuclear family – The smaller family unit of two generations – parent(s) and their children.

Nuclear imaging – Using a gamma camera and radionuclides to view abnormal function in the body, e.g. cancer cells.

Objective – This is a specific, clearly identified target to achieve.

Observation – In qualitative research, this procedure usually refers to watching people in their natural settings.

Open-ended interview – An informal interview in which the sequence and wording of the questions are not decided in advance.

Ophthalmic – Relating to the eye.

Organisational culture – The values, beliefs and assumptions that influence the practices and procedures or ways of working and 'atmosphere' of an organisation.

Organismic self – A version of the self that contains everything we experience, including things we are not aware of.

Osteoarthritis – A degenerative disease affecting the cartilage of the joints, often occurring after injury.

Paramountcy principle – The principle of putting the welfare of the child first in all decisions affecting them.

Parkinson's disease – A slowly progressing disease of the nervous system that results in involuntary tremors and the loss of muscular control and movement abilities.

Pathology – The scientific study of disease, but also a term used to describe something that is abnormal.

PET scan – Positron Emission Tomography, a diagnostic technique similar to a CAT scan, useful for diagnosing brain tumours, but expensive.

Philanthropy – The practice of helping people who are less well-off than oneself. It is associated with the charitable work of very wealthy people and played an important part in the emergence of voluntary organisations in the Victorian era.

Placebo – An inactive substance or procedure that resembles the experimental intervention being studied.

Placebo effect – The tendency of some participants to think they have been affected by a research intervention even though they haven't been. This occurs because they know about the aim of the research in which they are involved and are suggestible.

Population – The total of all persons who possess a common characteristic that is being studied (e.g. all poor children in Birmingham).

Positive reinforcement – This is any form of pleasant stimulus that has the effect of increasing the likely recurrence of a particular behaviour.

Post-industrial society – An economy based less on the manual production of goods but rather on non-manual work through the service, and office-based, occupations.

Poverty line – A term introduced by Seebohm Rowntree which set a level of income, below which people were said to be in poverty.

Prejudice – A strongly held attitude towards a particular group which will often persist even when shown to be unjustified or unfounded.

Prescription – In medical practice this refers to written instructions from a qualified doctor for the making-up and use of a medicine or treatment.

Pressure group – interest group organised to influence public, and especially government, policy.

Prevalence – The total number of cases of a specified disease occurring in a population at a particular point in time.

Primary care – This is 'first line' or 'first contact' care, usually provided by community-based health care workers such as general practitioners (GPs) or District Nurses. Typically, primary care involves the diagnosis of health symptoms, the treatment of 'everyday' and less serious complaints and referral of more complex cases to secondary care providers.

Primary Care Trust – Public sector organisations that monitor and manage the work of primary care providers in a local area.

Primary Health Care – Care provided by a care worker such as a GP, usually the first person to help a client.

Primary research – Research that produces new or 'fresh' data.

Private care/sector – Care services that are provided to people who are willing and able to pay for them. Organisations and individual practitioners who sell care services in this way are known as the 'private sector'.

Private practitioners – Care practitioners who are either self-employed or who are employed by a private sector care organisation.

Professional referral – A request by one care professional for care services to be provided by another care professional.

Provider organisation – A care organisation that delivers care services directly to service users.

Psychiatrist – A medical doctor who has specialist training and qualifications that allow them to work with people experiencing mental distress.

Psychodynamic approaches – Approaches that believe that our thoughts and feelings are the result of unconscious processes.

Psychology – The systematic study of how people think, feel and behave.

Punishment – This refers to the deliberate use or application of an unpleasant stimulus.

Purchaser organisation – An organisation that commissions or buys care services on behalf of an individual or group of people.

Qualitative – This term is used for methods of assessment that describe the outcomes in words rather than numbers.

Qualitative data – Non-numerical data, usually presented as 'talk' or 'text', though it can also include images and objects which provide some form of information or evidence.

Quality assurance – A general process of monitoring and evaluating whether specified standards of service quality have been achieved.

Quality standards – Statements of performance or outcomes that define an acceptable level of service.

Quantitative – The term used for methods of assessment that are numerical.

Quantitative data – Information presented in numerical form. Typically this involves some form of quantifiable measure.

Quasi-experiment – A research study that is based on, or mimics, the experimental method but which doesn't fulfil all of the criteria required in closely controlled experimental research.

Radionuclide – Low-level dose of a radioactive material.

Random sample – A sample of individuals selected from a population where all have an equal chance of being chosen.

Regulatory – This refers to monitoring and control.

Reinforcement – This refers to something (like a reward) that follows something we've done, which makes that behaviour more likely to happen again.

Relative poverty – Relative poverty occurs when people live below the standard of living normally accepted in a particular society.

Reliable results – Findings that can be confirmed by other scientists.

Research-based evidence – Findings that are based on data collected through systematic investigation.

Review – This refers to the process of checking to see how well an intervention has worked.

Rheumatism – A musculo-skeletal condition that causes pain in a person's muscles and joints and which can lead to deformity of the joints.

Rheumatoid arthritis – A degenerative disease affecting the joints where the body's immune system attacks itself.

Rogerian counselling – Person-centred counselling, in the style of Carl Rogers.

Role – The job, task or function that a person has.

Sample – A portion of some people in a population.

Schedule of reinforcement – This refers to how often a specific behaviour is reinforced.

Schemas – This refers to how we bring together and organise information about ourselves and things around us.

Schematic thinking – Thinking using schemas.

Science – A way of knowing, based upon testing the truthfulness of ideas against empirical evidence.

Scottish Parliament – The body that has central government responsibilities in Scotland.

Secondary care – Health care services that are provided by hospital-based specialists for people with more complex or emergency health care needs.

Secondary data – Existing data that has been collected and analysed by a previous researcher but which can be reanalysed and reused in a subsequent research study.

Secondary research – Typically, research based on the analysis of existing, secondary data or which focuses on finding this kind of data.

Secure attachment – This is where the young child feels safe and secure with their preferred carer.

Self-actualisation – The process of becoming a whole, complete person.

Self-referral – A direct request by an individual for health care services. Going to see a GP is an example of a self-referral.

Shaping behaviour – Building up complex patterns of behaviour gradually, in small steps.

Signs – Characteristics of a disease detectable by another person.

Social class – There are many competing definitions of social class. Central to all definitions is the idea that a person's position in society is determined by their economic circumstances that will then influence their life choices, opportunities and future prospects.

Social exclusion – A term used to describe a situation where people are unable to participate fully in society for a number of related reasons, often including poverty, unemployment, poor housing or homelessness, poor health and poor educational achievement.

Socialisation – This is the process of learning how our society works, its expectations and rules.

Social reinforcement – Any form of praise, attention and recognition that we get from others which encourages us to repeat desired behaviour.

Social stratification – The grouping of people together according to their perceived status or rank within the society.

Societal change – This refers to changes in the structure and processes of a society.

Sociology – The study of social structures and processes.

Statute – An Act of Parliament.

Statutory care/sector – Care services that have to be provided by law. They are usually provided by public or government-controlled care organisations such as NHS trusts.

Stereotype – Defining a group of people, e.g. black people or lone parents, as if they all possess the same personal characteristics, ignoring their individual differences.

Stigma – Negative attitudes which lead to the unfavourable treatment of particular groups.

Superego – The part of our mind that represents ideals and values; our conscience.

Survey – A method for obtaining information from a sample of a population.

Symptoms – Characteristics of a disease felt by the person that have no physical manifestation.

Symptom substitution – This happens when one behaviour (e.g. nail-biting) is extinguished, only to be replaced by another (e.g. bed-wetting).

Synthesised – Combined or brought together into a detailed summary.

Systematic review – A systematic analysis of other analyses.

Task-focused care – Forms of care that focus on carrying out a series of specified tasks for one or more service users, such as 'toileting everyone at 3 p.m.', regardless of the service users' individual care needs.

Team-building – The process of developing a group of employees into an effective work team.

Theory – The set of linked and abstract ideas we use to understand and explain things. Some theories allow us to predict and control events.

Third Way, The – An approach to welfare that tries to combine individual freedom and responsibility with a state providing for those most in need.

Time out – This is strategy for dealing with inappropriate behaviour that involves removing someone from all sources of social reinforcement until their inappropriate behaviour ends.

Transmission of disease – The passing of a disease from one person to another.

Token economy – Using tokens (stars, smiley faces) as reinforcement. The tokens have no value in themselves, but can be exchanged for something the person wants.

Total institutions – A large, highly organised residential establishment where people live their lives separate from the wider society, e.g. prison or army barracks or large psychiatric hospital.

Total Quality Management – A management philosophy that seeks to integrate all of the functions of an organisation (marketing, finance, care delivery, customer service, etc.) in a way that focuses on meeting customer needs and the organisation's objectives.

Transactional analysis (TA) – An approach to understanding behaviour through interpreting the interactions people have.

Typology – This is a classification system that identifies 'types' of something.

Ultrasound – A diagnostic technique that uses high-frequency sound to view soft tissues inside the body.

Unconditional positive regard – Acceptance and respect; being non-judgemental.

Unconscious – Thoughts and feelings that we are not aware of.

Underclass – A term coined by Gunnar Myrdal (1969) closely linked with the idea of social exclusion, normally used now to refer to the people in poverty who are excluded from fully participating in society by social and economic changes which are outside their control.

Unfair discrimination – The unjustified and less favourable treatment of a person or a group, perhaps as a result of prejudice.

Universal benefits – Welfare benefits to which people are entitled, regardless of their income or savings.

Urban living – A society where a high proportion of the population live and work in towns and cities rather than living and working off the land in agricultural communities.

Valid results – Findings that are based on the most appropriate research instruments.

Vector – An organism that transfers disease-causing micro-organisms from one person to another, e.g. mosquito or rat.

Vicarious reinforcement – Indirect reinforcement.

Victim blaming – Being held responsible for one's own misfortune.

Virus – Very small micro-organism with a simple structure.

Voluntary care/sector – Care services that are provided free of charge or for a small, subsidised fee by non-profit making organisations.

Welfare state – A term, first used during the 1940s, to refer to a system in which government took a primary responsibility for the health and welfare of the nation through the provision or monitoring of services.

Working hypothesis – An attempt to understand what is causing or contributing to a problem.

Bibliography

Acheson, D. (1998) Independent Inquiry into Inequalities in Health. HMSO, London.

Arksey H. (1994) 'Expert and lay participation in the construction of medical knowledge', Sociology of Health and Illness, Vol. 16, no. 4.

Bain D.J.G. (1977) 'Patient knowledge and the content of the consultation in general practice', Medical Education, 11: 347–50.

Becker, H. S., Geer, B., Hughes, E. C. and Strauss, A. L. (1961) Boys in White: Student Culture in Medical School. University of Chicago Press, Chicago.

Blaxter, (1990) Health and Lifestyle. Tavistock, London.

Brown, M (1990) An Introduction to Social Administration in Britain. Routledge, London.

Calnan, M. and Williams, S., 'Images of scientific medicine', Sociology of Health and Illness, Vol.14, no 2, 1992.

Cornwell, J. (2003) Hitler's Scientists: Science, War and the Devil's Pact. Penguin Books, New York.

Dekker F. W. et al. (1992) 'Quality of self-care of patients with asthma', Journal of Asthma, 29: 203–8.

Department of Health (2001) Research Governance Framework For Health and Social Care. Department of Health Publications, London.

Department of Health (2005) Research Governance Framework For Health and Social Care. Second Edition. Produced by COI for the Department of Health.

Goffman, E (1961) Asylums. Penguin, London.

Handy, C (1985) Understanding Organisations. Penguin, London

Haynes, R.B. et al. (1979) Compliance in Health Care. Johns Hopkins University Press, Baltimore.

Ley, P. (1989) 'Improving patients' understanding, recall, satisfaction and compliance', in A. Broome (ed.), Health Psychology. Chapman and Hall, London.

Mack, J. and Lansley, S. (1992) Breadline Britain 1990s: the Findings of the Television Series. London Weekend Television, London.

Mays, N. and Pope, C. (1995) 'Qualitative Research: Observational methods in health care settings', British Medical Journal, 311,182–184.

Ohna, S. E. (2004) 'Deaf in my own way: Identity, learning and narratives', Deafness and Education International, 6(1), 20–38.

Rutter, M. et al. (1998) 'Developmental catch up and deficit following adoption after severe global early privation', Journal of Child Psychology and Psychiatry, 39, 465–476.

Rosenfeld, E (1957) 'Institutional change in the Kibbutz', Social Problems 5, 110–136.

Schaffer, H. R. and Emerson, P. E.(1964) The Development of Social Attachments in Infancy. Monographs of the Society for Research in Child Development, 29 (3).

Torrance, H. (2004) 'Using action research to generate knowledge about educational practice'. In G. Thomas and R. Pring (eds) Evidence-Based Practice in Education (pp. 187–200). Open University Press, Maidenhead, Berkshire.

Tossell, D. and Webb D. (2000) Social Issues for Carers. Arnold, London.

Townsend, P., Davidson, N. and Whitehead, M. (eds) (1980) Inequalities in Health: the Black Report and the Health Divide. Penguin, Harmondsworth.

Walsh, M., Stephens, P. and Moore, S. (2000) Social Policy and Welfare. Stanley Thornes, Cheltenham.

WHO (1946) Constitution: Basic Documents. World Health Organization, Geneva.

WHO (1981) Development of Indicators for Monitoring Progress Towards Health for All by the Year 2000. World Health Organization, Geneva.

WHO (1996) Evaluating the Implementation of the Strategy for Health for All by the Year 2000. Indicators, definitions, bibliography. Unit of Health Situation Analysis and Projection. Division of Health Situation and Trend Assessment, World Health Organization, Geneva.

Numbers in **bold type** show the page on which the word is defined or used as a key word

Index

Index